The Principles and Ideologies of Clinical Pathology

The Principles and Ideologies of Clinical Pathology

Jhansi Rani Mallam

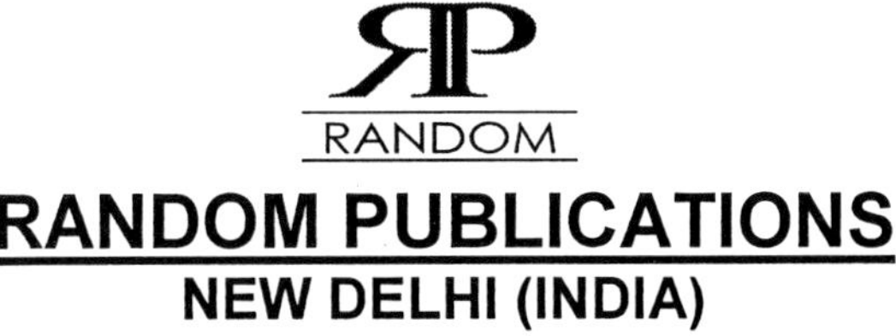

RANDOM PUBLICATIONS
NEW DELHI (INDIA)

The Principles and Ideologies of Clinical Pathology

ISBN 978-93-5111-802-2

Published in 2025 in India by

RANDOM PUBLICATIONS

4376-A/4B, Gali Murari Lal, Ansari Road
New Delhi-110 002
Phone: +9111-43580356, 23289044
E-mail: sales@randompublications.com
info@random publications.com, randomexports@gmail.com

Type Setting by: Friends Media, Delhi-110089
Digitally Printed at: Replika Press Pvt. Ltd.

Preface

Pathology, meaning is a significant component of the causal study of disease and a major field in modern medicine and diagnosis. The term pathology itself may be used broadly to refer to the study of disease in general, incorporating a wide range of bioscience research fields and medical practices, or more narrowly to describe work within the contemporary medical field of "general pathology," which includes a number of distinct but inter-related medical specialties which diagnose disease mostly through the analysis of tissue, cell, and body fluid samples. Used as a count noun, "a pathology" can also refer to the predicted or actual progression of particular diseases, and the affix path is sometimes used to indicate a state of disease in cases of both physical ailment and psychological conditions. Similarly, a pathological condition is one caused by disease, rather than occurring physiologically. A physician practicing pathology is called a pathologist.

Clinical pathology is a medical specialty that is concerned with the diagnosis of disease based on the laboratory analysis of bodily fluids, such as blood, urine, and tissue homogenates or extracts using the tools of chemistry, microbiology, hematology and molecular pathology. This specialty requires a medical residency and should not be confused with Biomedical science, which is not necessarily related to medicine. Clinical pathologists are often medical doctors. In some countries in South-America, Europe, Africa or Asia, this specialty can be practiced by non-physicians, such as Ph.D or Pharm.D after a variable number of years of residency.

– Author

Contents

1

Getting to Grips with Pathology

PATHOLOGY

Pathology, meaning "experience" or "suffering", "an account of" is a significant component of the causal study of disease and a major field in modern medicine and diagnosis. The term pathology itself may be used broadly to refer to the study of disease in general, incorporating a wide range of bioscience research fields and medical practices (including plant pathology and veterinary pathology), or more narrowly to describe work within the contemporary medical field of "general pathology," which includes a number of distinct but inter-related medical specialties which diagnose disease mostly through the analysis of tissue, cell, and body fluid samples. Used as a count noun, "a pathology" (plural, "pathologies") can also refer to the predicted or actual progression of particular diseases (as in the statement "the many different forms of cancer have diverse pathologies"), and the affix *path* is sometimes used to indicate a state of disease in cases of both physical ailment (as in cardiomyopathy) and psychological conditions (such as psychopathy). Similarly, a pathological condition is one caused by disease, rather than occurring physiologically. A physician practicing pathology is called a pathologist.

As a field of general inquiry and research, pathology addresses four components of disease: cause/etiology, mechanisms of development (pathogenesis), structural alterations of cells (morphologic changes), and the consequences of changes (clinical manifestations). In common medical practice, general pathology is mostly concerned with analyzing known clinical abnormalities that are markers or precursors for both infectious and non-infectious disease and is conducted by experts in one of two major specialties, anatomical pathology and clinical pathology. Further divisions in specialty exist on the basis of the involved sample types (comparing, for example, cytopathology, hematopathology, and histopathology), organs (as in renal pathology), and physiological systems (oral pathology), as well as on the basis of the focus of the examination (as with forensic pathology). The sense of the word *pathology* as a synonym of *disease* or *pathosis* is very common in health care. The persistence of this usage despite attempted proscription is discussed elsewhere.

The study of pathology, including the detailed examination of the body, including dissection and inquiry into specific maladies, dates back to antiquity. Rudimentary understanding of many conditions was present in most early societies and is attested to in the records of the earliest historical societies, including those of the Middle East, India, and China. By the Hellenic period of ancient Greece, a concerted causal study of disease was underway, with many notable early physicians (such as Hippocrates, for whom the modern Hippocratic Oath is named) having developed methods of diagnosis and prognosis for a number of diseases.The medical practices of the Romans and those of the Byzantines continued from these Greek roots, but, as with many areas of scientific inquiry, growth in understanding of medicine stagnated some after the Classical Era, but continued to slowly develop throughout numerous cultures. Notably, many advances were made in the medieval era of Islam during which numerous texts of complex pathologies were developed, also based on the Greek tradition. Even so, growth in complex understanding of disease mostly languished until knowledge and experimentation again began to proliferate in the Renaissance, Enlightenment, and Baroque eras, following the resurgence of the empirical method at new centers of scholarship. By the 17th century, the study of microscopy was underway and examination of tissues had led British Royal Society member Robert Hooke to coin the word "cell", setting the stage for later germ theory.

Modern pathology began to develop as a distinct field of inquiry during the 19th Century through natural philosophers and physicians that studied disease and the informal study of what they termed "pathological anatomy" or "morbid anatomy". However, pathology as a formal area of specialty was not fully developed until the late 19th and early 20th centuries, with the advent of detailed study of microbiology. In the 19th century, physicians had begun to understand that disease-causing pathogens, or "germs" (a catch-all for disease-causing, or pathogenic, microbes, such as bacteria, viruses, fungi, amoebae, molds, protists, and prions) existed and were capable of reproduction and multiplication, replacing earlier beliefs in humors or even spiritual agents, that had dominated for much of the previous 1,500 years in European medicine. With the new understanding of causative agents, physicians began to compare the characteristics of one germ's symptoms as they developed within an affected individual to another germ's characteristics and symptoms. This realization led to the foundational understanding that diseases are able to replicate themselves, and that they can have many profound and varied effects on the human host. In order to determine causes of diseases, medical experts used the most common and widely accepted assumptions or symptoms of their times, a general principal of approach that persists into modern medicine.

Modern medicine was particularly advanced by further developments of the microscope to analyze tissues, to which Rudolf Virchow gave a significant contribution, leading to a slew of research developments. By the late 1920s to early 1930s pathology was deemed a medical specialty. Combined with developments in the understanding of general physiology, by the beginning of the 20th century, the study of pathology had begun to split into a number of rarefied fields and resulting in the development of large number of modern specialties within pathology and related disciplines of diagnostic medicine.

GENERAL MEDICAL PATHOLOGY

The modern practice of pathology is divided into a number of subdisciplines within the discrete but deeply interconnected aims of biological research and medical practice. Biomedical research into disease incorporates the work of vast variety of life science specialists, whereas, in most parts of the world, to be licensed to practice pathology as medical specialty, one has to complete medical school and secure a license to practice medicine. Structurally, the study of disease is divided into many different fields which study or diagnose markers for disease using methods and technologies particular to specific scales, organs and tissue types. The information in this section mostly concerns pathology as it regards common medical practice in these systems, but each of these specialties is also the subject of voluminous pathology research as regards the disease pathways of specific pathogens and disorders that affect the tissues of these discrete organs or structures.

ANATOMICAL PATHOLOGY

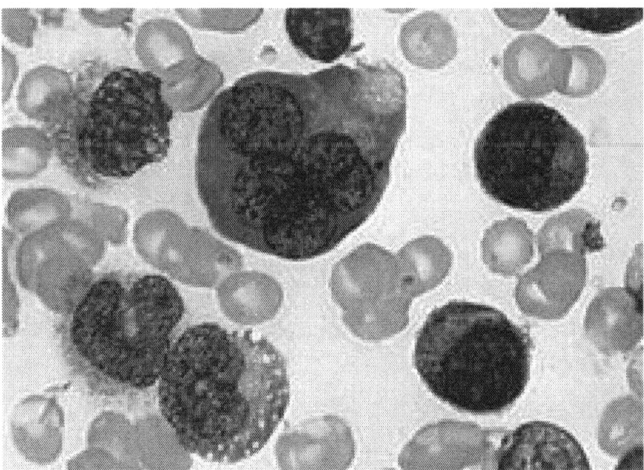

Fig. A bone marrow smear from a case of erythroleukemia showing a multinucleated erythroblast with megaloblastoid nuclear chromatin

Anatomical pathology (*Commonwealth*) or anatomic pathology (*United States*) is a medical specialty that is concerned with the diagnosis of disease based on the gross, microscopic, chemical, immunologic and molecular examination of organs, tissues, and whole bodies (as in a general examination or an autopsy). Anatomical pathology is itself divided into subfields, the main divisions being surgical pathology, cytopathology, and forensic pathology. Anatomical pathology is one of two main divisions of the medical practice of pathology, the other being clinical pathology, the diagnosis of disease through the laboratory analysis of bodily fluids and tissues. Sometimes, pathologists practice both anatomical and clinical pathology, a combination known as general pathology.

CYTOPATHOLOGY

Cytopathology (sometimes referred to as "cytology") is a branch of pathology that studies and diagnoses diseases on the cellular level. It is usually used to aid in the diagnosis of cancer, but also helps in the diagnosis of certain infectious diseases and other inflammatory conditions as well as thyroid lesions, diseases involving sterile body cavities (peritoneal, pleural, and cerebrospinal), and a wide range of other body sites. Cytopathology is generally used on samples of free cells or tissue fragments (in contrast to histopathology, which studies whole tissues) and cytopathologic tests are sometimes called smear tests because the samples may be smeared across a glass microscope slide for subsequent staining and microscopic examination. However, cytology samples may be prepared in other ways, including cytocentrifugation.

DERMATOPATHOLOGY

Dermatopathology is a subspecialty of anatomic pathology that focuses on the skin and the rest of the integumentary system as an organ. It is unique in that there are two routes which a physician can use to obtain thespecialization. All general pathologists and general dermatologists are trained in the pathology of the skin, so the term dermatopathologist denotes either of these who has reached a certainly level accreditation and experience; in the USA, either a general pathologist or a dermatologist can undergo a 1 to 2 year fellowship in the field of dermatopathology. The completion of this fellowship allows one to take a subspecialty board examination, and becomes a board certified dermatopathologist. Dermatologists are able to recognize most skin diseases based on their appearances, anatomic distributions, and behavior. Sometimes, however, those criteria do not allow a conclusive diagnosis to be made, and a skin biopsy is taken to be examined under the microscope using usual histological tests. In some cases, additional specialized testing needs to be performed on biopsies, including immunofluorescence, immunohistochemistry, electron microscopy, flow cytometry, and molecular-pathologic analysis. One of the greatest challenges of dermatopathology is its scope. More than 1500 different disorders of the skin exist, including cutaneous eruptions ("rashes") and neoplasms. Therefore, dermatopathologists must maintain a broad base of knowledge in clinical dermatology, and be familiar with several other specialty areas in Medicine.

FORENSIC PATHOLOGY

Forensic pathology focuses on determining the cause of death by post-mortem examination of a corpse or partial remains. An autopsy is typically performed by a coroner or medical examiner, often during criminal investigations; in this role, Coroners and medical examiners are also frequently asked to confirm the identity of a corpse. The requirements for becoming a licensed practitioner of forensic pathology varies from country to country (and even within a given nation) but typically a minimal requirement is a medical doctorate with a specialty in general or anatomical pathology with subsequent study in forensic medicine. The methods utilized by forensic scientists to determine death include examination of tissue specimens in order to identify the presence or absence of natural disease and other microscopic findings, interpretations of toxicology on body tissues and fluids to determine the chemical cause of overdoses, poisonings or other cases involving toxic agents, and the examinations of physical trauma. Forensic pathology is a major component in the trans-disciplinary field of forensic science.

HISTOPATHOLOGY

Histopathology refers to the microscopic examination of various forms of human tissue. Specifically, in clinical medicine, histopathology refers to the examination of a biopsy or surgical specimen by a pathologist, after the specimen has been processed and histological sections have been placed onto glass slides. This contrasts with the methods of cytopathology which utilizes free cells or tissue fragments. Histopathological examination of tissues starts with surgery, biopsy, or autopsy. The tissue is removed from the body of an organism and then placed in a fixative which stabilizes the tissues to prevent decay. The most common fixative is formalin, although frozen section fixing is also common. To see the tissue under a microscope, the sections are stained with one or more pigments. The aim of staining is to reveal cellular components; counterstains are used to provide contrast. Histochemistry refers to the science of using chemical reactions between laboratory chemicals and components within tissue. The histological slides are then interpreted diagnostically and the resulting pathology report describes the histological findings and the opinion of the pathologist. In the case of cancer, this represents the tissue diagnosis required for most treatment protocols.

NEUROPATHOLOGY

Neuropathology is the study of disease of nervous system tissue, usually in the form of either surgical biopsies or sometimes whole brains in the case of autopsy. Neuropathology is a subspecialty of anatomic pathology, neurology, and neurosurgery. In many English-speaking countries, neuropathology is considered a subfield of anatomical pathology. A physician who specializes in neuropathology, usually by completing a fellowship after a residency in anatomical or general pathology, is called a neuropathologist. In day-to-day clinical practice, a neuropathologist is a consultant for other physicians. If a disease of the nervous system is suspected, and the diagnosis cannot be made by less invasive methods, a biopsy of nervous tissue is taken from the brain or spinal cord to aid in diagnosis. Biopsy is usually requested after a mass is detected by medical imaging. With autopsies, the principal work of the neuropathologist is to help in the post-mortem diagnosis of various conditions that affect the central nervous system. Biopsies can also consist of the skin. Epidermal nerve fiber density testing (ENFD) is a more recently developed neuropathology test in which a punch skin biopsy is taken to identify small fiber neuropathies by analyzing the nerve fibers of the skin. This test is becoming available in select labs as well as many universities; it replaces the traditional nerve biopsy test as less invasive.

PULMONARY PATHOLOGY

Pulmonary pathology is the subspecialty of anatomic (and especially surgical) pathology which deals with the diagnosis and characterization of neoplastic and non-neoplastic diseases of the lungs and thoracic pleura. Diagnostic specimens are often obtained via bronchoscopic transbronchial biopsy, CT-guided percutaneous biopsy, or video-assisted thoracic surgery. These tests can be necessary to diagnose between infection, inflammation, or fibrotic conditions.

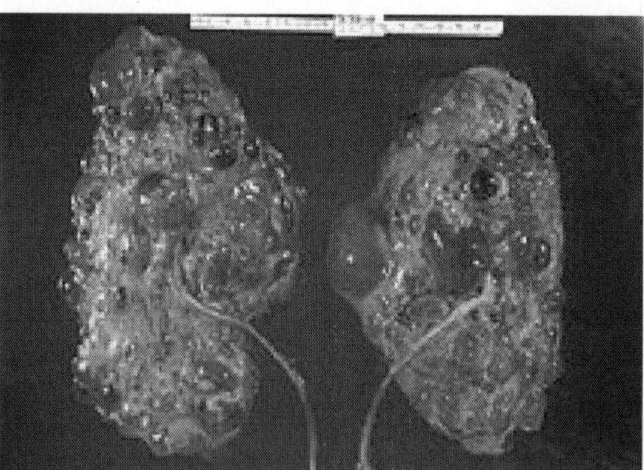

Fig. This tissue cross-section demonstrates the gross pathology of polycystic kidneys.

RENAL PATHOLOGY

Renal pathology is a subspecialty of anatomic pathology that deals with the diagnosis and characterization of disease of the kidneys. In a medical setting, renal pathologists work closely with nephrologists and transplant surgeons, who typically obtain diagnostic specimens via percutaneous renal biopsy. The renal pathologist must synthesize findings from traditional microscope histology, electron microscopy, and immunofluorescence to obtain a definitive diagnosis. Medical renal diseases may affect the glomerulus, the tubules and interstitium, the vessels, or a combination of these compartments.

SURGICAL PATHOLOGY

Surgical pathology is one of the primary areas of practice for most anatomical pathologists. Surgical pathology involves the gross and microscopic examination of surgical specimens, as well as biopsies submitted by surgeons and non-surgeons such as general internists, medical subspecialists, dermatologists, and interventional radiologists. Often an excised tissue sample is the best and most definitive evidence of disease (or lack thereof) in cases where tissue is surgically removed from a patient. These determinations are usually accomplished by a combination of gross (i.e., macroscopic) and histologic (i.e., microscopic) examination of the tissue, and may involve evaluations of molecular properties of the tissue by immunohistochemistry or other laboratory tests.

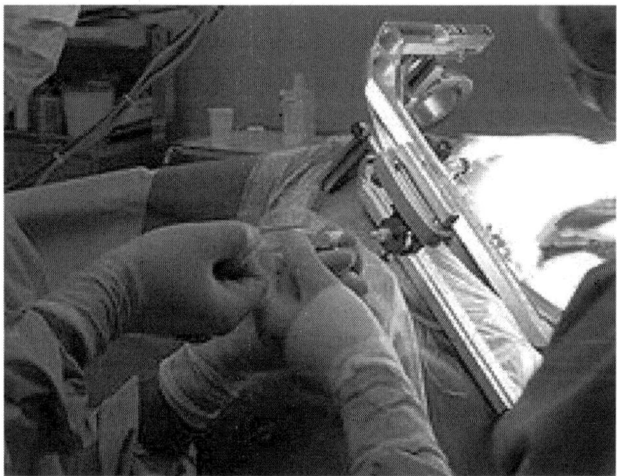

Fig. Brain biopsy under stereotaxy. A small part of the tumor is taken via a needle with a vacuum system.

There are two major types of specimens submitted for surgical pathology analysis: biopsies and surgical resections. A biopsy is a small piece of tissue removed primarily for the purposes of surgical pathology analysis, most often in order to render a definitive diagnosis. Types of biopsies include core biopsies, which are obtained through the use of large-bore needles, sometimes under the guidance of radiological techniques such as ultrasound, CT scan, or magnetic resonance imaging. Incisional biopsies are obtained through diagnostic surgical procedures that remove part of a suspicious lesion, whereas excisional biopsies remove the entire lesion, and are similar to therapeutic surgical resections. Excisional biopsies of skin lesions and gastrointestinal polyps are very common. The pathologist's interpretation of a biopsy is critical to establishing the diagnosis of a benign or malignant tumor, and can differentiate between different types and grades of cancer, as well as determining the activity of specific molecular pathways in the tumor.

Surgical resection specimens are obtained by the therapeutic surgical removal of an entire diseased area or organ (and occasionally multiple organs). These procedures are often intended as definitive surgical treatment of a disease in which the diagnosis is already known or strongly suspected, but pathological analysis of these specimens remains important in confirming the previous diagnosis.

CLINICAL PATHOLOGY

Clinical pathology is a medical specialty that is concerned with the diagnosis of disease based on the laboratory analysis of bodily fluids such as blood and urine, as well as tissues, using the tools of chemistry, clinical microbiology, hematology and molecular pathology. Clinical pathologists work in close collaboration with medical technologists, hospital administrations, and referring physicians. Clinical pathologists learn to administer a number of visual and microscopic tests and an especially large variety of tests of the biophysical properties of tissue samples involving Automated analysers and cultures. Sometimes the general term "laboratory medicine specialist" is used to refer to those working in clinical pathology, including medical doctors, Ph.D.s and doctors of pharmacology. Immunopathology, the study of an organism's immune response to infection, is sometimes considered to fall within the domain of clinical pathology.

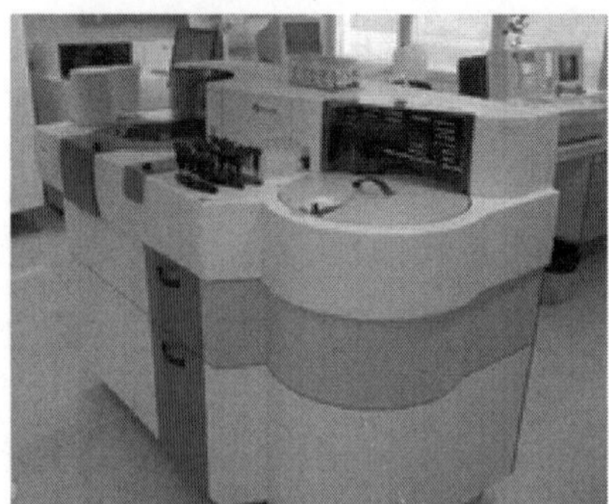

Fig. Clinical chemistry: an automated blood chemistry analyzer

HEMATOPATHOLOGY

Hematopathology is the study of diseases of blood cells (including constituents such as white blood cells, red blood cells, and platelets) and the tissues, and organs comprising the hematopoietic system. The term hematopoietic system refers to tissues and organs that produce and/or primarily host hematopoietic cells and includes bone marrow, the lymph nodes, thymus, spleen, and other lymphoid tissues. In the United States, hematopathology is a board certified subspecialty (licensed under the American Board of Pathology) practiced by those physicians who have completed a general pathology residency (anatomic, clinical, or combined) and an additional year of fellowship training in hematology. The hematopathologist reviews biopsies of lymph nodes, bone marrows and other tissues involved by an infiltrate of cells of the hematopoietic system. In addition, the hematopathologist may be in charge of flow cytometric and/or molecular hematopathology studies.

MOLECULAR PATHOLOGY

Molecular pathology is focused upon the study and diagnosis of disease through the examination of molecules within organs, tissues or bodily fluids. Molecular pathology is multidisciplinary by nature and shares some aspects of practice with both anatomic pathology and clinical pathology, molecular biology, biochemistry, proteomics and genetics. It is often applied in a context that is as much scientific as directly medical and encompasses the development of molecular and genetic approaches to the diagnosis and classification of human diseases, the design and validation of predictive biomarkers for treatment response and disease progression, and the susceptibility of individuals of different genetic constitution to particular disorders.

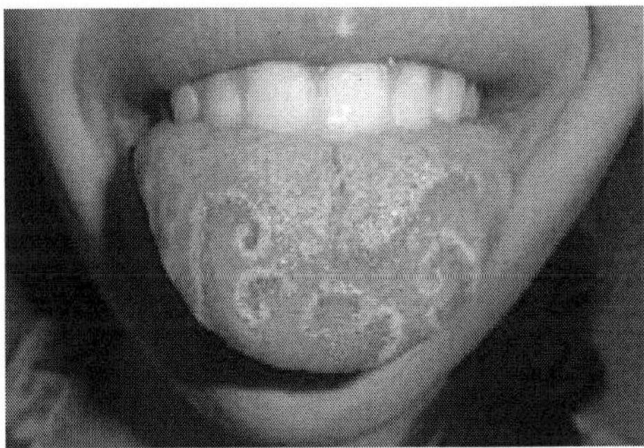

Fig. Many conditions, such as this case of geographic tongue, can be diagnosed partly on gross examination, but may be confirmed with tissue pathology.

The crossover between molecular pathology and epidemiology is represented by a related field "molecular pathological epidemiology". Molecular pathology is commonly used in diagnosis of cancer and infectious diseases. Techniques are numerous but include quantitative polymerase chain reaction (qPCR), multiplex PCR, DNA microarray, in situ hybridization, DNA sequencing, antibody based immunofluorescence tissue assays, molecular profiling of pathogens, and analysis of bacterial genes for antimicrobial resistance.

ORAL AND MAXILLOFACIAL PATHOLOGY

Oral and Maxillofacial Pathology is one of nine dental specialties recognized by the American Dental Association, and is sometimes considered a specialty of both dentistry and pathology. Oral Pathologists must complete three years of post doctoral training in an accredited program and subsequently obtain diplomate status from the American Board of Oral and Maxillofacial Pathology. The specialty focuses on the diagnosis, clinical management and investigation of diseases that affect the oral cavity and surrounding maxillofacial structures including but not limited to odontogenic, infectious, epithelial, salivary gland, bone and soft tissue pathologies. It also significantly intersects with the field of dental pathology. Although concerned with a broad variety of diseases of the oral cavity, they have roles distinct from otorhinolaryngologists ("ear, nose, and throat" specialists), and speech pathologists, the latter of which helps diagnose many neurological or neuromuscular conditions relevant to speech phonology or swallowing. Owing to the availability of the oral cavity to non-invasive examination, many conditions in the study of oral disease can be diagnosed, or at least suspected, from gross examination, but biopsies, cell smears, and other tissue analysis remain important diagnostic tools in oral pathology.

MEDICAL TRAINING AND ACCREDITATION

Individual nations vary some in the medical licensing required of pathologists. In the United States, pathologists are physicians (D.O. or M.D.) that have completed a four-year undergraduate program, four years of medical school training, and three to four years of postgraduate training in the form of a pathology residency.

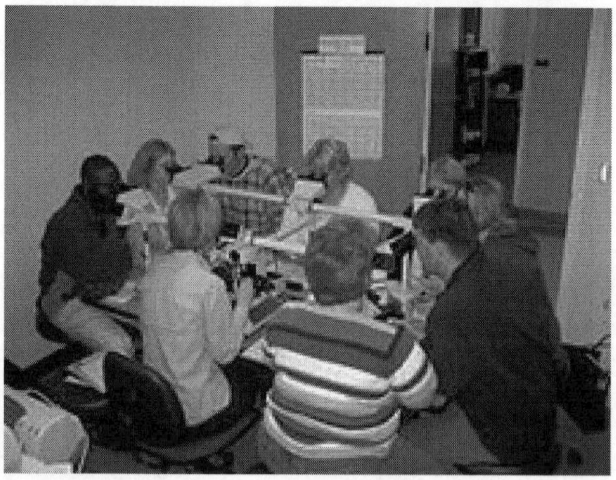

Fig. An anatomical pathology instructor uses a microscope with multiple eyepieces to instruct students in diagnostic microscopy.

Training may be within two primary specialties, as recognized by the American Board of Pathology: anatomical Pathology and clinical Pathology, each of which requires separate board certification. The American Osteopathic Board of Pathology also recognizes four primary specialties: anatomic pathology, dermatopathology, forensic pathology, and laboratory medicine. Pathologists may pursue specialised fellowship training within one or more subspecialties of either anatomical or clinical pathology. Some of these subspecialties permit additional board certification, while others do not.

In the United Kingdom, pathologists are physicians licensed by the UK General Medical Council. The training to become a pathologist is under the oversight of the Royal College of Pathologists. After four to six years of undergraduate medical study, trainees proceed to a two-year foundation program. Full-time training in histopathology currently lasts between five and five and a half years and includes specialist training in surgical pathology, cytopathology, and autopsy pathology. It is also possible to take a Royal College of Pathologists diploma in forensic pathology, dermatopathology, or cytopathology, recognising additional specialist training and expertise and to get specialist accreditation in forensic pathology, pediatric pathology, and neuropathology. All postgraduate medical training and education in the UK is overseen by the General Medical Council.

In France, Pathology is separate in two distinct specialties, anatomical pathology and clinical pathology. Residencies for both lasts four years. Residency in anatomical pathology is open to physicians only, while clinical pathology is open to both physicians and pharmacists. At the end of the second year of clinical pathology residency, residents can choose between general clinical pathology and a specialization in one of the disciplines, but they can not practice anatomical pathology, nor can anatomical pathology residents can not practice clinical pathology.

OVERLAP WITH OTHER DIAGNOSTIC MEDICINE

Although separate fields in terms of medical practice, there are a number of areas of inquiry in medicine and medical science which either overlap greatly with general pathology, work in tandem with it, or which contribute significantly to the understanding of the pathology of a given disease or its course in an individual. As a significant portion of all general pathology practice is concerned with cancer, the practice of oncology is deeply tied to, and dependent upon, the work of both anatomical and clinical pathologists. Biopsy, resection and blood tests are all examples of pathology work that is essential for the diagnoses of many kinds of cancer and for the staging of cancerous masses. In a similar fashion, the tissue and blood analysis techniques of general pathology are of central significance to the investigation of serious infectious disease and as such inform significantly upon the fields of epidemiology, etiology, immunology, and parasitology. General pathology methods are of great importance to biomedical research into disease, wherein they are sometimes referred to as "experimental" or "investigative" pathology.

Medical imaging is the process of generating visual representations of the interior of a body for clinical analysis and medical intervention, for the purpose of revealing details internal physiology in order to plan appropriate treatments for tissue infection and trauma. Medical imaging is also central in supplying the biometric data necessary to establish baseline features of anatomy and physiology so as to increase the accuracy with which early or fine-detail abnormalities are detected.

These diagnostic techniques are often performed in combination with general pathology procedures and are themselves often essential to developing new understanding of the pathogenesis of a given disease and tracking the progress of disease in specific medical cases.

Examples of important subdivisions in medical imaging include radiology (which uses the imaging technologies of X-ray radiography) magnetic resonance imaging, medical ultrasonography (or ultrasound), endoscopy, elastography, tactile imaging, thermography, medical photography, nuclear medicine and functional imaging techniques such as positron emission tomography. Though they do not strictly relay images, readings from diagnostics tests involving electroencephalography, magnetoencephalography, and electrocardiography often give hints as to the state and function of certain tissues in the brain and heart respectively.

PSYCHOPATHOLOGY

Psychopathology is the study of mental illness, particularly of severe disorders. Informed heavily by both psychology and neurology, its purpose is to classify mental illness, elucidate its underlying causes, and guide clinical psychiatric treatment accordingly. Although diagnosis and classification of mental norms and disorders is largely the purview of psychiatry—the results of which are guidelines such as the Diagnostic and Statistical Manual of Mental Disorders, which attempt to classify mental disease mostly on behavioural evidence, though not without controversy—the field is also heavily, and increasingly, informed upon by neuroscience and other of the biological cognitive sciences. Mental or social disorders or behaviours which are seen to be generally unhealthy or excessive in a given individual to the point where they cause harm or severe disruption to the sufferer's lifestyle are often given the handle of "pathological" (e.g. pathological gambling or pathological liar).

STUDY OF PATHOLOGY IN NON-HUMANS

Although the vast majority of lab work and research in pathology concerns the development of disease in humans, pathology is of significance throughout the biological sciences. Two main catch-all fields exist to represent most complex organisms capable of serving as host to a pathogen or other form of disease: veterinary pathology (concerned with all non-human species of kingdom of Animalia) and phytopathology, which studies disease in plants.

VETERINARY PATHOLOGY

Veterinary pathology covers a vast array of species, but with a significantly smaller number of practitioners, so understanding of disease in non-human animals, especially as regards veterinary practice, varies considerably by species. Nonetheless, significant amounts of pathology research are conducted on animals, for two primary reasons: 1) The origins of diseases are typically zoonotic in nature, and many infectious pathogens have animal vectors and, as such, understanding the mechanisms of action for these pathogens in non-human hosts is essential to the understanding and application of epidemiology and 2) those animals which share physiological and genetic traits with humans can be used as surrogates for the study of the disease and potential treatments as well as the effects of various synthetic products. For this reason, as well as their roles as livestock and companion animals, mammals generally have the largest body of research in veterinary pathology. Animal testing remains a controversial practice, even in cases where it is used to research treatment for human disease. As in human medical pathology, the practice of veterinary pathology is customarily divided into the two main fields of anatomical and clinical pathology.

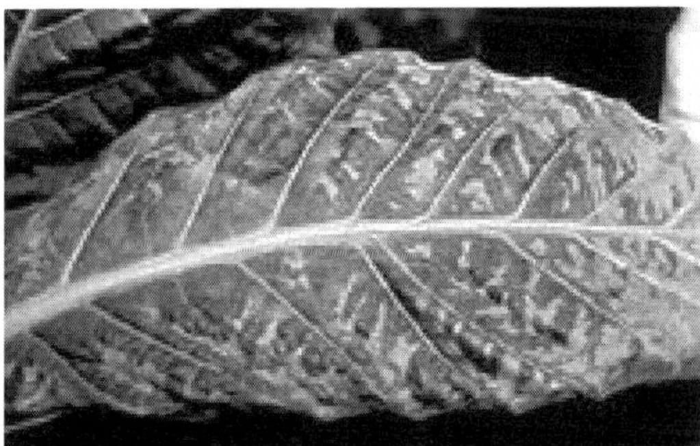

Fig. A tobacco plant infected with the tobacco mosaic virus

PHYTOPATHOLOGY

Although the pathogens and their mechanics differ greatly from those of animals, plants are subject to a wide variety of diseases, including those caused by fungi, oomycetes, bacteria, viruses, viroids, virus-like organisms, phytoplasmas, protozoa, nematodes and parasitic plants. Damage caused by insects, mites, vertebrate, and other small herbivores is not considered a part of the domain of plant pathology. The field is deeply connected to plant disease epidemiology and the horticulture of species that are of high importance to the human diet or other uses.

INFLAMMATION

Inflammation (Latin, *inflammatio*) is part of the complex biological response of body tissues to harmful stimuli, such as pathogens, damaged cells, or irritants.

Inflammation is a protective response that involves immune cells, blood vessels, and molecular mediators. The purpose of inflammation is to eliminate the initial cause of cell injury, clear out necrotic cells and tissues damaged from the original insult and the inflammatory process, and to initiate tissue repair.

The classical signs of acute inflammation are pain, heat, redness, swelling, and loss of function. Inflammation is a generic response, and therefore it is considered as a mechanism of innate immunity, as compared to adaptive immunity, which is specific for each pathogen.

Too little inflammation could lead to progressive tissue destruction by the harmful stimulus (e.g. bacteria) and compromise the survival of the organism. In contrast, chronic inflammation may lead to a host of diseases, such as hay fever, periodontitis, atherosclerosis, rheumatoid arthritis, and even cancer (e.g., gallbladder carcinoma). Inflammation is therefore normally closely regulated by the body.

Inflammation can be classified as either *acute* or *chronic*. *Acute inflammation* is the initial response of the body to harmful stimuli and is achieved by the increased movement of plasma and leukocytes (especially granulocytes) from the blood into the injured tissues. A series of biochemical events propagates and matures the inflammatory response, involving the local vascular system, the immune system, and various cells within the injured tissue. Prolonged inflammation, known as *chronic inflammation*, leads to a progressive shift in the type of cells present at the site of inflammation and is characterized by simultaneous destruction and healing of the tissue from the inflammatory process.

Inflammation is not a synonym for infection. Infection describes the interaction between the action of microbial invasion and the reaction of the body's inflammatory defensive response — the two components are considered together when discussing an infection, and the word is used to imply a microbial invasive cause for the observed inflammatory reaction. Inflammation on the other hand describes purely the body's immunovascular response, whatever the cause may be. But because of how often the two are correlated, words ending in the suffix *-itis* (which refers to inflammation) are sometimes informally described as referring to infection. For example, the word *urethritis* strictly means only "urethral inflammation", but clinical health care providers usually discuss urethritis as a urethral infection because urethral microbial invasion is the most common cause of urethritis.

It is useful to differentiate inflammation and infection as there are many pathological situations where inflammation is not driven by microbial invasion - for example, atherosclerosis, type III hypersensitivity, trauma, ischaemia. There are also pathological situations where microbial invasion does not result in classic inflammatory response—for example, parasitosis, eosinophilia.

CAUSES

Physical:

- Burns
- Frostbite
- Physical injury, blunt or penetrating
- Foreign bodies, including splinters, dirt and debris
- Trauma
- Ionizing radiation

Biological:

- Infection by pathogens
- Immune reactions due to hypersensitivity
- Stress

Chemical:

- Chemical irritants
- Toxins
- Alcohol

Psychological:

- Embarrassment
- Excitement

CARDINAL SIGNS

Acute inflammation is a short-term process, usually appearing within a few minutes or hours and begins to cease upon the removal of the injurious stimulus. It is characterized by five cardinal signs:

An acronym that may be used to remember the key symptoms is "PRISH" for Pain, Redness, Immobility (loss of function), Swelling and Heat.

The traditional names for signs of inflammation come from Latin:

- Dolor (pain)
- Calor (heat)
- Rubor (redness)
- Tumor (swelling)
- Functio laesa (loss of function)

The first four (classical signs) were described by Celsus (ca. 30 BC–38 AD), while *loss of function* was added later by Galen even though the attribution is disputed and the origination of the fifth sign has also been ascribed to Thomas Sydenham and Virchow.

Redness and heat are due to increased blood flow at body core temperature to the inflamed site; swelling is caused by accumulation of fluid; pain is due to the release of chemicals such as bradykinin and histamine that stimulate nerve endings. Loss of function has multiple causes.

Acute inflammation of the lung (pneumonia) does not cause pain unless the inflammation involves the parietal pleura, which does have pain-sensitive nerve endings.

PROCESS OF ACUTE INFLAMMATION

The process of acute inflammation is initiated by resident immune cells already present in the involved tissue, mainly resident macrophages, dendritic cells, histiocytes, Kupffer cells and mastocytes. These cells present on their surfaces certain receptors named *pattern recognition receptors* (PRRs), which recognise generic molecules that are broadly shared by pathogens but distinguishable from host molecules, collectively referred to as pathogen-associated molecular patterns (PAMPs). At the onset of an infection, burn, or other injuries, these cells undergo activation (one of their PRRs recognize a PAMP) and release inflammatory mediators responsible for the clinical signs of inflammation. Vasodilation and its resulting increased blood flow causes the redness (*rubor*) and increased heat (*calor*). Increased permeability of the blood vessels results in an exudation (leakage) of plasma proteins and fluid into the tissue (edema), which manifests itself as swelling (*tumor*). Some of the released mediators such as bradykinin increase the sensitivity to pain (hyperalgesia, *dolor*). The mediator molecules also alter the blood vessels to permit the migration of leukocytes, mainly neutrophils and macrophages, outside of the blood vessels (extravasation) into the tissue. The neutrophils migrate along a chemotactic gradient created by the local cells to reach the site of injury. The loss of function (*functio laesa*) is probably the result of a neurological reflex in response to pain. In addition to cell-derived mediators, several acellular biochemical cascade systems consisting of preformed plasma proteins act in parallel to initiate and propagate the inflammatory response. These include the complement system activated by bacteria and the coagulation and fibrinolysis systems activated by necrosis, e.g. a burn or a trauma.

The acute inflammatory response requires constant stimulation to be sustained. Inflammatory mediators are short-lived and are quickly degraded in the tissue. Hence, acute inflammation begins to cease once the stimulus has been removed.

VASCULAR COMPONENT

VASODILATION AND INCREASED PERMEABILITY

As defined, acute inflammation is an immunovascular response to an inflammatory stimulus. This means acute inflammation can be broader divided into a vascular phase that occurs first, followed by a cellular phase involving immune cells (more specifically myeloid granulocytes in the acute setting). The vascular component of acute inflammation involves the movement of plasma fluid, containing important proteins such as fibrin and immunoglobulins (antibodies), into inflamed tissue.

Upon contact with PAMPs, tissue macrophages and mastocytes release vasoactive amines such as histamine and serotonin, as well as eicosanoids such as prostaglandin E2 and leukotriene B4 to remodel the local vasculature. Macrophages and endothelial cells release nitric oxide. These mediators vasodilate and permeabilize the blood vessels, which results in the net distribution of blood plasma from the vessel into the tissue space. The increased collection of fluid into the tissue causes it to swell (edema). This exuded tissue fluid contain various antimicrobial mediators from the plasma such as complement, lysozyme, antibodies, which can immediately deal damage to microbes, and opsonise the microbes in preparation for the cellular phase. If the inflammatory stimulus is a lacerating wound, exuded platelets, coagulants, plasmin and kinins can clot the wounded area and provide haemostasis in the first instance. These clotting mediators also provide a structural staging framework at the inflammatory tissue site in the form of a fibrin lattice - as would construction scaffolding at a construction site - for the purpose of aiding phagocytic debridement and wound repair later on. Some of the exuded tissue fluid is also funneled by lymphatics to the regional lymph nodes, flushing bacteria along to start the recognition and attack phase of the adaptive immune system.

Acute inflammation is characterized by marked vascular changes, including vasodilation, increased permeability and increased blood flow, which are induced by the actions of various inflammatory mediators. Vasodilation occurs first at the arteriole level, progressing to the capillary level, and brings about a net increase in the amount of blood present, causing the redness and heat of inflammation. Increased permeability of the vessels results in the movement of plasma into the tissues, with resultant *stasis* due to the increase in the concentration of the cells within blood - a condition characterized by enlarged vessels packed with cells. Stasis allows leukocytes to marginate (move) along the endothelium, a process critical to their recruitment into the tissues. Normal flowing blood prevents this, as the shearing force along the periphery of the vessels moves cells in the blood into the middle of the vessel.

PLASMA CASCADE SYSTEMS

- The complement system, when activated, creates a cascade of chemical reactions that promotes opsonization, chemotaxis, and agglutination, and produces the MAC.
- The kinin system generates proteins capable of sustaining vasodilation and other physical inflammatory effects.

- The coagulation system or *clotting cascade*, which forms a protective protein mesh over sites of injury.
- The fibrinolysis system, which acts in opposition to the *coagulation system*, to counterbalance clotting and generate several other inflammatory mediators.

CELLULAR COMPONENT

The *cellular component* involves leukocytes, which normally reside in blood and must move into the inflamed tissue via *extravasation* to aid in inflammation. Some act as phagocytes, ingesting bacteria, viruses, and cellular debris. Others release enzymatic granules that damage pathogenic invaders. Leukocytes also release inflammatory mediators that develop and maintain the inflammatory response. In general, acute inflammation is mediated by granulocytes, whereas chronic inflammation is mediated by mononuclear cells such as monocytes and lymphocytes.

Leukocyte extravasation

Various leukocytes are critically involved in the initiation and maintenance of inflammation. These cells must be able to get to the site of injury from their usual location in the blood, therefore mechanisms exist to recruit and direct leukocytes to the appropriate place. The process of leukocyte movement from the blood to the tissues through the blood vessels is known as *extravasation*, and can be divided up into a number of broad steps:

1. Leukocyte margination and endothelial adhesion: Activated tissue macrophages release cytokines such as IL-1 and TNFá, which bind to their respective G protein-coupled receptors on the endothelial wall. Signal transduction induces the immediate expression of P-selectin on endothelial cell surfaces. This receptor binds weakly to carbohydrate ligands on leukocyte surfaces and causes them to "roll" along the endothelial surface as bonds are made and broken. Cytokines from injured cells induce the expression of E-selectin on endothelial cells, which functions similarly to P-selectin. Cytokines also induce the expression of integrin ligands such as ICAM-1 and VCAM-1 on endothelial cells, which further slow leukocytes down. These weakly bound leukocytes are free to detach if not activated by chemokines produced in injured tissue. Activation increases the affinity of bound integrin receptors for ICAM-1 and VCAM-1 on the endothelial cell surface, firmly binding the leukocytes to the endothelium.
2. Migration across the endothelium, known as *transmigration,* via the process of diapedesis: Chemokine gradients stimulate the adhered leukocytes to move between endothelial cells and pass the basement membrane into the tissues.

3. Movement of leukocytes within the tissue via chemotaxis: Leukocytes reaching the tissue interstitium bind to extracellular matrix proteins via expressed integrins and CD44 to prevent their loss from the site. Chemoattractants cause the leukocytes to move along a chemotactic gradient towards the source of inflammation.

Phagocytosis

Extravasated neutrophils in the cellular phase come into contact with microbes at the inflamed tissue. Phagocytes express cell-surface endocytic pattern recognition receptors (PRRs) that have affinity and efficacy against non-specific microbe-associated molecular patterns (PAMPs). Most PAMPs that bind to endocytic PRRs and initiate phagocytosis are cell wall components, including complex carbohydrates such as mannans and â-glucans, lipopolysaccharides (LPS), peptidoglycans, and surface proteins. Endocytic PRRs on phagocytes reflect these molecular patterns, with C-type lectin receptors binding to mannans and â-glucans, and scavenger receptors binding to LPS.

Upon endocytic PRR binding, actin-myosin cytoskeletal rearrangement adjacent to the plasma membrane occurs in a way that endocytoses the plasma membrane containing the PRR-PAMP complex, and the microbe. Phosphatidylinositol and Vps34-Vps15-Beclin1 signalling pathways have been implicated to traffic the endocytosed phagosome to intracellular lysosomes, where fusion of the phagosome and the lysosome produces a phagolysosome. The reactive oxygen species, superoxides and hypochlorite bleach within the phagolysosomes then kill microbes inside the phagocyte.

Phagocytic efficacy can be enhanced by opsonization. Plasma derived complement C3b and antibodies that exude into the inflamed tissue during the vascular phase bind to and coat the microbial antigens. As well as endocytic PRRs, phagocytes also express opsonin receptors Fc receptor and complement receptor 1 (CR1), which bind to antibodies and C3b, respectively. The co-stimulation of endocytic PRR and opsonin receptor increases the efficacy of the phagocytic process, enhancing the lysosomal elimination of the infective agent.

MORPHOLOGIC PATTERNS

Specific patterns of acute and chronic inflammation are seen during particular situations that arise in the body, such as when inflammation occurs on an epithelial surface, or pyogenic bacteria are involved.

- Granulomatous inflammation: Characterised by the formation of granulomas, they are the result of a limited but diverse number of diseases, which include among others tuberculosis, leprosy, sarcoidosis, and syphilis.

- Fibrinous inflammation: Inflammation resulting in a large increase in vascular permeability allows fibrin to pass through the blood vessels. If an appropriate *procoagulative* stimulus is present, such as cancer cells, a fibrinous exudate is deposited. This is commonly seen in serous cavities, where the conversion of fibrinous exudate into a scar can occur between serous membranes, limiting their function. The deposit sometimes forms a pseudomembrane sheet. During inflammation of the intestine (Pseudomembranous colitis), pseudomembranous tubes can be formed.
- Purulent inflammation: Inflammation resulting in large amount of pus, which consists of neutrophils, dead cells, and fluid. Infection by pyogenic bacteria such as staphylococci is characteristic of this kind of inflammation. Large, localised collections of pus enclosed by surrounding tissues are called abscesses.
- Serous inflammation: Characterised by the copious effusion of non-viscous serous fluid, commonly produced by mesothelial cells of serous membranes, but may be derived from blood plasma. Skin blisters exemplify this pattern of inflammation.
- Ulcerative inflammation: Inflammation occurring near an epithelium can result in the necrotic loss of tissue from the surface, exposing lower layers. The subsequent excavation in the epithelium is known as an ulcer.

INFLAMMATORY DISORDERS

Inflammatory abnormalities are a large group of disorders that underlie a vast variety of human diseases. The immune system is often involved with inflammatory disorders, demonstrated in both allergic reactions and some myopathies, with many immune system disorders resulting in abnormal inflammation. Non-immune diseases with etiological origins in inflammatory processes include cancer, atherosclerosis, and ischaemic heart disease.

A large variety of proteins are involved in inflammation, and any one of them is open to a genetic mutation which impairs or otherwise dysregulates the normal function and expression of that protein.

Examples of disorders associated with inflammation include:

- Acne vulgaris
- Asthma
- Autoimmune diseases
- Autoinflammatory diseases
- Celiac disease
- Chronic prostatitis
- Glomerulonephritis
- Hypersensitivities

- Inflammatory bowel diseases
- Pelvic inflammatory disease
- Reperfusion injury
- Rheumatoid arthritis
- Sarcoidosis
- Transplant rejection
- Vasculitis
- Interstitial cystitis

Atherosclerosis

Atherosclerosis, formerly considered a bland lipid storage disease, actually involves an ongoing inflammatory response. Recent advances in basic science have established a fundamental role for inflammation in mediating all stages of this disease from initiation through progression and, ultimately, the thrombotic complications of atherosclerosis. These new findings provide important links between risk factors and the mechanisms of atherogenesis. Clinical studies have shown that this emerging biology of inflammation in atherosclerosis applies directly to human patients. Elevation in markers of inflammation predicts outcomes of patients with acute coronary syndromes, independently of myocardial damage. In addition, low-grade chronic inflammation, as indicated by levels of the inflammatory marker C-reactive protein, prospectively defines risk of atherosclerotic complications, thus adding to prognostic information provided by traditional risk factors. Moreover, certain treatments that reduce coronary risk also limit inflammation. In the case of lipid lowering with statins, this anti-inflammatory effect does not appear to correlate with reduction in low-density lipoprotein levels. These new insights into inflammation in atherosclerosis not only increase our understanding of this disease but also have practical clinical applications in risk stratification and targeting of therapy for this scourge of growing worldwide importance.

Allergies

An allergic reaction, formally known as type 1 hypersensitivity, is the result of an inappropriate immune response triggering inflammation. A common example is hay fever, which is caused by a hypersensitive response by skin mast cells to allergens. Pre-sensitised mast cells respond by degranulating, releasing vasoactive chemicals such as histamine. These chemicals propagate an excessive inflammatory response characterised by blood vessel dilation, production of pro-inflammatory molecules, cytokine release, and recruitment of leukocytes. Severe inflammatory response may mature into a systemic response known as anaphylaxis. Other hypersensitivity reactions (*type 2* and *type 3*) are mediated by antibody reactions and induce inflammation by attracting leukocytes that damage surrounding tissue.

Myopathies

Inflammatory myopathies are caused by the immune system inappropriately attacking components of muscle, leading to signs of muscle inflammation. They may occur in conjunction with other immune disorders, such as systemic sclerosis, and include dermatomyositis, polymyositis, and inclusion body myositis.

Leukocyte defects

Due to the central role of leukocytes in the development and propagation of inflammation, defects in leukocyte functionality often result in a decreased capacity for inflammatory defense with subsequent vulnerability to infection. Dysfunctional leukocytes may be unable to correctly bind to blood vessels due to surface receptor mutations, digest bacteria (Chediak-Higashi syndrome), or produce microbicides (chronic granulomatous disease). In addition, diseases affecting the bone marrow may result in abnormal or few leukocytes.

Pharmacological

Certain drugs or exogenous chemical compounds are known to affect inflammation. Vitamin A deficiency causes an increase in inflammatory responses, and anti-inflammatory drugs work specifically by inhibiting the enzymes that produce inflammatory eicosanoids. Certain illicit drugs such as cocaine and ecstasy may exert some of their detrimental effects by activating transcription factors intimately involved with inflammation (e.g. NF-êB).

Cancer

Inflammation orchestrates the microenvironment around tumours, contributing to proliferation, survival and migration. Cancer cells use selectins, chemokines and their receptors for invasion, migration and metastasis. On the other hand, many cells of the immune system contribute to cancer immunology, suppressing cancer. Molecular intersection between receptors of steroid hormones, which have important effects on cellular development, and transcription factors that play key roles in inflammation, such as NF-êB, may mediate some of the most critical effects of inflammatory stimuli on cancer cells.

This capacity of a mediator of inflammation to influence the effects of steroid hormones in cells, is very likely to affect carcinogenesis on the one hand; on the other hand, due to the modular nature of many steroid hormone receptors, this interaction may offer ways to interfere with cancer progression, through targeting of a specific protein domain in a specific cell type. Such an approach may limit side effects that are unrelated to the tumor of interest, and may help preserve vital homeostatic functions and developmental processes in the organism. According to a review of 2009, recent data suggests that cancer-related inflammation (CRI) may lead to accumulation of random genetic alterations in cancer cells.

Resolution of inflammation

The inflammatory response must be actively terminated when no longer needed to prevent unnecessary "bystander" damage to tissues. Failure to do so results in chronic inflammation, and cellular destruction. Resolution of inflammation occurs by different mechanisms in different tissues. Mechanisms that serve to terminate inflammation include:

- Short half-life of inflammatory mediators *in vivo*.
- Production and release of Transforming growth factor (TGF) beta from macrophages
- Production and release of Interleukin 10 (IL-10)
- Production of anti-inflammatory lipoxins
- Downregulation of pro-inflammatory molecules, such as leukotrienes.
- Upregulation of anti-inflammatory molecules such as the Interleukin 1 receptor antagonist or the soluble tumor necrosis factor receptor (TNFR)
- Apoptosis of pro-inflammatory cells
- Desensitization of receptors.
- Increased survival of cells in regions of inflammation due to their interaction with the extracellular matrix (ECM)
- Downregulation of receptor activity by high concentrations of ligands
- Cleavage of chemokines by matrix metalloproteinases (MMPs) might lead to production of anti-inflammatory factors.
- Production of resolvins, protectins or maresins.
- Acute inflammation normally resolves by mechanisms that have remained somewhat elusive. Emerging evidence now suggests that an active, coordinated program of resolution initiates in the first few hours after an inflammatory response begins. After entering tissues, granulocytes promote the switch of arachidonic acid–derived prostaglandins and leukotrienes to lipoxins, which initiate the termination sequence. Neutrophil recruitment thus ceases and programmed death by apoptosis is engaged. These events coincide with the biosynthesis, from omega-3 polyunsaturated fatty acids, of resolvins and protectins, which critically shorten the period of neutrophil infiltration by initiating apoptosis. As a consequence, apoptotic neutrophils undergo phagocytosis by macrophages, leading to neutrophil clearance and release of anti-inflammatory and reparative cytokines such as transforming growth factor-â1. The anti-inflammatory program ends with the departure of macrophages through the lymphatics.—/*Charles Serhan*

Connection to depression

There is evidence for a link between inflammation and depression. Inflammatory processes can be triggered by negative cognitions or their consequences, such as stress, violence, or deprivation. Thus, negative cognitions can cause inflammation that can, in turn, lead to depression. In addition there is increasing evidence that inflammation can cause depression because of the increase of cytokines, setting the brain into a "sickness mode". Classical symptoms of being physically sick like lethargy show a large overlap in behaviors that characterize depression. Levels of cytokines tend to increase sharply during depressive episodes in manics and drop off during remission. Furthermore, it has been shown in clinical trials that anti-inflammatory medicines taken in addition to antidepressants not only significantly improves symptoms but also increases the proportion of subjects positively responding to treatment. Inflammations that lead to serious depression could be caused by common infections such as those caused by a virus, bacteria or even parasites.

SYSTEMIC EFFECTS

An infectious organism can escape the confines of the immediate tissue via the circulatory system or lymphatic system, where it may spread to other parts of the body. If an organism is not contained by the actions of acute inflammation it may gain access to the lymphatic system via nearby lymph vessels. An infection of the lymph vessels is known as lymphangitis, and infection of a lymph node is known as lymphadenitis. When lymph nodes cannot destroy all pathogens, the infection spreads further. A pathogen can gain access to the bloodstream through lymphatic drainage into the circulatory system.

When inflammation overwhelms the host, systemic inflammatory response syndrome is diagnosed. When it is due to infection, the term sepsis is applied, with the terms bacteremia being applied specifically for bacterial sepsis and viremia specifically to viral sepsis. Vasodilation and organ dysfunction are serious problems associated with widespread infection that may lead to septic shock and death.

Acute-phase proteins

Inflammation also induces high systemic levels of acute-phase proteins. In acute inflammation, these proteins prove beneficial, however in chronic inflammation they can contribute to amyloidosis. These proteins include C-reactive protein, serum amyloid A, and serum amyloid P, which cause a range of systemic effects including:

- Fever
- Increased blood pressure
- Decreased sweating
- Malaise

- Loss of appetite
- Somnolence

Leukocyte numbers

Inflammation often affects the numbers of leukocytes present in the body:

- Leukocytosis is often seen during inflammation induced by infection, where it results in a large increase in the amount of leukocytes in the blood, especially immature cells. Leukocyte numbers usually increase to between 15 000 and 20 000 cells per microliter, but extreme cases can see it approach 100 000 cells per microliter. Bacterial infection usually results in an increase of neutrophils, creating neutrophilia, whereas diseases such as asthma, hay fever, and parasite infestation result in an increase in eosinophils, creating eosinophilia.
- Leukopenia can be induced by certain infections and diseases, including viral infection, *Rickettsia* infection, some protozoa, tuberculosis, and some cancers.

Systemic inflammation and obesity

With the discovery of interleukins (IL), the concept of systemic inflammation developed. Although the processes involved are identical to tissue inflammation, systemic inflammation is not confined to a particular tissue but involves the endothelium and other organ systems.

Chronic inflammation is widely observed in obesity. The obese commonly have many elevated markers of inflammation, including:

- IL-6 (Interleukin-6)
- IL-8 (Interleukin-8)
- IL-18 (Interleukin-18)
- TNF-á (Tumor necrosis factor-alpha)
- CRP (C-reactive protein)
- Insulin
- Blood glucose
- Leptin

Low-grade chronic inflammation is characterized by a two- to threefold increase in the systemic concentrations of cytokines such as TNF-á, IL-6, and CRP. Waist circumference correlates significantly with systemic inflammatory response. A predominant factor in this correlation is due to the autoimmune response triggered by adiposity, whereby immune cells may mistake fatty deposits for intruders. The body attacks fat similar to bacteria and fungi. When expanded fat cells leak or break open, macrophages mobilize to clean up and embed into the adipose tissue. Then macrophages release inflammatory chemicals, including TNF-á and (IL-6). TNF's primary role is to regulate the immune cells and induce inflammation. White blood cells then assist by releasing more cytokines. This link between adiposity and inflammation has been shown to produce 10-35% of IL-6 in a resting individual, and this production increases with increasing adiposity.

During clinical studies, inflammatory-related molecule levels were reduced and increased levels of anti-inflammatory molecules were seen within four weeks after patients began a very low calorie diet. The association of systemic inflammation with insulin resistance and atherosclerosis is the subject of intense research.

In the obese mouse models, inflammation and macrophage-specific genes are upregulated in white adipose tissue (WAT). There were also signs of dramatic increase in circulating insulin level, adipocyte lipolysis and formation of multinucleate giant cells. The fat-derived protein called angiopoietin-like protein 2 (Angptl2) elevates in fat tissues. Higher than normal Angptl2 level in fat tissues develop inflammation as well as insulin and leptin resistance. Stored fat secretes Leptin to signal satiety. Leptin resistance plays a role in the process where appetite overrules the message of satiety. Angptl2 then starts an inflammatory cascade causing blood vessels to remodel and attract macrophages. Angptl2 is an adipocyte-derived inflammatory mediator linking obesity to systemic insulin resistance. It is possible that, as an inflammatory marker, leptin responds specifically to adipose-derived inflammatory cytokines.

C-reactive protein (CRP) is generated at a higher level in obese people. It raises when there is inflammation throughout the body. Mild elevation in CRP increase risk of heart attacks, strokes, high blood pressure, muscle weakness and fragility.

Systemic inflammation and overeating

Hyperglycemia induces IL-6 production from endothelial cells and macrophages. Meals high in saturated fat, as well as meals high in calories have been associated with increases in inflammatory markers. While the inflammatory responses are acute and arise in response to overeating, the response may become chronic if the overeating is chronic.

Bente Klarlund Pedersen wrote in 2013 that interstitial abdominal adiposity (also referred to as accumulated intra-abdominal fat) is a major and possibly primary factor in increasing systemic risk for multiple inflammatory diseases. However, she indicates that this is mediated via TNF-á, rather than Interleukin 6, which she identified as a myokine in 2003. Dr. Pedersen concludes: "Until the beginning of this millennium, it was commonly thought that the increase in IL-6 during exercise was a consequence of an immune response due to local damage in the working muscles and it was hypothesized that macrophages were responsible for this increase. However, an early study demonstrated that IL-6 mRNA in monocytes did not increase as a result of exercise. Further work confirmed this finding at the protein level. In addition, the liver clears, rather than secretes, IL-6 during exercise. The finding that the nuclear transcription rate for IL-6 and the IL-6mRNA levels were rapidly and markedly increased after the onset of exercise suggested that a factor associated with contraction was responsible for the increase in IL-6 transcriptional rate within the nuclei from myocytes.... We recently reported that insulin-resistant individuals demonstrated IL-6 resistance. Accordingly, we suspect that muscle disuse may lead to IL-6 resistance. The elevated circulating levels of IL-6 that accompany obesity and physical inactivity may represent a compensatory mechanism. This would be in line with the well-known facts that insulin resistance is accompanied by hyperinsulinemia and that chronic high circulating levels of leptin may reflect leptin resistance."

Dr. Pedersen continues (in the same article): "Abdominal adiposity is associated with CVD, type 2 diabetes, dementia, colon cancer, and breast cancer, as well as all-cause mortality independently of body mass index, that is, also in people with a normal body weight. Thus, it appears that the health consequences of abdominal adiposity and physical inactivity are very similar. It is well known that both physical inactivity and abdominal adiposity are associated with persistent systemic low-grade inflammation. Models of lipodystrophy suggest that if the subcutaneous fat becomes inflamed and adipocytes undergo apoptosis/ necrosis, the fat storing capacity is impaired and fat will, as a consequence, be deposited as ectopic fat. One obvious explanation to the differential outcome of accumulating fat subcutaneously or as ectopic fat could be that when fat is stored in "the wrong places," it will stimulate an inflammatory response. Evidence exists that visceral fat is more inflamed than subcutaneous fat and constitutes an important source of systemic inflammation.... Accumulating data suggest that although TNF-á is not the pathogenetic factor, it plays a direct role in the metabolic syndrome.

In short, patients with diabetes have a high protein expression of TNF-á in skeletal muscle and increased TNF-á levels in plasma, and it is likely that adipose tissue, which produces TNF-á, is the main source of the circulating TNF-á. In vitro studies demonstrate that TNF-á has direct inhibitory effects on insulin signaling. In addition, TNF-á infusion in healthy humans induces insulin resistance in skeletal muscle, without an effect on EGP [endogenous glucose production]. It has also been proposed that TNF-á causes insulin resistance indirectly *in vivo* by increasing the release of FFAs from adipose tissue. TNF-á increases lipolysis in human and 3T3-L1 adipocytes. However, TNF-á has no effect on muscle fatty acid oxidation, but increases fatty acid incorporation into diacylglycerol, which may be involved in the development of the TNF-á-induced insulin resistance in skeletal muscle. In addition, evidence suggests that TNF-á plays a direct role in linking insulin resistance to vascular disease. Moreover, in CVDs, activated immune cells also play major roles, particularly in the etiology of atherosclerosis. Importantly, also tumor initiation, promotion, and progression is stimulated by systemic elevation of proinflammatory cytokines."

OUTCOMES

The outcome in a particular circumstance will be determined by the tissue in which the injury has occurred and the injurious agent that is causing it. Here are the possible outcomes to inflammation:

1. *Resolution* The complete restoration of the inflamed tissue back to a normal status. Inflammatory measures such as vasodilation, chemical production, and leukocyte infiltration cease, and damaged parenchymal cells regenerate. In situations where limited or short-lived inflammation has occurred this is usually the outcome.
2. *Fibrosis* Large amounts of tissue destruction, or damage in tissues unable to regenerate, cannot be regenerated completely by the body. Fibrous scarring occurs in these areas of damage, forming a scar composed primarily of collagen. The scar will not contain any specialized structures, such as parenchymal cells, hence functional impairment may occur.
3. *Abscess formation* A cavity is formed containing pus, an opaque liquid containing dead white blood cells and bacteria with general debris from destroyed cells.
4. *Chronic inflammation* In acute inflammation, if the injurious agent persists then chronic inflammation will ensue. This process, marked by inflammation lasting many days, months or even years, may lead to the formation of a chronic wound. Chronic inflammation is characterised by the dominating presence of macrophages in the injured tissue. These cells are powerful defensive agents of the body, but the toxins they release (including reactive oxygen species) are injurious to the organism's own tissues as well as invading agents. As a consequence, chronic inflammation is almost always accompanied by tissue destruction.

EXERCISE AND INFLAMMATION

Exercise-induced acute inflammation

Acute inflammation of the muscle cells, as understood in exercise physiology, can result after induced eccentric and concentric muscle training. Participation in eccentric training and conditioning, including resistance training and activities that emphasize eccentric lengthening of the muscle including downhill running on a moderate to high incline can result in considerable soreness within 24 to 48 hours, even though blood lactate levels, previously thought to cause muscle soreness, were much higher with level running. This delayed onset muscle soreness (DOMS) results from structural damage to the contractile filaments and z-disks, which has been noted especially in marathon runners whose muscle fibers revealed remarkable damage to the muscle fibers after both training and marathon competition. The onset and timing of this gradient damage to the muscle parallels the degree of muscle soreness experienced by the runners.

Z-disks are the point of contact for the contractile proteins. They provide structural support for transmission of force when muscle fibers are activated to shorten. However, in marathon runners and those who subscribe to the overload principle to enhance their muscles, show moderate Z-disk streaming and major disruption of thick and thin filaments in parallel groups of sarcomeres as a result of the force of eccentric actions or stretching of tightened muscle fibers.

This disruption of muscle fibers triggers white blood cells to increase following induced muscle soreness, leading to the inflammatory response observation from induced muscle soreness. Elevations in plasma enzymes, myoglobinemia, and abnormal muscle histology and ultrastructure are concluded to be associated with inflammatory response. High tension in the contractile-elastic system of muscle results in structural damage to the muscle fiber and plasmalemma and its epimysium, perimysium, and/or endomysium. The mysium damage disrupts calcium homeostasis in injured fibers and fiber bundles, resulting in necrosis that peaks about 48 hours after exercise. The products of macrophage activity and intracellular contents (such as histamines, kinins, and K^{+}) accumulate outside cells. These substances then stimulate free nerve endings in the muscle; a process that appears accentuated by eccentric exercise, in which large forces are distributed over a relatively small cross-sectional area of the muscle.

Post-inflammatory muscle growth and repair

There is a known relationship between inflammation and muscle growth. For instance, high doses of anti-inflammatory medicines (e.g., NSAIDs) are able to blunt muscle growth.

It has been further theorized that the acute localized inflammatory responses to muscular contraction during exercise, as described above, are a necessary precursor to muscle growth. As a response to muscular contractions, the acute inflammatory response initiates the breakdown and removal of damaged muscle tissue. Muscles can synthesize cytokines in response to contractions, such that the cytokines Interleukin-1 beta (IL-1â), TNF-á, and IL-6 are expressed in skeletal muscle up to 5 days after exercise.

In particular, the increase in levels of IL-6 (Interleukin 6), a myokine, can reach up to one hundred times that of resting levels. Depending on volume, intensity, and other training factors, the IL-6 increase associated with training initiates about 4 hours after resistance training and remains elevated for up to 24 hours.

These acute increases in cytokines, as a response to muscle contractions, help initiate the process of muscle repair and growth by activating satellite cells within the inflamed muscle. Satellite cells are crucial for skeletal muscle adaption to exercise. They contribute to hypertrophy by providing new myonuclei and repair damaged segments of mature myofibers for successful regeneration following injury- or exercise-induced muscle damage; high-level powerlifters can have up to 100% more satellite cells than untrained controls.

A rapid and transient localization of the IL-6 receptor and increased IL-6 expression occurs in satellite cells following contractions. IL-6 has been shown to mediate hypertrophic muscle growth both *in vitro* and *in vivo*. Unaccustomed exercise can increase IL-6 by up to sixfold at 5 hours post-exercise and threefold 8 days after exercise. Also telling is the fact that NSAIDs can decrease satellite cell response to exercise, thereby reducing exercise-induced protein synthesis.

The increase in cytokines (myokines) after resistance exercise coincides with the decrease in levels of myostatin, a protein that inhibits muscle differentiation and growth. The cytokine response to resistance exercise and moderate-intensity running occur differently, with the latter causing a more prolonged response, especially at the 12-24 hour mark.

Developing research has demonstrated that many of the benefits of exercise are mediated through the role of skeletal muscle as an endocrine organ. That is, contracting muscles release multiple substances known as myokines, including but not limited to those cited in the above description, which promote the growth of new tissue, tissue repair, and various anti-inflammatory functions, which in turn reduce the risk of developing various inflammatory diseases. The new view that muscle is an endocrine organ is transforming our understanding of exercise physiology and with it, of the role of inflammation in adaptation to stress.

Chronic inflammation and muscle loss

Both chronic and extreme inflammation are associated with disruptions of anabolic signals initiating muscle growth. Chronic inflammation has been implicated as part of the cause of the muscle loss that occurs with aging. Increased protein levels of myostatin have been described in patients with diseases characterized by chronic low-grade inflammation. Increased levels of TNF-á can suppress the AKT/mTOR pathway, a crucial pathway for regulating skeletal muscle hypertrophy, thereby increasing muscle catabolism. Cytokines may antagonize the anabolic effects of Insulin-like growth factor 1 (IGF-1). In the case of sepsis, an extreme whole body inflammatory state, the synthesis of both myofibrillar and sarcoplasmic proteins are inhibited, with the inhibition taking place preferentially in fast-twitch muscle fibers. Sepsis is also able to prevent leucine from stimulating muscle protein synthesis. In animal models, when inflammation is created, mTOR loses its ability to be stimulated by muscle growth.

Exercise as a treatment for inflammation

Regular physical activity is reported to decrease markers of inflammation, although the correlation is imperfect and seems to reveal differing results contingent upon training intensity. For instance, while baseline measurements of circulating inflammatory markers do not seem to differ greatly between healthy trained and untrained adults, long-term training may help reduce chronic low-grade inflammation. On the other hand, levels of the anti-inflammatory myokine IL-6 (Interleukin 6) remained elevated longer into the recovery period following an acute bout of exercise in patients with inflammatory diseases, relative to the recovery of healthy controls. It may well be that low-intensity training can reduce resting pro-inflammatory markers (CRP, IL-6), while moderate-intensity training has milder and less-established anti-inflammatory benefits. There is a strong relationship between exhaustive exercise and chronic low-grade inflammation. Marathon running may enhance IL-6 levels as much as 100 times over normal and increases total leuckocyte count and neturophil mobilization.

Regarding the above, IL-6 had previously been classified as a proinflammatory cytokine. Therefore, it was first thought that the exercise-induced IL-6 response was related to muscle damage. However, it has become evident that eccentric exercise is not associated with a larger increase in plasma IL-6 than exercise involving concentric "nondamaging" muscle contractions. This finding clearly demonstrates that muscle damage is not required to provoke an increase in plasma IL-6 during exercise. As a matter of fact, eccentric exercise may result in a delayed peak and a much slower decrease of plasma IL-6 during recovery.

Recent work has shown that both upstream and downstream signalling pathways for IL-6 differ markedly between myocytes and macrophages. It appears that unlike IL-6 signalling in macrophages, which is dependent upon activation of the NFêB signalling pathway, intramuscular IL-6 expression is regulated by a network of signalling cascades, including the Ca2+/NFAT and glycogen/p38 MAPK pathways. Thus, when IL-6 is signalling in monocytes or macrophages, it creates a pro-inflammatory response, whereas IL-6 activation and signalling in muscle is totally independent of a preceding TNF-response or NFêB activation, and is anti-inflammatory.

Several studies show that markers of inflammation are reduced following longer-term behavioural changes involving both reduced energy intake and a regular program of increased physical activity, and that, in particular, IL-6 was miscast as an inflammatory marker. For example, the anti-inflammatory effects of IL-6 have been demonstrated by IL-6 stimulating the production of the classical anti-inflammatory cytokines IL-1ra and IL-10.

As such, individuals pursuing exercise as a means to treat the causal factors underlying chronic inflammation are pursuing a course of action strongly supported by current research, as an inactive lifestyle is strongly associated with the development and progression of multiple inflammatory diseases. Note that cautions regarding over-exertion may apply in certain cases, as discussed above, though this concern rarely applies to the general population.

Signal-to-noise theory

Given that localized acute inflammation is a necessary component for muscle growth, and that chronic low-grade inflammation is associated with a disruption of anabolic signals initiating muscle growth, it has been theorized that a signal-to-noise model may best describe the relationship between inflammation and muscle growth. By keeping the "noise" of chronic inflammation to a minimum, the localized acute inflammatory response signals a stronger anabolic response than could be achieved with higher levels of chronic inflammation.

INFECTION

Infection is the invasion of an organism's body tissues by disease-causing agents, their multiplication, and the reaction of host tissues to these organisms and the toxins they produce.

Infectious disease, also known as transmissible disease or communicable disease, is illness resulting from an infection.

Infections are caused by infectious agents including viruses, viroids, prions, bacteria, nematodes such as parasitic roundworms and pinworms, arthropods such as ticks, mites, fleas, and lice, fungi such as ringworm, and other macroparasites such as tapeworms and other helminths.

Hosts can fight infections using their immune system. Mammalian hosts react to infections with an innate response, often involving inflammation, followed by an adaptive response. Specific medications used to treat infections include antibiotics, antivirals, antifungals, antiprotozoals, and antihelminthics. Infectious diseases resulted in 9.2 million deaths in 2013 (about 17% of all deaths). The branch of medicine that focuses on infections is referred to as Infectious Disease.

CLASSIFICATION

Bacterial infections are classified by the causative agent, as well as the symptoms and medical signs produced. Symptomatic infections are *apparent,* whereas an infection that is active but does not produce noticeable symptoms may be called *inapparent, silent, subclinical* or occult. An infection that is inactive or dormant is called a *latent infection*. A short-term infection is an *acute* infection. A long-term infection is a chronic infection.

Primary versus opportunistic

Among the vast varieties of microorganisms, relatively few cause disease in otherwise healthy individuals. Infectious disease results from the interplay between those few pathogens and the defenses of the hosts they infect. The appearance and severity of disease resulting from any pathogen, depends upon the ability of that pathogen to damage the host as well as the ability of the host to resist the pathogen.

Clinicians therefore classify infectious microorganisms or microbes according to the status of host defenses - either as *primary pathogens* or as *opportunistic pathogens*:

- Primary pathogens cause disease as a result of their presence or activity within the normal, healthy host, and their intrinsic virulence (the severity of the disease they cause) is, in part, a necessary consequence of their need to reproduce and spread. Many of the most common primary pathogens of humans only infect humans, however many serious diseases are caused by organisms acquired from the environment or which infect non-human hosts.
- Opportunistic pathogens can cause an infectious disease in a host with depressed resistance. Opportunistic infection may be caused by microbes ordinarily in contact with the host, such as pathogenic bacteria or fungi in the gastrointestinal or the upper respiratory tract, and they may also result from (otherwise innocuous) microbes acquired from other hosts (as in *Clostridium difficile* colitis) or from the environment as a result of traumatic introduction (as in surgical wound infections or compound fractures). An opportunistic disease requires impairment of host defenses, which may occur as a result of genetic defects (such as Chronic granulomatous disease), exposure to antimicrobial drugs or immunosuppressive chemicals (as might occur following poisoning or cancer chemotherapy), exposure to ionizing radiation, or as a result of an infectious disease with immunosuppressive activity (such as with measles, malaria or HIV disease). Primary pathogens may also cause more severe disease in a host with depressed resistance than would normally occur in an immunosufficient host.

Occult infection

Occult infection is a hidden infection first recognized by secondary manifestations. Dr. Fran Giampietro discovered this type, and coined the term "occult infection" in the late 1930s.

Infectious or not

One way of proving that a given disease is "infectious", is to satisfy Koch's postulates (first proposed by Robert Koch), which demands that the infectious agent be identified only in patients and not in healthy controls, and that patients who contract the agent also develop the disease. These postulates were first used in the discovery that Mycobacteria species cause tuberculosis. Koch's postulates can not be applied ethically for many human diseases because they require experimental infection of a healthy individual with a pathogen produced as a pure culture. Often, even clearly infectious diseases do not meet the infectious criteria. For example, *Treponema pallidum*, the causative spirochete of syphilis, cannot be cultured *in vitro* - however the organism can be cultured in rabbit testes.

It is less clear that a pure culture comes from an animal source serving as host than it is when derived from microbes derived from plate culture. Epidemiology is another important tool used to study disease in a population. For infectious diseases it helps to determine if a disease outbreak is sporadic (occasional occurrence), endemic (regular cases often occurring in a region), epidemic (an unusually high number of cases in a region), or pandemic (a global epidemic).

Contagiousness

Infectious diseases are sometimes called contagious disease when they are easily transmitted by contact with an ill person or their secretions (e.g., influenza). Thus, a contagious disease is a subset of infectious disease that is especially infective or easily transmitted. Other types of infectious/transmissible/communicable diseases with more specialized routes of infection, such as vector transmission or sexual transmission, are usually not regarded as "contagious," and often do not require medical isolation (sometimes loosely called quarantine) of victims. However, this specialized connotation of the word "contagious" and "contagious disease" (easy transmissibility) is not always respected in popular use.

By anatomic location

Infections can be classified by the anatomic location or organ system infected, including:

- Urinary tract infection
- Skin infection
- Respiratory tract infection
- Odontogenic infection (an infection that originates within a tooth or in the closely surrounding tissues)
- Vaginal infections
- Intra-amniotic infection

In addition, locations of inflammation where infection is the most common cause include pneumonia, meningitis and salpingitis.

SIGNS AND SYMPTOMS

The symptoms of an infection depend on the type of disease. Some signs of infection affect the whole body generally, such as fatigue, loss of appetite, weight loss, fevers, night sweats, chills, aches and pains. Others are specific to individual body parts, such as skin rashes, coughing, or a runny nose.

In certain cases, infectious diseases may be asymptomatic for much or even all of their course in a given host. In the latter case, the disease may only be defined as a "disease" (which by definition means an illness) in hosts who secondarily become ill after contact with an asymptomatic carrier. An infection is not synonymous with an infectious disease, as some infections do not cause illness in a host.

Bacterial or viral

Bacterial and viral infections can both cause the same kinds of symptoms. It can be difficult to distinguish which is the cause of a specific infection. It's important to distinguish, because viral infections cannot be cured by antibiotics.

Comparison of viral and bacterial infection

Comparison of viral and bacterial infection		
Characteristic	Viral infection	Bacterial infection
Typical symptoms	In general, viral infections are systemic. This means they involve many different parts of the body or more than one body system at the same time; i.e. a runny nose, sinus congestion, cough, body aches etc. They can be local at times as in viral conjunctivitis or "pink eye" and herpes. Only a few viral infections are painful, like herpes. The pain of viral infections is often described as itchy or burning.	The classic symptoms of a bacterial infection are localized redness, heat, swelling and pain. One of the hallmarks of a bacterial infection is local pain, pain that is in a specific part of the body. For example, if a cut occurs and is infected with bacteria, pain occurs at the site of the infection. Bacterial throat pain is often characterized by more pain on one side of the throat. An ear infection is more likely to be diagnosed as bacterial if the pain occurs in only one ear. A cut that produces pus and milky-colored liquid is most likely infected.
Cause	Pathogenic viruses	Pathogenic bacteria

PATHOPHYSIOLOGY

There is a general chain of events that applies to infections. For infections to occur, a given chain of events must occur. The chain of events involves several steps—which include the infectious agent, reservoir, entering a susceptible host, exit and transmission to new hosts. Each of the links must be present in a chronological order for an infection to develop. Understanding these steps helps health care workers target the infection and prevent it from occurring in the first place.

Colonization

Infection begins when an organism successfully colonizes by entering the body, growing and multiplying. Most humans are not easily infected. Those who are weak, sick, malnourished, have cancer or are diabetic have increased susceptibility to chronic or persistent infections. Individuals who have a suppressed immune system are particularly susceptible to opportunistic infections. Entrance to the host at host-pathogen interface, generally occurs through the mucosa in orifices like the oral cavity, nose, eyes, genitalia, anus, or the microbe can enter through open wounds. While a few organisms can grow at the initial site of entry, many migrate and cause systemic infection in different organs. Some pathogens grow within the host cells (intracellular) whereas others grow freely in bodily fluids.

Wound colonization refers to nonreplicating microorganisms within the wound, while in infected wounds, replicating organisms exist and tissue is injured. All multicellular organisms are colonized to some degree by extrinsic organisms, and the vast majority of these exist in either a mutualistic or commensal relationship with the host. An example of the former is the anaerobic bacteria species, which colonizes the mammalian colon, and an example of the latter is various species of staphylococcus that exist on human skin. Neither of these colonizations are considered infections. The difference between an infection and a colonization is often only a matter of circumstance. Non-pathogenic organisms can become pathogenic given specific conditions, and even the most virulent organism requires certain circumstances to cause a compromising infection. Some colonizing bacteria, such as *Corynebacteria sp.* and *viridans streptococci*, prevent the adhesion and colonization of pathogenic bacteria and thus have a symbiotic relationship with the host, preventing infection and speeding wound healing.

The variables involved in the outcome of a host becoming inoculated by a pathogen and the ultimate outcome include:

- the route of entry of the pathogen and the access to host regions that it gains
- the intrinsic virulence of the particular organism
- the quantity or load of the initial inoculant
- the immune status of the host being colonized

As an example, the staphylococcus species remains harmless on the skin, but, when present in a normally sterile space, such as in the capsule of a joint or the peritoneum, multiplies without resistance and creates a burden on the host. It can be difficult to know which chronic wounds are infected. Despite the huge number of wounds seen in clinical practice, there are limited quality data for evaluated symptoms and signs. A review of chronic wounds in the Journal of the American Medical Association's "Rational Clinical Examination Series" quantified the importance of increased pain as an indicator of infection. The review showed that the most useful finding is an increase in the level of pain [likelihood ratio (LR) range, 11-20] makes infection much more likely, but the absence of pain (negative likelihood ratio range, 0.64-0.88) does not rule out infection (summary LR 0.64-0.88).

Disease

Disease can arise if the host's protective immune mechanisms are compromised and the organism inflicts damage on the host. Microorganisms can cause tissue damage by releasing a variety of toxins or destructive enzymes. For example, Clostridium tetani releases a toxin that paralyzes muscles, and staphylococcus releases toxins that produce shock and sepsis. Not all infectious agents cause disease in all hosts. For example, less than 5% of individuals infected with polio develop disease. On the other hand, some infectious agents are highly virulent. The prion causing mad cow disease and Creutzfeldt–Jakob disease invariably kills all animals and people that are infected.

Persistent infections occur because the body is unable to clear the organism after the initial infection. Persistent infections are characterized by the continual presence of the infectious organism, often as latent infection with occasional recurrent relapses of active infection. There are some viruses that can maintain a persistent infection by infecting different cells of the body. Some viruses once acquired never leave the body. A typical example is the herpes virus, which tends to hide in nerves and become reactivated when specific circumstances arise.

Persistent infections cause millions of deaths globally each year. Chronic infections by parasites account for a high morbidity and mortality in many underdeveloped countries.

Transmission

For infecting organisms to survive and repeat the infection cycle in other hosts, they (or their progeny) must leave an existing reservoir and cause infection elsewhere. Infection transmission can take place via many potential routes:

- Droplet contact, also known as the *respiratory route*, and the resultant infection can be termed airborne disease. If an infected person coughs or sneezes on another person the microorganisms, suspended in warm, moist droplets, may enter the body through the nose, mouth or eye surfaces.
- Fecal-oral transmission, wherein foodstuffs or water become contaminated (by people not washing their hands before preparing

food, or untreated sewage being released into a drinking water supply) and the people who eat and drink them become infected. Common fecal-oral transmitted pathogens include *Vibrio cholerae*, *Giardia* species, rotaviruses, *Entameba histolytica*, *Escherichia coli*, and tape worms. Most of these pathogens cause gastroenteritis.

- Sexual transmission, with the resulting disease being called sexually transmitted disease
- Oral transmission; Diseases that are transmitted primarily by oral means may be caught through direct oral contact such as kissing, or by indirect contact such as by sharing a drinking glass or a cigarette.
- Transmission by direct contact; Some diseases that are transmissible by direct contact include athlete's foot, impetigo and warts
- Vertical transmission'; directly from the mother to an embryo, fetus or baby during pregnancy or childbirth. It can occur when the mother gets an infection as an intercurrent disease in pregnancy.
- Iatrogenic transmission, due to medical procedures such as injection or transplantation of infected material.

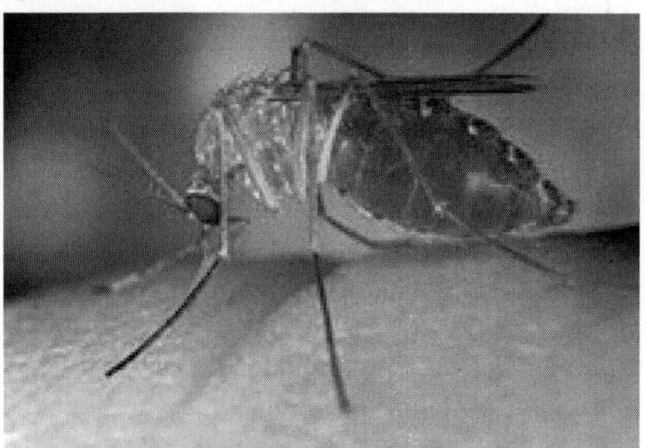

Fig. Culex mosquitos (*Culex quinquefasciatus* shown) are biological vectors that transmit West Nile Virus.

- Vector-borne transmission, transmitted by a vector, which is an organism that does not cause disease itself but that transmits infection by conveying pathogens from one host to another.

The relationship between *virulence versus transmissibility* is complex; if a disease is rapidly fatal, the host may die before the microbe can be passed along to another host.

DIAGNOSIS

Diagnosis of infectious disease sometimes involves identifying an infectious agent either directly or indirectly. In practice most minor infectious diseases such as warts, cutaneous abscesses, respiratory system infections and diarrheal diseases are diagnosed by their clinical presentation. Conclusions about the cause of the disease are based upon the likelihood that a patient came in contact with a particular agent, the presence of a microbe in a community, and other epidemiological considerations. Given sufficient effort, all known infectious agents can be specifically identified. The benefits of identification, however, are often greatly outweighed by the cost, as often there is no specific treatment, the cause is obvious, or the outcome of an infection is benign.

Diagnosis of infectious disease is nearly always initiated by medical history and physical examination. More detailed identification techniques involve the culture of infectious agents isolated from a patient. Culture allows identification of infectious organisms by examining their microscopic features, by detecting the presence of substances produced by pathogens, and by directly identifying an organism by its genotype. Other techniques (such as X-rays, CAT scans, PET scans or NMR) are used to produce images of internal abnormalities resulting from the growth of an infectious agent. The images are useful in detection of, for example, a bone abscess or a spongiform encephalopathy produced by a prion.

Symptomatic diagnostics

The diagnosis is aided by the presenting symptoms in any individual with an infectious disease, yet it usually needs additional diagnostic techniques to confirm the suspicion. Some signs are specifically characteristic and indicative of a disease and are called pathognomonic signs; but these are rare. Not all infections are symptomatic.

In children the presence of cyanosis, rapid breathing, poor peripheral perfusion, or a petechial rash increases the risk of a serious infection by greater than 5 fold. Other important indicators include parental concern, clinical instinct, and temperature greater than 40 °C.

Microbial culture

Microbiological culture is a principal tool used to diagnose infectious disease. In a microbial culture, a growth medium is provided for a specific agent. A sample taken from potentially diseased tissue or fluid is then tested for the presence of an infectious agent able to grow within that medium. Most pathogenic bacteria are easily grown on nutrient agar, a form of solid medium that supplies carbohydrates and proteins necessary for growth of a bacterium, along with copious amounts of water. A single bacterium will grow into a visible mound on the surface of the plate called a colony, which may be separated from other colonies or melded together into a "lawn".

The size, color, shape and form of a colony is characteristic of the bacterial species, its specific genetic makeup (its strain), and the environment which supports its growth. Other ingredients are often added to the plate to aid in identification. Plates may contain substances that permit the growth of some bacteria and not others, or that change color in response to certain bacteria and not others. Bacteriological plates such as these are commonly used in the clinical identification of infectious bacterium. Microbial culture may also be used in the identification of viruses: the medium in this case being cells grown in culture that the virus can infect, and then alter or kill. In the case of viral identification, a region of dead cells results from viral growth, and is called a "plaque". Eukaryotic parasites may also be grown in culture as a means of identifying a particular agent.

In the absence of suitable plate culture techniques, some microbes require culture within live animals. Bacteria such as *Mycobacterium leprae* and *Treponema pallidum* can be grown in animals, although serological and microscopic techniques make the use of live animals unnecessary. Viruses are also usually identified using alternatives to growth in culture or animals. Some viruses may be grown in embryonated eggs. Another useful identification method is Xenodiagnosis, or the use of a vector to support the growth of an infectious agent. Chagas disease is the most significant example, because it is difficult to directly demonstrate the presence of the causative agent, *Trypanosoma cruzi* in a patient, which therefore makes it difficult to definitively make a diagnosis. In this case, xenodiagnosis involves the use of the vector of the Chagas agent *T. cruzi*, an uninfected triatomine bug, which takes a blood meal from a person suspected of having been infected. The bug is later inspected for growth of *T. cruzi* within its gut.

Microscopy

Another principal tool in the diagnosis of infectious disease is microscopy. Virtually all of the culture techniques discussed above rely, at some point, on microscopic examination for definitive identification of the infectious agent. Microscopy may be carried out with simple instruments, such as the compound light microscope, or with instruments as complex as an electron microscope. Samples obtained from patients may be viewed directly under the light microscope, and can often rapidly lead to identification. Microscopy is often also used in conjunction with biochemical staining techniques, and can be made exquisitely specific when used in combination with antibody based techniques. For example, the use of antibodies made artificially fluorescent (fluorescently labeled antibodies) can be directed to bind to and identify a specific antigens present on a pathogen. A fluorescence microscope is then used to detect fluorescently labeled antibodies bound to internalized antigens within clinical samples or cultured cells. This technique is especially useful in the diagnosis of viral diseases, where the light microscope is incapable of identifying a virus directly.

Other microscopic procedures may also aid in identifying infectious agents. Almost all cells readily stain with a number of basic dyes due to the electrostatic attraction between negatively charged cellular molecules and the positive charge on the dye. A cell is normally transparent under a microscope, and using a stain increases the contrast of a cell with its background. Staining a cell with a dye such as Giemsa stain or crystal violet allows a microscopist to describe its size, shape, internal and external components and its associations with other cells.

The response of bacteria to different staining procedures is used in the taxonomic classification of microbes as well. Two methods, the Gram stain and the acid-fast stain, are the standard approaches used to classify bacteria and to diagnosis of disease. The Gram stain identifies the bacterial groups Firmicutes and Actinobacteria, both of which contain many significant human pathogens. The acid-fast staining procedure identifies the Actinobacterial genera *Mycobacterium* and *Nocardia*.

Biochemical tests

Biochemical tests used in the identification of infectious agents include the detection of metabolic or enzymatic products characteristic of a particular infectious agent. Since bacteria ferment carbohydrates in patterns characteristic of their genus and species, the detection of fermentation products is commonly used in bacterial identification. Acids, alcohols and gases are usually detected in these tests when bacteria are grown in selective liquid or solid media.

The isolation of enzymes from infected tissue can also provide the basis of a biochemical diagnosis of an infectious disease. For example, humans can make neither RNA replicases nor reverse transcriptase, and the presence of these enzymes are characteristic of specific types of viral infections. The ability of the viral protein hemagglutinin to bind red blood cells together into a detectable matrix may also be characterized as a biochemical test for viral infection, although strictly speaking hemagglutinin is not an *enzyme* and has no metabolic function.

Serological methods are highly sensitive, specific and often extremely rapid tests used to identify microorganisms. These tests are based upon the ability of an antibody to bind specifically to an antigen. The antigen, usually a protein or carbohydrate made by an infectious agent, is bound by the antibody. This binding then sets off a chain of events that can be visibly obvious in various ways, dependent upon the test. For example, "Strep throat" is often diagnosed within minutes, and is based on the appearance of antigens made by the causative agent, *S. pyogenes*, that is retrieved from a patients throat with a cotton swab. Serological tests, if available, are usually the preferred route of identification, however the tests are costly to develop and the reagents used in the test often require refrigeration. Some serological methods are extremely costly, although when commonly used, such as with the "strep test", they can be inexpensive.

Complex serological techniques have been developed into what are known as Immunoassays. Immunoassays can use the basic antibody – antigen binding as the basis to produce an electro - magnetic or particle radiation signal, which can be detected by some form of instrumentation. Signal of unknowns can be compared to that of standards allowing quantitation of the target antigen. To aid in the diagnosis of infectious diseases, immunoassays can detect or measure antigens from either infectious agents or proteins generated by an infected organism in response to a foreign agent. For example, immunoassay A may detect the presence of a surface protein from a virus particle. Immunoassay B on the other hand may detect or measure antibodies produced by an organism's immune system which are made to neutralize and allow the destruction of the virus.

Instrumentation can be used to read extremely small signals created by secondary reactions linked to the antibody – antigen binding. Instrumentation can control sampling, reagent use, reaction times, signal detection, calculation of results, and data management to yield a cost effective automated process for diagnosis of infectious disease.

Molecular diagnostics

Technologies based upon the polymerase chain reaction (PCR) method will become nearly ubiquitous gold standards of diagnostics of the near future, for several reasons. First, the catalog of infectious agents has grown to the point that virtually all of the significant infectious agents of the human population have been identified. Second, an infectious agent must grow within the human body to cause disease; essentially it must amplify its own nucleic acids in order to cause a disease. This amplification of nucleic acid in infected tissue offers an opportunity to detect the infectious agent by using PCR. Third, the essential tools for directing PCR, primers, are derived from the genomes of infectious agents, and with time those genomes will be known, if they are not already.

Thus, the technological ability to detect any infectious agent rapidly and specifically are currently available. The only remaining blockades to the use of PCR as a standard tool of diagnosis are in its cost and application, neither of which is insurmountable. The diagnosis of a few diseases will not benefit from the development of PCR methods, such as some of the clostridial diseases (tetanus and botulism). These diseases are fundamentally biological poisonings by relatively small numbers of infectious bacteria that produce extremely potent neurotoxins. A significant proliferation of the infectious agent does not occur, this limits the ability of PCR to detect the presence of any bacteria.

Indication of tests

There is usually an indication for a specific identification of an infectious agent only when such identification can aid in the treatment or prevention of the disease, or to advance knowledge of the course of an illness prior to the development of effective therapeutic or preventative measures. For example, in the early 1980s, prior to the appearance of AZT for the treatment of AIDS, the course of the disease was closely followed by monitoring the composition of patient blood samples, even though the outcome would not offer the patient any further treatment options. In part, these studies on the appearance of HIV in specific communities permitted the advancement of hypotheses as to the route of transmission of the virus. By understanding how the disease was transmitted, resources could be targeted to the communities at greatest risk in campaigns aimed at reducing the number of new infections. The specific serological diagnostic identification, and later genotypic or molecular identification, of HIV also enabled the development of hypotheses as to the temporal and geographical origins of the virus, as well as a myriad of other hypothesis.

The development of molecular diagnostic tools have enabled physicians and researchers to monitor the efficacy of treatment with anti-retroviral drugs. Molecular diagnostics are now commonly used to identify HIV in healthy people long before the onset of illness and have been used to demonstrate the existence of people who are genetically resistant to HIV infection.

Thus, while there still is no cure for AIDS, there is great therapeutic and predictive benefit to identifying the virus and monitoring the virus levels within the blood of infected individuals, both for the patient and for the community at large.

PREVENTION

Techniques like hand washing, wearing gowns, and wearing face masks can help prevent infections from being passed from the surgeon to the patient or vice versa. Frequent hand washing remains the most important defense against the spread of unwanted organisms. Nutrition must be improved and one has to make changes in life style- such as avoiding the use of illicit drugs, using a condom, and entering an exercise program. Cooking foods well and avoiding foods that have been left outside for a long time is also important.

Antimicrobial substances used to prevent transmission of infections include:

- antiseptics, which are applied to living tissue/skin
- disinfectants, which destroy microorganisms found on non-living objects.
- antibiotics, called prophylactic when given as prevention rather as treatment of infection. However, long term use of antibiotics leads to resistance and chances of developing opportunistic infections like clostridium difficile colitis. Thus, avoiding using antibiotics longer than necessary helps preventing such infectious diseases.

One of the ways to prevent or slow down the transmission of infectious diseases is to recognize the different characteristics of various diseases. Some critical disease characteristics that should be evaluated include virulence, distance traveled by victims, and level of contagiousness. The human strains of Ebola virus, for example, incapacitate their victims extremely quickly and kill them soon after.

As a result, the victims of this disease do not have the opportunity to travel very far from the initial infection zone. Also, this virus must spread through skin lesions or permeable membranes such as the eye. Thus, the initial stage of Ebola is not very contagious since its victims experience only internal hemorrhaging. As a result of the above features, the spread of Ebola is very rapid and usually stays within a relatively confined geographical area. In contrast, the Human Immunodeficiency Virus (HIV) kills its victims very slowly by attacking their immune system. As a result, many of its victims transmit the virus to other individuals before even realizing that they are carrying the disease. Also, the relatively low virulence allows its victims to travel long distances, increasing the likelihood of an epidemic.

Another effective way to decrease the transmission rate of infectious diseases is to recognize the effects of small-world networks. In epidemics, there are often extensive interactions within hubs or groups of infected individuals and other interactions within discrete hubs of susceptible individuals. Despite the low interaction between discrete hubs, the disease can jump to and spread in a susceptible hub via a single or few interactions with an infected hub. Thus, infection rates in small-world networks can be reduced somewhat if interactions between individuals within infected hubs are eliminated (Figure 1). However, infection rates can be drastically reduced if the main focus is on the prevention of transmission jumps between hubs.

The use of needle exchange programs in areas with a high density of drug users with HIV is an example of the successful implementation of this treatment method. Another example is the use of ring culling or vaccination of potentially susceptible livestock in adjacent farms to prevent the spread of the foot-and-mouth virus in 2001.

A general method to prevent transmission of vector-borne pathogens is pest control.

Immunity

Infection with most pathogens does not result in death of the host and the offending organism is ultimately cleared after the symptoms of the disease have waned. This process requires immune mechanisms to kill or inactivate the inoculum of the pathogen. Specific acquired immunity against infectious diseases may be mediated by antibodies and/or T lymphocytes. Immunity mediated by these two factors may be manifested by:

- a direct effect upon a pathogen, such as antibody-initiated complement-dependent bacteriolysis, opsonoization, phagocytosis and killing, as occurs for some bacteria,
- neutralization of viruses so that these organisms cannot enter cells,
- or by T lymphocytes which will kill a cell parasitized by a microorganism.

The immune system response to a microorganism often causes symptoms such as a high fever and inflammation, and has the potential to be more devastating than direct damage caused by a microbe.

Resistance to infection (immunity) may be acquired following a disease, by asymptomatic carriage of the pathogen, by harboring an organism with a similar structure (crossreacting), or by vaccination. Knowledge of the protective antigens and specific acquired host immune factors is more complete for primary pathogens than for opportunistic pathogens.

Immune resistance to an infectious disease requires a critical level of either antigen-specific antibodies and/or T cells when the host encounters the pathogen. Some individuals develop natural serum antibodies to the surface polysaccharides of some agents although they have had little or no contact with the agent, these natural antibodies confer specific protection to adults and are passively transmitted to newborns.

Host genetic factors

The clearance of the pathogens, either treatment-induced or spontaneous, it can be influenced by the genetic variants carried by the individual patients. For instance, for genotype 1 hepatitis C treated with Pegylated interferon-alpha-2a or Pegylated interferon-alpha-2b (brand names Pegasys or PEG-Intron) combined with ribavirin, it has been shown that genetic polymorphisms near the human IL28B gene, encoding interferon lambda 3, are associated with significant differences in the treatment-induced clearance of the virus. This finding, originally reported in Nature, showed that genotype 1 hepatitis C patients carrying certain genetic variant alleles near the IL28B gene are more possibly to achieve sustained virological response after the treatment than others. Later report from Nature demonstrated that the same genetic variants are also associated with the natural clearance of the genotype 1 hepatitis C virus.

TREATMENTS

When infection attacks the body, *anti-infective* drugs can suppress the infection. Four types of *anti-infective* or drugs exist: antibacterial (antibiotic), antiviral, antitubercular, and antifungal. Depending on the severity and the type of infection, the antibiotic may be given by mouth, injection or may be applied topically. Severe infections of the brain are usually treated with intravenous antibiotics. Sometimes, multiple antibiotics are used to decrease the risk of resistance and increase efficacy. Antibiotics only work for bacteria and do not affect viruses. Antibiotics work by slowing down the multiplication of bacteria or killing the bacteria. The most common classes of antibiotics used in medicine include penicillin, cephalosporins, aminoglycosides, macrolides, quinolones and tetracyclines.

EPIDEMIOLOGY

In 2010 about 10 million people died of an infectious disease.

The World Health Organization collects information on global deaths by International Classification of Disease (ICD) code categories. The following table lists the top infectious disease by number of deaths in 2002. 1993 data is included for comparison.

Worldwide mortality due to infectious diseases					
Rank	Cause of death	Deaths 2002 (in millions)	Percentage of all deaths	Deaths 1993 (in millions)	1993 Rank
N/A	All infectious diseases	14.7	25.9%	16.4	32.2%
1	Lower respiratory infections	3.9	6.9%	4.1	1
2	HIV/AIDS	2.8	4.9%	0.7	7
3	Diarrheal diseases	1.8	3.2%	3.0	2
4	Tuberculosis (TB)	1.6	2.7%	2.7	3
5	Malaria	1.3	2.2%	2.0	4
6	Measles	0.6	1.1%	1.1	5
7	Pertussis	0.29	0.5%	0.36	7
8	Tetanus	0.21	0.4%	0.15	12
9	Meningitis	0.17	0.3%	0.25	8
10	Syphilis	0.16	0.3%	0.19	11
11	Hepatitis B	0.10	0.2%	0.93	6
12-17	Tropical diseases (6)	0.13	0.2%	0.53	9, 10, 16-18
Note: Other causes of death include maternal and perinatal conditions (5.2%), nutritional deficiencies (0.9%),noncommunicable conditions (58.8%), and injuries (9.1%).					

The top three single agent/disease killers are HIV/AIDS, TB and malaria. While the number of deaths due to nearly every disease have decreased, deaths due to HIV/AIDS have increased fourfold. Childhood diseases include pertussis, poliomyelitis, diphtheria, measles and tetanus. Children also make up a large percentage of lower respiratory and diarrheal deaths. In 2012, approximately 3.1 million people have died due to lower respiratory infections, making it the number 4 leading cause of death in the world.

Historic pandemics

A pandemic (or global epidemic) is a disease that affects people over an extensive geographical area.

- Plague of Justinian, from 541 to 750, killed between 50% and 60% of Europe's population.

- The Black Death of 1347 to 1352 killed 25 million in Europe over 5 years. The plague reduced the world population from an estimated 450 million to between 350 and 375 million in the 14th century.
- The introduction of smallpox, measles, and typhus to the areas of Central and South America by European explorers during the 15th and 16th centuries caused pandemics among the native inhabitants. Between 1518 and 1568 disease pandemics are said to have caused the population of Mexico to fall from 20 million to 3 million.
- The first European influenza epidemic occurred between 1556 and 1560, with an estimated mortality rate of 20%.
- Smallpox killed an estimated 60 million Europeans during the 18th century (approximately 400,000 per year). Up to 30% of those infected, including 80% of the children under 5 years of age, died from the disease, and one-third of the survivors went blind.
- In the 19th century, tuberculosis killed an estimated one-quarter of the adult population of Europe; by 1918 one in six deaths in France were still caused by TB.
- The Influenza Pandemic of 1918 (or the Spanish Flu) killed 25-50 million people (about 2% of world population of 1.7 billion). Today Influenza kills about 250,000 to 500,000 worldwide each year.

Emerging diseases

In most cases, microorganisms live in harmony with their hosts via mutual or commensal interactions. Diseases can emerge when existing parasites become pathogenic or when new pathogenic parasites enter a new host.

1. Coevolution between parasite and host can lead to hosts becoming resistant to the parasites or the parasites may evolve greater virulence, leading to immunopathological disease.
2. Human activity is involved with many emerging infectious diseases, such as environmental change enabling a parasite to occupy new niches. When that happens, a pathogen that had been confined to a remote habitat has a wider distribution and possibly a new host organism. Parasites jumping from nonhuman to human hosts are known as zoonoses. Under disease invasion, when a parasite invades a new host species, it may become pathogenic in the new host.

Several human activities have led to the emergence of zoonotic human pathogens, including viruses, bacteria, protozoa, and rickettsia, and spread of vector-borne diseases:

- Encroachment on wildlife habitats. The construction of new villages and housing developments in rural areas force animals to live in dense populations, creating opportunities for microbes to mutate and emerge.

- Changes in agriculture. The introduction of new crops attracts new crop pests and the microbes they carry to farming communities, exposing people to unfamiliar diseases.
- The destruction of rain forests. As countries make use of their rain forests, by building roads through forests and clearing areas for settlement or commercial ventures, people encounter insects and other animals harboring previously unknown microorganisms.
- Uncontrolled urbanization. The rapid growth of cities in many developing countries tends to concentrate large numbers of people into crowded areas with poor sanitation. These conditions foster transmission of contagious diseases.
- Modern transport. Ships and other cargo carriers often harbor unintended "passengers", that can spread diseases to faraway destinations. While with international jet-airplane travel, people infected with a disease can carry it to distant lands, or home to their families, before their first symptoms appear.

HISTORY

Ideas of contagion became more popular in Europe during the Renaissance, particularly through the writing of the Italian physician Girolamo Fracastoro.

Anton van Leeuwenhoek (1632–1723) advanced the science of microscopy by being the first to observe microorganisms, allowing for easy visualization of bacteria.

In the mid-19th century John Snow and William Budd did important work demonstrating the contagiousness of typhoid and cholera through contaminated water. Both are credited with decreasing epidemics of cholera in their towns by implementing measures to prevent contamination of water.

Louis Pasteur proved beyond doubt that certain diseases are caused by infectious agents, and developed a vaccine for rabies.

Robert Koch, provided the study of infectious diseases with a scientific basis known as Koch's postulates.

Edward Jenner, Jonas Salk and Albert Sabin developed effective vaccines for smallpox and polio, which would later result in the eradication and near-eradication of these diseases, respectively.

Alexander Fleming discovered the world's first antibiotic Penicillin which Florey and Chain then developed.

Gerhard Domagk developed sulphonamides, the first broad spectrum synthetic antibacterial drugs.

Medical specialists

The medical treatment of infectious diseases falls into the medical field of Infectious Disease and in some cases the study of propagation pertains to the field of Epidemiology. Generally, infections are initially diagnosed by primary care physicians or internal medicine specialists. For example, an "uncomplicated" pneumonia will generally be treated by the internist or the pulmonologist (lung physician).The work of the infectious diseases specialist therefore entails working with both patients and general practitioners, as well as laboratory scientists, immunologists, bacteriologists and other specialists.

An infectious disease team may be alerted when:

- The disease has not been definitively diagnosed after an initial workup
- The patient is immunocompromised (for example, in AIDS or after chemotherapy);
- The infectious agent is of an uncommon nature (e.g. tropical diseases);
- The disease has not responded to first line antibiotics;
- The disease might be dangerous to other patients, and the patient might have to be isolated

SOCIETY AND CULTURE

A number of studies have reported associations between pathogen load in an area and human behavior. Higher pathogen load is associated with decreased size of ethnic and religious groups in an area. This may be due high pathogen load favoring avoidance other groups which may reduce pathogen transmission or a high pathogen load preventing the creation of large settlements and armies which enforce a common culture. Higher pathogen load is also associated with more restricted sexual behavior which may reduce pathogen transmission. It also associated with higher preferences for health and attractiveness in mates. Higher fertility rates and shorter or less parental care per child is another association which may be a compensation for the higher mortality rate. There is also an association with polygyny which may be due to higher pathogen load making selecting males with a high genetic resistance increasingly important. Higher pathogen load is also associated with more collectivism and less individualism which may limit contacts with outside groups and infections. There are alternative explanations for at least some of the associations although some of these explanations may in turn ultimately be due to pathogen load. Thus, polygny may also be due to a lower male:female ratio in these areas but this may ultimately be due to male infants having increased mortality from infectious diseases. Another example is that poor socioeconomic factors may ultimately in part be due to high pathogen load preventing economic development.

FOSSIL RECORD

Evidence of infection in fossil remains is a subject of interest for paleopathologists, scientists who study occurrences of injuries and illness in extinct life forms. Signs of infection have been discovered in the bones of carnivorous dinosaurs. When present, however, these infections seem to tend to be confined to only small regions of the body. A skull attributed to the early carnivorous dinosaur *Herrerasaurus ischigualastensis* exhibits pit-like wounds surrounded by swollen and porous bone. The unusual texture of the bone around the wounds suggests they were afflicted by a short-lived, non-lethal infection. Scientists who studied the skull speculated that the bite marks were received in a fight with another *Herrerasaurus*. Other carnivorous dinosaurs with documented evidence of infection include *Acrocanthosaurus*, *Allosaurus*, *Tyrannosaurus* and a tyrannosaur from the Kirtland Formation. The infections from both tyrannosaurs were received by being bitten during a fight, like the *Herrerasaurus* specimen.

IMMUNOLOGY

Immunology is a branch of biomedical science that covers the study of all aspects of the immune system in all organisms. It deals with the physiological functioning of the immune system in states of both health and diseases; malfunctions of the immune system in immunological disorders (autoimmune diseases, hypersensitivities, immune deficiency, transplant rejection); the physical, chemical and physiological characteristics of the components of the immune system *in vitro*, *in situ* and *in vivo*. Immunology has applications in several disciplines of science, and as such is further divided.

Even before the concept of immunity (from *immunis*, Latin for "exempt") was developed, numerous early physicians characterized organs that would later prove to be part of the immune system. The key primary lymphoid organs of the immune system are the thymus and bone marrow, and secondary lymphatic tissues such as spleen, tonsils, lymph vessels, lymph nodes, adenoids, and skin and liver. When health conditions warrant, immune system organs including the thymus, spleen, portions of bone marrow, lymph nodes and secondary lymphatic tissues can be surgically excised for examination while patients are still alive.

Many components of the immune system are actually cellular in nature and not associated with any specific organ but rather are embedded or circulating in various tissues located throughout the body.

CLASSICAL IMMUNOLOGY

Classical immunology ties in with the fields of epidemiology and medicine. It studies the relationship between the body systems, pathogens, and immunity. The earliest written mention of immunity can be traced back to the plague of Athens in 430 BCE. Thucydides noted that people who had recovered from a previous bout of the disease could nurse the sick without contracting the illness a second time. Many other ancient societies have references to this phenomenon, but it was not until the 19th and 20th centuries before the concept developed into scientific theory.

The study of the molecular and cellular components that comprise the immune system, including their function and interaction, is the central science of immunology. The immune system has been divided into a more primitive innate immune system and, in vertebrates, an acquired or adaptive immune system. The latter is further divided into humoral (or antibody) and cell-mediated components.

The humoral (antibody) response is defined as the interaction between antibodies and antigens. Antibodies are specific proteins released from a certain class of immune cells known as B lymphocytes, while antigens are defined as anything that elicits the generation of antibodies ("anti"body "gen"erators). Immunology rests on an understanding of the properties of these two biological entities and the cellular response to both.

Immunological research continues to become more specialized, pursuing non-classical models of immunity and functions of cells, organs and systems not previously associated with the immune system (Yemeserach 2010).

CLINICAL IMMUNOLOGY

Clinical immunology is the study of diseases caused by disorders of the immune system (failure, aberrant action, and malignant growth of the cellular elements of the system). It also involves diseases of other systems, where immune reactions play a part in the pathology and clinical features.

The diseases caused by disorders of the immune system fall into two broad categories:

- immunodeficiency, in which parts of the immune system fail to provide an adequate response (examples include chronic granulomatous disease and primary immune diseases);
- autoimmunity, in which the immune system attacks its own host's body (examples include systemic lupus erythematosus, rheumatoid arthritis, Hashimoto's disease and myasthenia gravis).

Other immune system disorders include various hypersensitivities (such as in asthma and other allergies) that respond inappropriately to otherwise harmless compounds.

The most well-known disease that affects the immune system itself is AIDS, an immunodeficiency characterized by the suppression of CD4+ ("helper") T cells, dendritic cells and macrophages by the Human Immunodeficiency Virus (HIV).

Clinical immunologists also study ways to prevent the immune system's attempts to destroy allografts (transplant rejection).

DEVELOPMENTAL IMMUNOLOGY

The body's capability to react to antigen depends on a person's age, antigen type, maternal factors and the area where the antigen is presented. Neonates are said to be in a state of physiological immunodeficiency, because both their innate and adaptive immunological responses are greatly suppressed. Once born, a child's immune system responds favorably to protein antigens while not as well to glycoproteins and polysaccharides. In fact, many of the infections acquired by neonates are caused by low virulence organisms like *Staphylococcus* and *Pseudomonas*. In neonates, opsonic activity and the ability to activate the complement cascade is very limited.

For example, the mean level of C3 in a newborn is approximately 65% of that found in the adult. Phagocytic activity is also greatly impaired in newborns. This is due to lower opsonic activity, as well as diminished up-regulation of integrin and selectin receptors, which limit the ability of neutrophils to interact with adhesion molecules in the endothelium. Their monocytes are slow and have a reduced ATP production, which also limits the newborn's phagocytic activity. Although, the number of total lymphocytes is significantly higher than in adults, the cellular and humoral immunity is also impaired. Antigen-presenting cells in newborns have a reduced capability to activate T cells. Also, T cells of a newborn proliferate poorly and produce very small amounts of cytokines like IL-2, IL-4, IL-5, IL-12, and IFN-g which limits their capacity to activate the humoral response as well as the phagocitic activity of macrophage. B cells develop early during gestation but are not fully active.

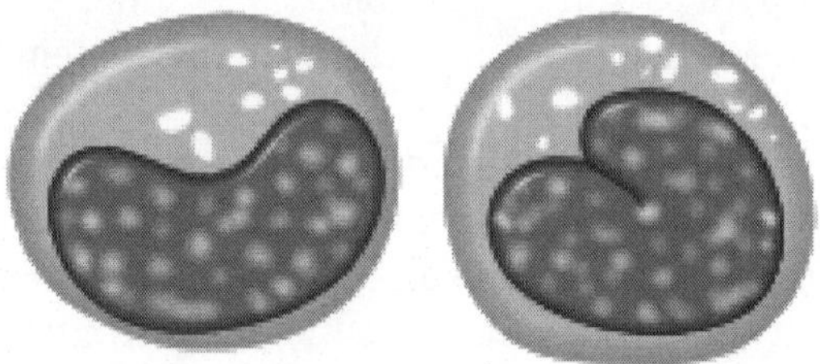

Fig. Artist's impression of monocytes.

Maternal factors also play a role in the body's immune response. At birth, most of the immunoglobulin present is maternal IgG. Because IgM, IgD, IgE and IgA don't cross the placenta, they are almost undetectable at birth. Some IgA is provided by breast milk.

These passively-acquired antibodies can protect the newborn for up to 18 months, but their response is usually short-lived and of low affinity. These antibodies can also produce a negative response. If a child is exposed to the antibody for a particular antigen before being exposed to the antigen itself then the child will produce a dampened response. Passively acquired maternal antibodies can suppress the antibody response to active immunization. Similarly the response of T-cells to vaccination differs in children compared to adults, and vaccines that induce Th1 responses in adults do not readily elicit these same responses in neonates. Between six to nine months after birth, a child's immune system begins to respond more strongly to glycoproteins, but there is usually no marked improvement in their response to polysaccharides until they are at least one year old. This can be the reason for distinct time frames found in vaccination schedules.

During adolescence, the human body undergoes various physical, physiological and immunological changes triggered and mediated by hormones, of which the most significant in females is 17-â-oestradiol (an oestrogen) and, in males, is testosterone. Oestradiol usually begins to act around the age of 10 and testosterone some months later. There is evidence that these steroids act directly not only on the primary and secondary sexual characteristics but also have an effect on the development and regulation of the immune system, including an increased risk in developing pubescent and post-pubescent autoimmunity. There is also some evidence that cell surface receptors on B cells and macrophages may detect sex hormones in the system.

The female sex hormone 17-â-oestradiol has been shown to regulate the level of immunological response, while some male androgens such as testosterone seem to suppress the stress response to infection. Other androgens, however, such as DHEA, increase immune response. As in females, the male sex hormones seem to have more control of the immune system during puberty and post-puberty than during the rest of a male's adult life. Physical changes during puberty such as thymic involution also affect immunological response.

IMMUNOTHERAPY

The use of immune system components to treat a disease or disorder is known as immunotherapy. Immunotherapy is most commonly used in the context of the treatment of cancers together with chemotherapy (drugs) and radiotherapy (radiation). However, immunotherapy is also often used in the immunosuppressed (such as HIV patients) and people suffering from other immune deficiencies or autoimmune diseases. Like IL2,IL10,GM-CSF B,INF a .

DIAGNOSTIC IMMUNOLOGY

The specificity of the bond between antibody and antigen has made it an excellent tool in the detection of substances in a variety of diagnostic techniques. Antibodies specific for a desired antigen can be conjugated with an isotopic (radio) or fluorescent label or with a color-forming enzyme in order to detect it. However, the similarity between some antigens can lead to false positives and other errors in such tests by antibodies cross-reacting with antigens that aren't exact matches.

CANCER IMMUNOLOGY

The study of the interaction of the immune system with cancer cells can lead to diagnostic tests and therapies with which to find and fight cancer.

REPRODUCTIVE IMMUNOLOGY

This area of the immunology is devoted to the study of immunological aspects of the reproductive process including fetus acceptance. The term has also been used by fertility clinics to address fertility problems, recurrent miscarriages, premature deliveries and dangerous complications such as pre-eclampsia.

THEORETICAL IMMUNOLOGY

Immunology is strongly experimental in everyday practice but is also characterized by an ongoing theoretical attitude. Many theories have been suggested in immunology from the end of the nineteenth century up to the present time.

The end of the 19th century and the beginning of the 20th century saw a battle between "cellular" and "humoral" theories of immunity. According to the cellular theory of immunity, represented in particular by Elie Metchnikoff, it was cells – more precisely, phagocytes – that were responsible for immune responses. In contrast, the humoral theory of immunity, held, among others, by Robert Koch and Emil von Behring, stated that the active immune agents were soluble components (molecules) found in the organism's "humors" rather than its cells.

In the mid-1950s, Frank Burnet, inspired by a suggestion made by Niels Jerne, formulated the clonal selection theory (CST) of immunity. On the basis of CST, Burnet developed a theory of how an immune response is triggered according to the self/nonself distinction: "self" constituents (constituents of the body) do not trigger destructive immune responses, while "nonself" entities (pathogens, an allograft) trigger a destructive immune response. The theory was later modified to reflect new discoveries regarding histocompatibility or the complex "two-signal" activation of T cells. The self/nonself theory of immunity and the self/nonself vocabulary have been criticized, but remain very influential.

More recently, several theoretical frameworks have been suggested in immunology, including "autopoietic" views, "cognitive immune" views, the "danger model" (or "danger theory", and the "discontinuity" theory. The danger model, suggested by Polly Matzinger and colleagues, has been very influential, arousing many comments and discussions.

IMMUNOLOGIST

According to the American Academy of Allergy, Asthma, and Immunology (AAAAI), "an immunologist is a research scientist who investigates the immune system of vertebrates (including the human immune system). Immunologists include research scientists (PhDs) who work in laboratories. Immunologists also include physicians who, for example, treat patients with immune system disorders. Some immunologists are physician-scientists who combine laboratory research with patient care."

Career in immunology

Bioscience is the overall major in which undergraduate students who are interested in general well-being take in college. Immunology is a branch of bioscience for undergraduate programs but the major gets specified as students move on for graduate program in immunology. The aim of immunology is to study the health of humans and animals through effective yet consistent research, (AAAAI, 2013). The most important thing about being immunologists is the research because it is the biggest portion of their jobs.

Most graduate immunology schools follow the AAI courses immunology which are offered throughout numerous schools in the United States. For example, in New York State, there are several universities that offer the AAI courses immunology: Albany Medical College, Cornell University, Icahn School of Medicine at Mount Sinai, New York University Langone Medical Center, University at Albany (SUNY), University at Buffalo (SUNY), University of Rochester Medical Center and Upstate Medical University (SUNY). The AAI immunology courses include an Introductory Course and an Advance Course. The Introductory Course is a course that gives students an overview of the basics of immunology.

In addition, this Introductory Course gives students more information to complement general biology or science training. It also has two different parts: Part I is an introduction to the basic principles of immunology and Part II is a clinically-oriented lecture series. On the other hand, the Advanced Course is another course for those who are willing to expand or update their understanding of immunology. It is advised for students who want to attend the Advanced Course to have a background of the principles of immunology. Most schools require students to take electives in other to complete their degrees. A Master's degree requires two years of study following the attainment of a bachelor's degree. For a doctoral programme it is required to take two additional years of study.

The expectation of occupational growth in immunology is an increase of 36 percent from 2010 to 2020. The median annual wage was $76,700 in May 2010. However, the lowest 10 percent of immunologists earned less than $41,560, and the top 10 percent earned more than $142,800, (Bureau of Labor Statistics, 2013). The practice of immunology itself is not specified by the U.S. Department of Labor but it belongs to the practice of life science in general.

NEOPLASM

Neoplasm (from Ancient Greek íÝïò- *neo* "new" and ðëÜóìá *plasma* "formation, creation") is an abnormal growth of tissue, and when also forming a mass is commonly referred to as a tumor or tumour. This abnormal growth (neoplasia) usually but not always forms a mass.

The World Health Organization (WHO) classifies neoplasms into four main groups: benign neoplasms, in situ neoplasms, malignant neoplasms, and neoplasms of uncertain or unknown behavior. Malignant neoplasms are also simply known as cancers. Prior to the abnormal growth of tissue, as neoplasia, cells often undergo an abnormal pattern of growth, such as metaplasia or dysplasia. However, metaplasia or dysplasia do not always progress to neoplasia.

TYPES

A neoplasm can be benign, potentially malignant (pre-cancer), or malignant (cancer).

- Benign tumors include uterine fibroids and melanocytic nevi (skin moles). They are circumscribed and localized and do not transform into cancer.
- Potentially-malignant neoplasms include carcinoma in situ. They are localised, do not invade and destroy but in time, may transform into a cancer.
- Malignant neoplasms are commonly called cancer. They invade and destroy the surrounding tissue, may form metastases and untreated or unresponsive to treatment, will prove fatal.
- Secondary neoplasm refers to any of a class of cancerous tumor that is either a metastatic offshoot of a primary tumor, or an apparently unrelated tumor that increases in frequency following certain cancer treatments such as chemotherapy or radiotherapy.
- Rarely there can be a metastatic neoplasm with no known site of the primary cancer and this is classed as a cancer of unknown primary origin

Clonality

Neoplastic tumors are often heterogeneous and contain more than one type of cell, but their initiation and continued growth is usually dependent on a single population of neoplastic cells. These cells are presumed to be clonal – that is, they are derived from the same cell, and all carry the same genetic or epigenetic anomaly – evident of clonality. For lymphoid neoplasms, e.g. lymphoma and leukemia, clonality is proven by the amplification of a single rearrangement of their immunoglobulin gene (for B cell lesions) or T cell receptor gene (for T cell lesions). The demonstration of clonality is now considered to be necessary to identify a lymphoid cell proliferation as neoplastic.

It is tempting to define neoplasms as clonal cellular proliferations but the demonstration of clonality is not always possible. Therefore, clonality is not required in the definition of neoplasia.

Neoplasia vs. tumor

Tumor (Latin for *swelling*, one of the cardinal signs of inflammation) originally meant any form of swelling, neoplastic or not. Current English, however, both medical and non-medical, uses *tumor* as a synonym of *neoplasm*.

Some neoplasms do not form a tumor. These include leukemia and most forms of carcinoma in situ.

A tumor (American English) or tumour (British English) is commonly used as a synonym for a neoplasm (a solid or fluid-filled cystic lesion that may or may not be formed by an abnormal growth of *neoplastic* cells) that appears enlarged in size.*Tumor* is not synonymous with cancer. While cancer is by definition malignant, a tumor can be benign, precancerous, or malignant.

The terms "mass" and "nodule" are often used synonymously with "tumor". Generally speaking, however, the term "tumor" is used generically, without reference to the physical size of the lesion. More specifically, the term "mass" is often used when the lesion has a maximal diameter of at least 20 millimeters (mm) in greatest direction, while the term "nodule" is usually used when the size of the lesion is less than 20 mm in its greatest dimension (25.4 mm = 1 inch).

CAUSES

A neoplasm can be caused by an abnormal proliferation of tissues, which can be caused by genetic mutations. Not all types of neoplasms cause a tumorous overgrowth of tissue, however (such as leukemia or carcinoma in situ).

Recently, tumor growth has been studied using mathematics and continuum mechanics. Vascular tumors (formed from blood vessels) are thus looked at as being amalgams of a solid skeleton formed by sticky cells and an organic liquid filling the spaces in which cells can grow. Under this type of model, mechanical stresses and strains can be dealt with and their influence on the growth of the tumor and the surrounding tissue and vasculature elucidated. Recent findings from experiments that use this model show that active growth of the tumor is restricted to the outer edges of the tumor, and that stiffening of the underlying normal tissue inhibits tumor growth as well.

Benign conditions that are *not* associated with an abnormal proliferation of tissue (such as sebaceous cysts) can also present as tumors, however, but have no malignant potential. Breast cysts (as occur commonly during pregnancy and at other times) are another example, as are other encapsulated glandular swellings (thyroid, adrenal gland, pancreas).

Encapsulated hematomas, encapsulated necrotic tissue (from an insect bite, foreign body, or other noxious mechanism), keloids (discrete overgrowths of scar tissue) and granulomas may also present as tumors.

Discrete localized enlargements of normal structures (ureters, blood vessels, intrahepatic or extrahepatic biliary ducts, pulmonary inclusions, or gastrointestinal duplications) due to outflow obstructions or narrowings, or abnormal connections, may also present as a tumor. Examples are arteriovenous fistulae or aneurysms (with or without thrombosis), biliary fistulae or aneurysms, sclerosing cholangitis, cysticercosis or hydatid cysts, intestinal duplications, and pulmonary inclusions as seen with cystic fibrosis. It can be dangerous to biopsy a number of types of tumor in which the leakage of their contents would potentially be catastrophic. When such types of tumors are encountered, diagnostic modalities such as ultrasound, CT scans, MRI, angiograms, and nuclear medicine scans are employed prior to (or during) biopsy and/or surgical exploration/excision in an attempt to avoid such severe complications.

The nature of a tumor is determined by imaging, by surgical exploration, and/or by a pathologist after examination of the tissue from a biopsy or a surgical specimen.

MALIGNANT NEOPLASMS

DNA damage

DNA damage is considered to be the primary underlying cause of malignant neoplasms known as cancers. Its central role in progression to cancer is illustrated in the figure in this section, in the box near the top. (The central features of DNA damage, epigenetic alterations and deficient DNA repair in progression to cancer are shown in red.) DNA damage is very common. Naturally occurring DNA damages (mostly due to cellular metabolism and the properties of DNA in water at body temperatures) occur at a rate of more than 60,000 new damages, on average, per human cell, per day. Additional DNA damages can arise from exposure to exogenous agents. Tobacco smoke causes increased exogenous DNA damage, and these DNA damages are the likely cause of lung cancer due to smoking. UV light from solar radiation causes DNA damage that is important in melanoma. *Helicobacter pylori* infection produces high levels of reactive oxygen species that damage DNA and contributes to gastric cancer. Bile acids, at high levels in the colons of humans eating a high fat diet, also cause DNA damage and contribute to colon cancer. Katsurano et al. indicated that macrophages and neutrophils in an inflamed colonic epithelium are the source of reactive oxygen species causing the DNA damages that initiate colonic tumorigenesis. Some sources of DNA damage are indicated in the boxes at the top of the figure in this section.

Individuals with a germ line mutation causing deficiency in any of 34 DNA repair genes are at increased risk of cancer. Some germ line mutations in DNA repair genes cause up to 100% lifetime chance of cancer (e.g. p53 mutations). These germ line mutations are indicated in a box at the left of the figure with an arrow indicating their contribution to DNA repair deficiency.

About 70% of malignant neoplasms have no hereditary component and are called "sporadic cancers". Only a minority of sporadic cancers have a deficiency in DNA repair due to mutation in a DNA repair gene. However, a majority of sporadic cancers have deficiency in DNA repair due to epigenetic alterations that reduce or silence DNA repair gene expression. For example, of 113 sequential colorectal cancers, only four had a missense mutation in the DNA repair gene MGMT, while the majority had reduced MGMT expression due to methylation of the MGMT promoter region (an epigenetic alteration). Five reports present evidence that between 40% and 90% of colorectal cancers have reduced MGMT expression due to methylation of the MGMT promoter region.

Similarly, out of 119 cases of mismatch repair-deficient colorectal cancers that lacked DNA repair gene PMS2 expression, PMS2 was deficient in 6 due to mutations in the PMS2 gene, while in 103 cases PMS2 expression was deficient because its pairing partner MLH1 was repressed due to promoter methylation (PMS2 protein is unstable in the absence of MLH1). In the other 10 cases, loss of PMS2 expression was likely due to epigenetic overexpression of the microRNA, miR-155, which down-regulates MLH1.

In further examples, epigenetic defects were found at frequencies of between 13%-100% for the DNA repair genes BRCA1, WRN, FANCB, FANCF, MGMT, MLH1, MSH2, MSH4, ERCC1, XPF, NEIL1 and ATM. These epigenetic defects occurred in various cancers (e.g. breast, ovarian, colorectal and head and neck). Two or three deficiencies in expression of ERCC1, XPF and/or PMS2 occur simultaneously in the majority of the 49 colon cancers evaluated by Facista et al. Epigenetic alterations causing reduced expression of DNA repair genes is shown in a central box at the third level from the top of the figure in this section, and the consequent DNA repair deficiency is shown at the fourth level.

When expression of DNA repair genes is reduced, DNA damages accumulate in cells at a higher than normal level, and these excess damages cause increased frequencies of mutation and/or epimutation. Mutation rates strongly increase in cells defective in DNA mismatch repair or in homologous recombinational repair (HRR).

During repair of DNA double strand breaks, or repair of other DNA damages, incompletely cleared sites of repair can cause epigenetic gene silencing. DNA repair deficiencies (level 4 in the figure) cause increased DNA damages (level 5 in the figure) which result in increased somatic mutations and epigenetic alterations (level 6 in the figure).

Field defects, normal appearing tissue with multiple alterations (and discussed in the section below), are common precursors to development of the disordered and improperly proliferating clone of tissue in a malignant neoplasm. Such field defects (second level from bottom of figure) may have multiple mutations and epigenetic alterations.

Once a cancer is formed, it usually has genome instability. This instability is likely due to reduced DNA repair or excessive DNA damage. Because of such instability, the cancer continues to evolve and to produce sub clones. For example, a renal cancer, sampled in 9 areas, had 40 ubiquitous mutations, demonstrating tumour heterogeneity (i.e. present in all areas of the cancer), 59 mutations shared by some (but not all areas), and 29 "private" mutations only present in one of the areas of the cancer.

Production and accumulation of DNA mutations

DNA mutation is the basis for cell transformation in cancer-development. Misrepair-accumulation aging theory suggests that Misrepair of DNA is the main source of DNA mutations in somatic cells. Since the surviving rate of a cell through DNA Misrepair is low, accumulation of DNA Misrepairs (mutations) can only take place in the cells and their offspring cells, which can proliferate. Cell transformation is a slow and long process, because the accumulation of DNA mutations needs to proceed over many generations of cells. This is why we have increasing rate of cancer-development with age and why tumors mainly develop in regenerable tissues.

Field defects

Various other terms have been used to describe this phenomenon, including "field effect", "field cancerization", and "field carcinogenesis". The term "field cancerization" was first used in 1953 to describe an area or "field" of epithelium that has been preconditioned by (at that time) largely unknown processes so as to predispose it towards development of cancer. Since then, the terms "field cancerization" and "field defect" have been used to describe pre-malignant tissue in which new cancers are likely to arise.

Field defects are important in progression to cancer. However, in most cancer research, as pointed out by Rubin "The vast majority of studies in cancer research has been done on well-defined tumors in vivo, or on discrete neoplastic foci in vitro. Yet there is evidence that more than 80% of the somatic mutations found in mutator phenotype human colorectal tumors occur before the onset of terminal clonal expansion. Similarly, Vogelstein et al. point out that more than half of somatic mutations identified in tumors occurred in a pre-neoplastic phase (in a field defect), during growth of apparently normal cells. Likewise, epigenetic alterations present in tumors may have occurred in pre-neoplastic field defects.

An expanded view of field effect has been termed "etiologic field effect", which encompasses not only molecular and pathologic changes in pre-neoplastic cells but also influences of exogenous environmental factors and molecular changes in the local microenvironment on neoplastic evolution from tumor initiation to patient death. In the colon, a field defect probably arises by natural selection of a mutant or epigenetically altered cell among the stem cells at the base of one of the intestinal crypts on the inside surface of the colon. A mutant or epigenetically altered stem cell may replace the other nearby stem cells by natural selection. Thus, a patch of abnormal tissue may arise. The figure in this section includes a photo of a freshly resected and lengthwise-opened segment of the colon showing a colon cancer and four polyps. Below the photo there is a schematic diagram of how a large patch of mutant or epigenetically altered cells may have formed, shown by the large area in yellow in the diagram. Within this first large patch in the diagram (a large clone of cells), a second such mutation or epigenetic alteration may occur so that a given stem cell acquires an advantage compared to other stem cells within the patch, and this altered stem cell may expand clonally forming a secondary patch, or sub-clone, within the original patch. This is indicated in the diagram by four smaller patches of different colors within the large yellow original area. Within these new patches (sub-clones), the process may be repeated multiple times, indicated by the still smaller patches within the four secondary patches (with still different colors in the diagram) which clonally expand, until stem cells arise that generate either small polyps or else a malignant neoplasm (cancer).

In the photo, an apparent field defect in this segment of a colon has generated four polyps (labeled with the size of the polyps, 6mm, 5mm, and two of 3mm, and a cancer about 3 cm across in its longest dimension). These neoplasms are also indicated, in the diagram below the photo, by 4 small tan circles (polyps) and a larger red area (cancer). The cancer in the photo occurred in the cecal area of the colon, where the colon joins the small intestine (labeled) and where the appendix occurs (labeled). The fat in the photo is external to the outer wall of the colon. In the segment of colon shown here, the colon was cut open lengthwise to expose the inner surface of the colon and to display the cancer and polyps occurring within the inner epithelial lining of the colon.

If the general process by which sporadic colon cancers arise is the formation of a pre-neoplastic clone that spreads by natural selection, followed by formation of internal sub-clones within the initial clone, and sub-sub-clones inside those, then colon cancers generally should be associated with, and be preceded by, fields of increasing abnormality reflecting the succession of premalignant events. The most extensive region of abnormality (the outermost yellow irregular area in the diagram) would reflect the earliest event in formation of a malignant neoplasm.

In experimental evaluation of specific DNA repair deficiencies in cancers, many specific DNA repair deficiencies were also shown to occur in the field defects surrounding those cancers. The Table, below, gives examples for which the DNA repair deficiency in a cancer was shown to be caused by an epigenetic alteration, and the somewhat lower frequencies with which the same epigenetically caused DNA repair deficiency was found in the surrounding field defect.

Frequency of epigenetic changes in DNA repair genes in sporadic cancers and in adjacent field defects				
Cancer	Gene	Frequency in Cancer	Frequency in Field Defect	Ref.
Colorectal	MGMT	46%	34%	
Colorectal	MGMT	47%	11%	
Colorectal	MGMT	70%	60%	
Colorectal	MSH2	13%	5%	
Colorectal	ERCC1	100%	40%	
Colorectal	PMS2	88%	50%	
Colorectal	XPF	55%	40%	
Head and Neck	MGMT	54%	38%	
Head and Neck	MLH1	33%	25%	
Head and Neck	MLH1	31%	20%	
Stomach	MGMT	88%	78%	
Stomach	MLH1	73%	20%	
Esophagus	MLH1	77%-100%	23%-79%	

Some of the small polyps in the field defect shown in the photo of the opened colon segment may be relatively benign neoplasms. Of polyps less than 10mm in size, found during colonoscopy and followed with repeat colonoscopies for 3 years, 25% were unchanged in size, 35% regressed or shrank in size while 40% grew in size.

Genome instability

Cancers are known to exhibit genome instability or a mutator phenotype. The protein-coding DNA within the nucleus is about 1.5% of the total genomic DNA. Within this protein-coding DNA (called the exome), an average cancer of the breast or colon can have about 60 to 70 protein altering mutations, of which about 3 or 4 may be "driver" mutations, and the remaining ones may be "passenger" mutations However, the average number of DNA sequence mutations in the entire genome (including non-protein-coding regions) within a breast cancer tissue sample is about 20,000. In an average melanoma tissue sample (where melanomas have a higher exome mutation frequency) the total number of DNA sequence mutations is about 80,000. This compares to the very low mutation frequency of about 70 new mutations in the entire genome between generations (parent to child) in humans.

The high frequencies of mutations in the total nucleotide sequences within cancers suggest that often an early alteration in the field defects giving rise to a cancer (e.g. yellow area in the diagram in this section) is a deficiency in DNA repair. The large field defects surrounding colon cancers (extending to at about 10 cm on each side of a cancer) were shown by Facista et al. to frequently have epigenetic defects in 2 or 3 DNA repair proteins (ERCC1, XPF and/or PMS2) in the entire area of the field defect. Deficiencies in DNA repair cause increased mutation rates. A deficiency in DNA repair, itself, can allow DNA damages to accumulate, and error-prone translesion synthesis past some of those damages may give rise to mutations. In addition, faulty repair of these accumulated DNA damages may give rise to epimutations. These new mutations and/or epimutations may provide a proliferative advantage, generating a field defect. Although the mutations/epimutations in DNA repair genes do not, themselves, confer a selective advantage, they may be carried along as passengers in cells when the cells acquire additional mutations/epimutations that do provide a proliferative advantage.

ETYMOLOGY

The term tumor is derived from the Latin "tumere" to swell. It is similar to the Old French *tumour* (contemporary French: *tumeur*). In the Commonwealth the spelling "tumour" is commonly used, whereas in the U.S. it is usually spelled "tumor". In its medical sense it has traditionally meant an abnormal swelling of the flesh. The Roman medical encyclopedist Celsus (ca 30 BC–38 AD) described the four cardinal signs of acute inflammation as *tumor*, *dolor*, *calor*, and *rubor* (swelling, pain, increased heat, and redness). His treatise, De Medicina, was the first medical book printed in 1478 following the invention of the movable-type printing press.

In contemporary English, the word tumor is often used as a synonym for a cystic (liquid-filled) growth or solid neoplasm (cancerous or non-cancerous), with other forms of swelling often referred to as *swellings*. Related terms are common in the medical literature, where the nouns tumefaction and tumescence (derived from the adjective tumefied), are current medical terms for non-neoplastic swelling. This type of swelling is most often caused by inflammation caused by trauma, infection, and other factors. Tumors may be caused by conditions other than an overgrowth of neoplastic cells, however. Cysts (such as sebaceous cysts) are also referred to as tumors, even though they have no neoplastic cells. This is standard in medical billing terminology (especially when billing for a growth whose pathology has yet to be determined).

2

What is Clinical Pathology

Pathologists are referred to sometimes ironically as *doctors of dead persons*. This has roots in the common idea that pathologists are only responsible for doing autopsies and providing clues for the possible cause(s) of death. What accentuate such misconceptions are the equipment and methods of pathologic examinations. A pathologist never uses the usual tools of ordinary physical examinations such as stethoscopes or sphygmomanometers. He or she has also no direct encounter with patients. There is very little similarity between the image that people have in mind of a physician and of a pathologist. In this chapter, we try to provide a realistic image about the territories of working of a pathologist.

We begin this chapter with a brief definition of the science of pathology and the history of contemporary surgical pathology. Then the reader can find general information about the frequent types of specimens that are handled by pathologists as well as the ordinary diagnostic methods that are applied by them for making an accurate diagnosis. This section is followed by a brief review of the ancillary and more sophisticated diagnostic methods in the field of pathology. In the next section, we will introduce a list of basic definitions that are used frequently by pathologists to describe specifically the different groups of pathologic processes. Finally, we provide some examples of the limitations in the field of diagnostic pathology.

PATHOLOGY AS A MEDICAL AND RESEARCH DISCIPLINE

In the study of medicine, pathology functions as a bridge between basic and applied medical sciences and in this way it plays a very substantial role not only in the understanding of the pathophysiologic basis of diseases but also in translating it into the practical management of patients and disease samples. There are two basic schools of thought about the practice of pathology. In most European countries, a pathologist deals principally with microscopic evaluation of tissue specimens (small biopsy samples as well as large resection specimens) and cytological material. As an adjunct to this histologic and cytological evaluation, a pathologist uses some ancillary methods (such as immunohistochemistry (IHC) or molecular and genetic examinations) formore accurate diagnosis, classification, and prognostication of diseases. In the United States, a pathologist is, in addition, responsible for all laboratory investigations that are elsewhere covered by disciplines such as microbiology and laboratory medicine. These analyses are carried out on body fluids (blood, serous fluids, urine, feces, etc.), secretions of organs (exocrine secretions of pancreas), or other materials that are taken out from or expectorated by a patient (sputum, coverings of skin ulcers, etc.).

They cover a broad spectrum of diagnostic methods apart from microscopy, including microbiologic, serologic, biochemical, and microscopic examinations. In this chapter, wherever we use the term *pathology*, it refers mainly to the macroscopic and microscopic evaluation as well as molecular assessments of tissue samples.

HISTORICAL PERSPECTIVES

The microscopic analysis of cells and tissue (e.g., cytology and histology) appeared for the first time in the nineteenth century as an important method for research and diagnosis in the field of medicine. Generally, Xavier Bichat is considered in most publications as the founder of pathology. The branch of histopathology appeared some years later, with M¨uller publishing a book on the structural characteristics of cancer cells and their growth. Virchow, a student of M¨uller, introduced the important correlations between cells, which are the smallest units of vital organisms and tissues, disease states, and related diseasemechanisms. He became famous worldwide for his cellular pathology studies and his claim that every disease originates from diseased cells or, according to him, "Omnis cellula e cellula."

This statement is valid also today in the era of molecular pathology. The introduction of more innovative techniques, such as the microtome in the year 1839, enabled the pathologist to have better and thinner sections from tissues and had a great influence on the development of pathology. Gradually, the application of frozen section examination found its place in the routine practice of pathology for rapid as well as intraoperative evaluation of the suspected tissues.

Another important development was the invention of standard hematoxylin and eosin (H&E) staining in the year 1875. The Carl Zeiss Company developed the first fluorescence microscope in the year 1965 in G¨ottingen. During the 1980s, the immunohistochemical analysis of tissues developed rapidly, which even today continues to be an invaluable diagnostic tool in pathology laboratories around the world. Cytopathology is one of the important branches of pathology. By this method, it is possible to analyze all body fluids for the presence of tumor cells and evidences of inflammatory changes. In the middle of the nineteenth century, Virchow introduced the cell as the basic functional element of the body and hence the basic element in the development of diseases. This way he deserves to be considered as the founder of cytopathology. But the development of cytopathology as a diagnostic tool took, in fact, more time. The first important development took place under the influence of the Greek physician Papanicolaou. He introduced in the year 1928 a method of staining cytology smears, which was named after him as the Pap test. His knowledge and works had a great influence on the routine performance of gynecologic cytology and led to a considerable reduction in mortality due to uterine cervical carcinoma by early diagnosis.

SPECIMENS

BIOPSIES, RESECTIONS, AND CYTOLOGY

One of the main duties of a pathologist is to provide the clinicians with a precise tissue-based diagnosis, particularly in cases with a complicated disease process or in situations in which there are uncertainties with the clinical diagnosis. In these situations, the pathologists receive a small biopsy sample from a relatively large lesion or organ. Most of the time the questions asked are as follows:

- Is there any pathologic change in this specimen?
- If yes, is it a preneoplastic, neoplastic, or non-neoplastic lesion?
- If it is a (pre)neoplastic lesion, is there any sign of dysplasia or malignancy?
- If yes, which type of tumor is it? Is it invasive or noninvasive? What is the grade of the tumor?
- If it is a non-neoplastic lesion, which type of disease process can it be? Is it an inflammatory process? Is it an infectious disease? If yes, is there any sign of the responsible infectious agent? If no, which type of inflammatory reaction can it be?

The notable improvement of endoscopic devices and imaging techniques has enabled physicians to gain access to the mucosal coverings of most internal organs and to take samples from them. Accordingly, pathologists encounter these days more frequently small biopsy samples. The most frequent areas of endoscopic samplings are mucosal coverings of the upper and lower intestinal tracts, respiratory tract, acoustic sinuses, female genital tract, urinary tract, and joint spaces.

The same set of questions can be answered by pathologists using other types of specimens that are obtained for cytologic examinations. The fluid accumulations in serosal spaces (pleura and abdominal spaces), secretions of some organs (nipple discharge), expectorated sputum, and voided urine can contain single as well as small aggregates of detached epithelial cells or suspended inflammatory cells, whose morphologic evaluation can serve as a basis for diagnosis. After collection, these fluids are centrifuged. The supernatant fluid, which is usually cell-poor or near completely acellular, can be used for chemical or serologic laboratory examinations. By preparing a direct smear, staining, and microscopically evaluating the cell-rich sediment, a pathologist or cytopathologist can provide an appreciable amount of diagnostic information. It is also possible to prepare a cell block from the sediment and to examine their sections microscopically. Other alternative methods to obtain specimens for cytologic examinations are brushing and washing of the mucosal (respiratory tract, esophagus) and serosal surfaces (washing cytology of Douglas pouch) or extracting fine tissue particles by aspiration using a narrow (fine pore size) needle.

Fine needle aspiration (FNA) is a rapid and relatively noninvasive method of sampling, particularly when the target organ is superficial or palpable (thyroid, breast). With the guidance of sonography or computerized tomography (CT), FNA or fine needle biopsy (FNB) can also be used safely to obtain material from more deeply located organs such as pancreas, mediastinal structures, lungs, and liver. Alternatively, pathologists receive large specimens, for example, resections, which can be different in size and extent from a part of an organ to complete removal of one or many organs together as well as limb amputations.

Not infrequently, the reason for such an extensive operation is tissue necrosis and gangrene due to problems of blood supply (ischemia). But most of the time, such a large resection is performed for the complete removal of a malignant tumor as in curative surgery or for the reduction of the size of a tumor as in palliative surgery. Particularly in the case of curative surgeries, a pathologist should thoroughly examine the specimen at both themacroscopic andmicroscopic levels. The frequently asked questions about such specimens relate to the reconfirmation of diagnosis, grading of the tumor (i.e., degree of malignancy), the extent of tumor infiltration, and the evaluation of resection margins (i.e., if they are tumor-free or affected by the tumor). There are many different recommendations and guidelines for standardization of sampling and for reporting tumor resections.

CONVENTIONAL DIAGNOSTIC METHODS IN PATHOLOGY

After taking a tissue sample from a patient by any of the above-mentioned methods, it is necessary to fix it. Fixation is a way of treating a tissue using specific kinds of chemicals, usually in the form of fluids. The process of tissue decay and organ destruction begins as soon as the tissue is detached from the body and has lost its source of blood supply. It is a self-destruction and autolytic process that can continue up to the complete destruction of the sample. In the case of inappropriate and untimely fixation, the tissue consistency will be lost and it will not be possible to examine the tissue at both the macroscopic and microscopic levels. In some cases, it is very important that the pathologist provides the clinicians with some information about the characteristics and composition of the constituting cells at the molecular level. Such molecular evaluations are exceedingly difficult if not impossible to carry out on improperly fixed samples. The most universally used fixative solution in most of the pathology laboratories around the world is buffered 4% formalin solution.

(A)

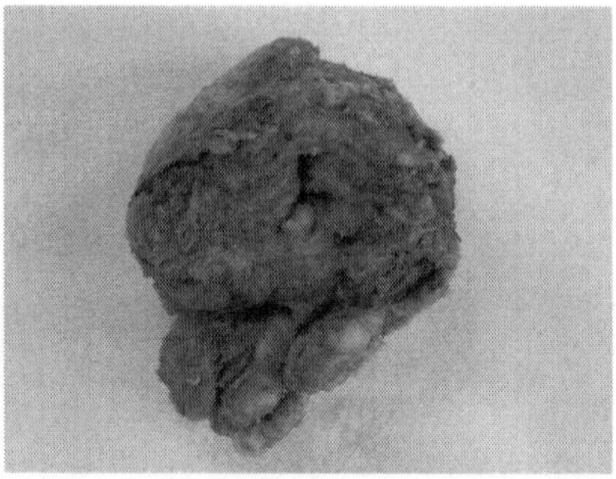

(B)

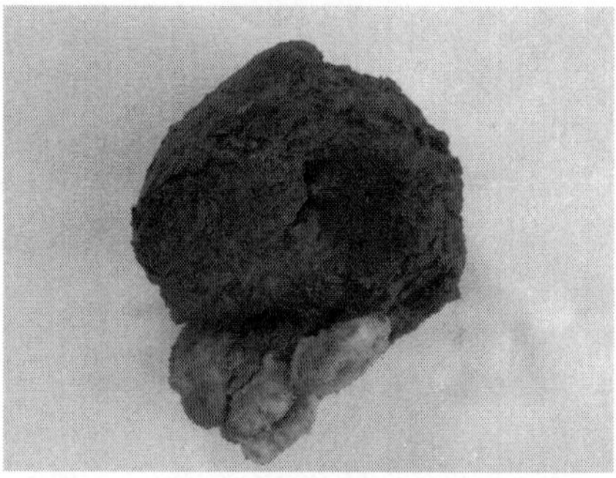

(c)

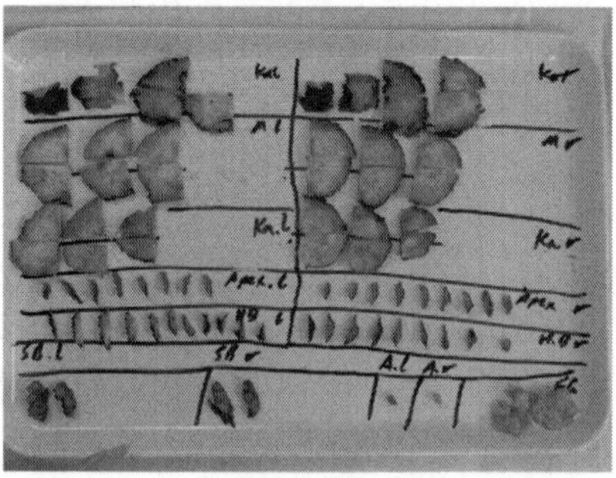

Fig. A radical prostatectomy specimen with both seminal vesicles (a). The outer surface of prostate (resection margin) is marked with blue ink. Such an approach makes the decision about the presence of tumor infiltration at resection margins easier (b). The specimen is completely sectioned in a systematic fashion in small pieces. All tissue fragments are processed and examined microscopically (c).(A)

There are many other fixatives that can be used in specific situations. Most of them suffer from one or more drawbacks such as high costs, problems with disposal, need for specific methods of tissue processing after fixation, too long a fixation time, and effects on the results of immunohistochemical or molecular examinations.

CYTOLOGY

As described above, the specimens that are received for cytologic examinations are usually in the form of an aspirated, expectorated, or washed fluid. One or more smears are usually prepared from the sediment of a centrifuged fluid. Depending on the desired staining method, these smears can be fixed by chemicals or are air-dried. The rest of the sediment can be processed similarly as for a tissue sample by transferring the cells into a network of protein material, for example, protein glycerin or plasma, followed by coagulation with thrombin. The cells are then fixed in formalin followed by paraffin embedding just like a tissue sample. If these cell blocks contain a sufficient number of cells, they serve as a very helpful reserve for further examinations such as immunohistochemical or sometimes molecular genetic tests.

(A)

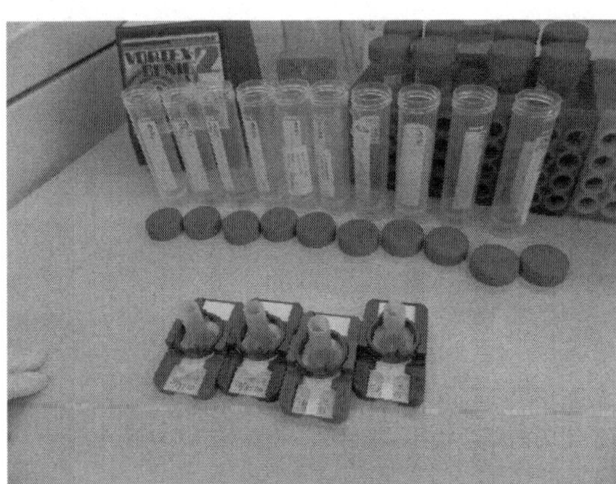

(B)

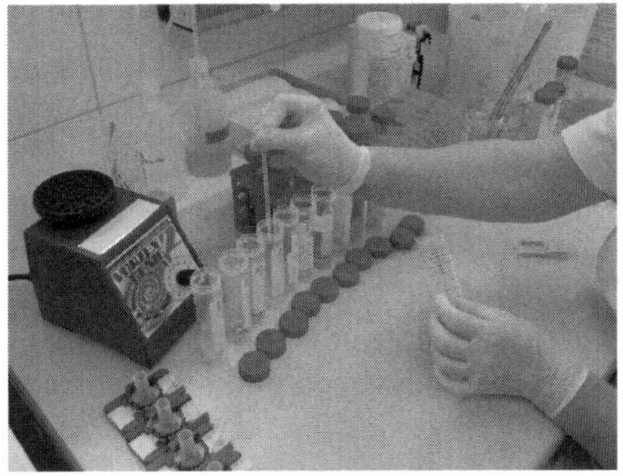

(c)

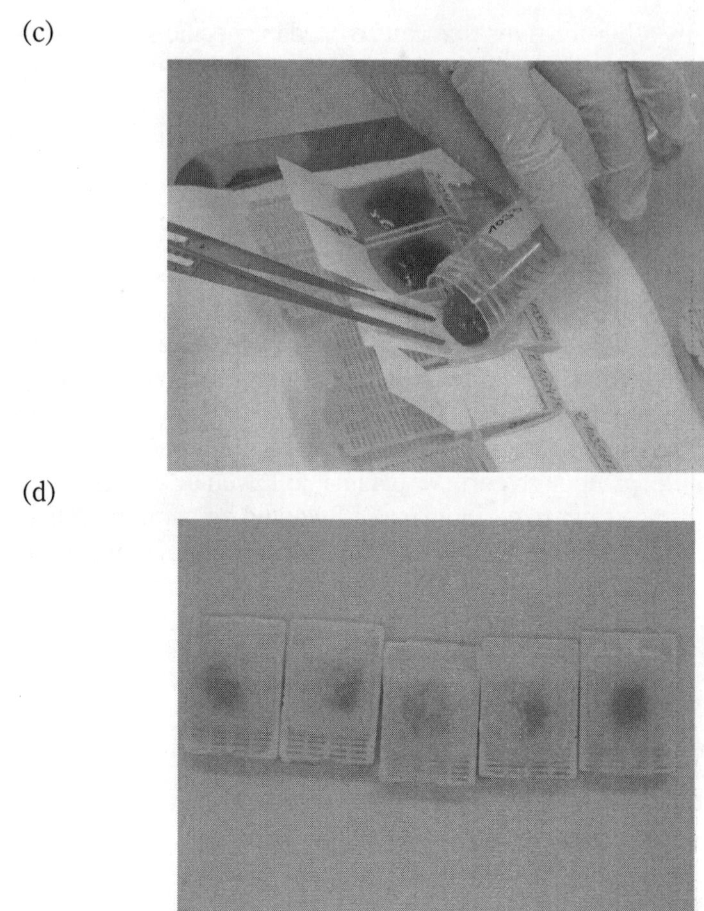

(d)

Fig. Preparation of cell block from liquid samples. The fluid is centrifuged. A part of the sediment is used for the preparation of cytologic smears by cytocentrifugation (a). The remaining sediment is coagulated by adding plasma and thrombin (b). The coagulated sediment is drained into a plastic basket and processed as a tissue fragment in a tissue processor (c). The paraffin blocks that were prepared from a liquid sample are ready for sectioning by a microtome (d).

HISTOLOGY

Immediately after submission to a pathology laboratory, every tissue sample is given a numerical code. Different methods of labeling, such as bar coding, can be used for coding the samples. The process of tissue examination by a pathologist begins by naked eye examination. A lot of information can be obtained after a careful macroscopic tissue examination or grossing. For small biopsy samples, these pieces of information are usually limited to the dimensions, as well as the number, color, and amount of the sample. It provides basic information regarding the adequacy of the specimen for further evaluations. In the case of some specific types of specimens, it is the duty of the pathologist to examine the small specimens by a hand lens or by a low-power microscope before subjecting it to complete formalin fixation and ordinary tissue processing. The best example is the renal needle biopsy. By low-power microscopic examination, the pathologist can tell the clinician whether he or she was successful in obtaining an adequate amount of renal tissue. On the other hand, the pathologist may need to divide the sample appropriately into three portions. Each portion is then handled differently for different methods of examination, that is, fresh tissue for immunofluorescent examination, fixation in glutaraldehyde for electron microscopy, and fixation in buffered formalin for conventional tissue microscopy and specific chemical staining. The last option represents the standard procedure that is applicable in all cases. The most important role of grossing is in the evaluation of large resection samples. It is evident that microscopic evaluation of a whole resection sample, for example, the complete removal of an organ or extremity, is neither possible nor necessary.

There are specific guidelines from which a pathologist can obtain information on how a resection specimen should be sampled and examined for microscopy. In most cases, these resection samples are those that contain a malignant tumor. In this situation, the clinicians might want to know the extent of the tumor and the completeness of its removal. The macroscopic examination defines the exact location, size, shape, and configuration of the tumor, the depth of local invasion (in tumors of luminal structures such as intestinal tract), the relationship with adjacent normal tissue, and the distance from surgical resection margins. It is also necessary to look for lymph nodes to examine them for possible metastatic foci. According to the guidelines, a pathologist takes small tissue fragments from the tumor, resection margins, and lymph nodes, which should not be less than a minimum recommended number. In some types of specimens, for example, radical prostatectomy specimens, it is recommended to completely embed the specimen in thin sections. To maintain the orientation during the microscopic examination, it is sometimes necessary to paint the specific areas such as resection margins by the different colors of specific dyes. The prepared tissue slices are then placed in a plastic cassette. On this cassette, the code number of the specimen and if necessary the specific code of the area of sampling are written or typed. Now the tissue slices are ready to be processed.

Tissue processing is a vital step for preparing the tissue slices for microscopic examinations. This task is performed automatically by a "tissue processor." The device consists of vessels containing specific chemical compounds (mainly alcohol and xylene) at a previously determined and graded concentration. The processing of tissue is enhanced and accelerated in new-generation tissue processors by the application of microwave energy or vacuum. The tissue processing ends with embedding the tissue in a paraffin block. Now the tissue is ready to be cut to obtain thin slices for microscopic examinations. Using specific sharp blades and a precisely designed device, it is possible to cut the paraffin blocks into very thin sections (preferably 3–5 m in thickness). The sections are placed on a glass slide, stained, and finally cover by a cover slip. They are now ready for microscopic examination by a pathologist.

MICROSCOPY

Aphysician collects the necessary information by examining a patient and observing the signs and symptoms of the disease. Then he or she makes a list of differential diagnoses and tries to reduce the size of this table by the application of specific laboratory tests. The final target is to reach an accurate diagnosis. Pathology as a practice has similar components. By careful examination of the microscopic changes on a slide, a pathologist tries to gather specific morphologic signs and symptoms (in this situation the key morphologic findings) in order to have a list of differential diagnoses. The basic forms of pathologic changes (with few exceptions) more and less resemble each other in the different organs and body tissues. For example, an acute or a chronic inflammatory reaction is accompanied almost always by a predominantly neutrophilic or lympho-plasmacytic inflammatory cell infiltration, respectively. The basic microscopic examinations are performed almost always in the first step on H&E stained slides. By using two different acidic (eosin) and basic (hematoxylin) stains, the basophilic components of the cell structure (mainly RNA and DNA) gain a deep blue color and the acidophilic components (cell cytoplasm and interstitial stromal materials) gain a pale to deep pink appearance. Some specific cell components or specific cell types can be amphophilic (neither eosinophilic nor basophilic). Although the basic structure of the tissue and basic forms of pathologic processes are in most cases easily appreciable during this primary microscopic evaluation, it is sometimes necessary to stain new tissue sections to answer specific questions. Some examples of chemical-specific tissue stains are as follows:

- *Periodic acid-Schiff* (*PAS*): Using this stain, we can see a better reaction of chemicals or structures with a high content of carbohydrates or glycoproteins. It shows better intracytoplasmic or interstitial accumulations of mucinous secretions (for example, in mucin-secreting adenocarcinomas). Some specific forms of microorganisms, for example, fungi, are better recognizable by this type of staining. A pathologist can find more easily the megakaryocytes in a closely packed and hypercellular bone marrow tissue. It is also a very good staining of the basement membrane in different epithelial coverings, and its application plays a crucial role in the microscopic investigation of glomerular diseases in the field of renal pathology.

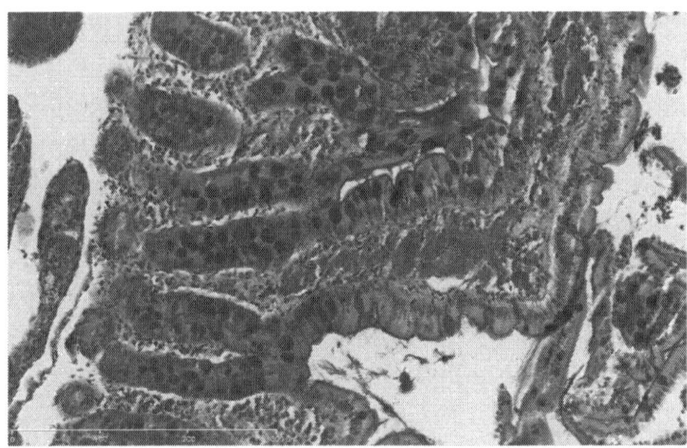

Fig. Collection of macrophages with deeply PAS-positive cytoplasm in the lamina propria of a duodenum mucosa biopsy is a characteristic feature of Whipple's disease.

- *Giemsa*: It is one of the basic special stains and is regularly used in the microscopic examination of lymphoid and hematopoietic tissues (lymph node or bonemarrow biopsies). In addition to providing better nuclear morphology, application of this staining is a single histologic method for the evaluation of tissue infiltration by mast cells. Most of the microorganisms, particularly bacteria, are better recognizable by this method of staining. A modified Giemsa staining is routinely used in gastricmucosa biopsies for the evaluation of *Helicobacter pylori* infection.
- *Masson trichrome*: It provides a better evaluation of the extent and severity of tissue fibrosis. In liver pathology, its routine application is one of the bases of diagnosis of advanced liver fibrosis or liver cirrhosis. Its application inmedical renal biopsies as adjunct to other specific chemical stains (such as Jones staining) is extremely useful in judging the presence of fibrinoid necrosis, glomerulosclerosis, and abnormal depositions in the mesangial spaces and basement membrane.
- *Iron staining*: Iron depositions in tissue are recognized in routine H&E staining as coarse dark-brown crystalloid materials. Although an experienced pathologist can recognize iron deposition by noticing the background histologic features and morphologic characteristics, in the liver tissue, for instance, it can be often mistaken for the intracellular bilirubin (a product of hepatocytes) or lipofuscin (a final metabolite of fat in senescent or hypoxic injured cells). In one of the specific iron staining methods (Prussian blue), the iron crystals gain a deep blue stain, while the other two remain unstained. The same staining can help a pathologist to differentiate between iron-laden intra-alveolar macrophages (i.e., heart failure cells) from pigment-laden macrophages with ingested coal particles. The estimation of

iron stores in bone marrow specimens is important to differentiate pathologic situations with increased iron stores (for example, myelodysplastic syndromes, sideroblastic anemia, and anemia of chronic disease) from situations with low iron stores (such as iron deficiency or chronic hemorrhagic anemia).

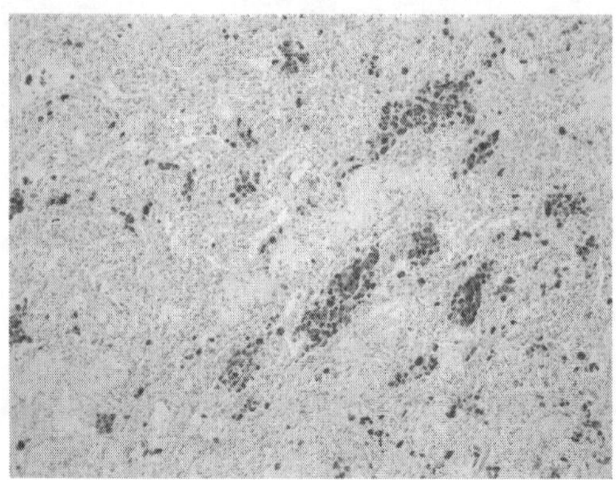

Fig. Iron staining of a lung tissue shows large number of intra-alveolar iron-containing macrophages (blue stained cells). This is an indication of recurrent and chronic intra-alveolar hemorrhage due to blood congestion. Such a situation happens, for example, in patients suffering from heart failure. Accordingly, these cells are called *heart failure cells*.

INTRAOPERATIVE ASSESSMENT (FROZEN SECTION EXAMINATION(

Preparation of formalin-fixed paraffin-embedded (FFPE) tissues is the usual method of tissue processing before microscopic examination, but it is not the only one. In some instances, the pathologists receive the sample in a fresh state (without any fixative or other chemical additives). The interested part(s) of the sample can be embedded in special media and rapidly frozen by immersing the sample in liquid nitrogen. Using a microtome mounted inside a freezer (cryocut microtome), thin tissue sections are prepared and stained. Such type of examination is called *frozen section examination* and is usually performed for the following purposes:

- *Intraoperative consultation*: To provide surgeons with an accurate diagnosis or as accurately as possible, the impression about the nature of a pathologic change to avoid a second surgical intervention and reducing the risks of reoperation. In this way, the pathologists are usually asked about the biologic (benign or malignant) behavior of the sampled tissue. This method of diagnosis was more frequent in earlier years. Nowadays, it is performed less frequently because of improvements in preoperative diagnostic methods and nonoperative invasive sampling techniques. Even in cases with confirmed diagnosis of cancer, a pathologist can be asked to determine the extent of a tumor or its grade. These types of information can influence the extent and method of surgery. Another application of frozen section examination during a surgery of a malignant neoplastic process is the evaluation of surgical margins.

- *Adequacy of sampling*: Even when the pathologist is not specifically asked by a surgeon to provide an accurate intraoperative diagnosis, by using this method the former can assess the adequacy of sampling for further examinations.
- *Molecular testing*: Although some specific types of tissue fixative solutions have been shown to protect the tissue structures, fixation with most of the commercially available and routinely used fixatives can hamper molecular testing.Well known is themasking of many antigenic epitopes and false negative immunohistochemical results in FFPE tissues.On the other hand, some sensitive molecules such asRNA can be damaged (partially or completely) during chemical fixation. Particularly for research purposes, there is a trend to archive a small, rapidly frozen tissue fragment.
- *Specific chemical staining*: Some basic chemical components of the tissue structure, such as fat, can easily dissolve in the chemicals that are used for tissue processing. For qualitative and semiquantitative assessment of these materials, there is also a need for fresh frozen samples. A good example is the confirmation of fatty deposition in some genetic metabolic storage diseases to differentiate them from other intracellular accumulations, such as watery changes.

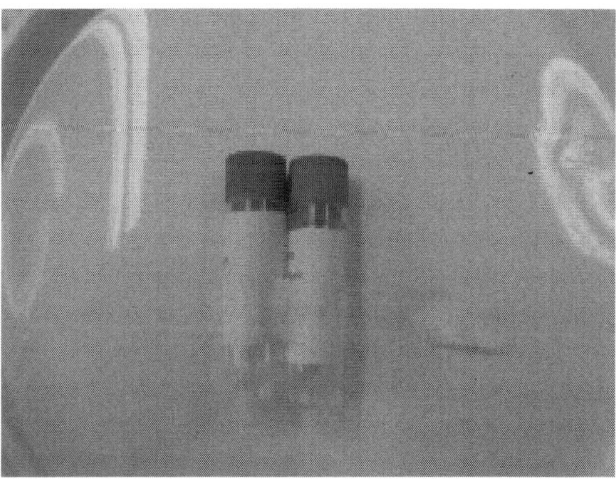

Fig. Two small vessels with patient identification are attached to the tissue container. The specimen has been sent in fresh state (without fixative solution). In patients with a macroscopically identifiable tumor, small fractions of tumor and nontumoral tissue are sampled, transferred into red-top and green-top vessels, respectively, and kept in a "70 æ%C freezer for further research or diagnostic molecular examinations.

WHY PATHOLOGISTS DO NOT LIKE FROZEN TISSUE EXAMINATION?

For many reasons, the assessment of a frozen tissue during a surgery is not a favored way of tissue examination for most pathologists. Some of the reasons are as follows:

- An intraoperative consultation is an emergency situation. That means that, during the preparation of sections and microscopic examination for an intraoperative consultation, all the normal working activities have to be stopped. This takes a relatively long time, which affects the daily practice.
- The quality of tissue sections that are prepared during an intraoperative consultation is usually not comparable with that of the slides that are processed in the normal way by FFPE. Seeing such slides is sometimes similar to seeing through fogged glasses. Taking decisions that have a great influence on the patients' situation by examining frozen sections is a very difficult and sometimes risky task. A pathologist can defer his diagnosis until the examination of permanent sections, but such a delay is not acceptable for many clinicians and surgeons.
- Some tissue samples, particularly those rich in fat, are difficult to cut after freezing. Preparing an appropriate interpretable section from these samples is not a simple task.
- The results of frozen sections examination can be partially or sometimes totally different from those of tissue examination on permanent paraffin-embedded blocks. This can have legal as well as moral consequences.

MICRODISSECTION

The purpose of microdissection is to provide a group of cells consisting as pure as possible of target cells for a specific examination. This method is particularly important for some diagnostic molecular assessments. For example, during the assessment of microsatellite instability in colon carcinoma, it is necessary to compare the length of microsatellite DNA polymorphism in normal and tumoral tissues. For this reason, these two cell elements have to be examined separately. The simplest way for microdissection is to look for normal and neoplastic cell components on a routinely stained H&E slide and marking the area occupied by neoplasm on the slide. This area can then be extrapolated on a thicker and unstained section from the paraffin block. The demarcated area is dissected using a sharp knife, suspended in specific solutions, and then examined by a desired method (for example, by polymerase chain reaction (PCR)). For more accurate assessments and especially for research purposes, it is also possible to use more accuratemethods of microdissection that will let the scientists even to cut a single or a small and purified group of desired cells. One of these methods is laser capture microdissection.

NONCONVENTIONAL (ANCILLARY) DIAGNOSTIC METHODS IN PATHOLOGY (MOLECULAR ASSESSMENT OF TISSUES)

Themolecular methods of tissue assessment can be divided into two broad groups. The first group of assessments is performed on tissue sections and provides information that is interpretable in conjunction with the location of the reaction. The results of these methods provide a color signal that can be seen under ordinary light microscopes (i.e., IHC) or by specifically designed microscopes such as fluorescence microscopes (for example, fluorescent *in situ* hybridization or FISH). The examiner can judge whether the reaction is mainly in the tumoral or normal cells. He or she can also evaluate the reaction in relation to the location of the reaction in different parts of the cell structure, for example, nucleus, cytoplasm, or cell membrane. These groups of tests are accordingly categorized as *in situ* methods. In the second large group of molecular testing, the subject of examination is an extracted and usually amplified sequence of the DNA of tumoral or normal cells. As in these methods there is no possibility for assessing the relation of results with morphologic parameters, they are categorized as non-*in situ* methods.

IN SITU REACTIONS

Immunofluorescence (IF)

It is a simple, fast, and usually cheap method of *in situ* molecular assessment. Briefly, a microscopic section of a frozen tissue is exposed to an antibody. In case the tissue section contains the material of interest, a specific antigen–antibody reaction ensues. Any excess unbound antibody is washed away. In the next step, the tissue section is exposed to a secondary antibody which is conjugated with a fluorescence material. A specific antigen–antibody reaction is detected by looking at the slides under a fluorescent light. By using two different fluorophores, it is possible to carry out simultaneously two different immunofluorescence (IF) examinations on a single slide. There are some drawbacks for IF. Before describing these drawbacks, it is worth pointing out that, despite the following problems, IF has kept its role in the assessment of abnormal glomerular depositions in the field of nephropathology:

- The results of IF examinations on FFPE tissues are usually unsatisfactory. It should be carried out on fresh frozen tissues. As in the normal workflow of a pathology laboratory, most of the samples are FFPE, they cannot be used appropriately for IF examinations.
- IF needs a specific type of microscope and a dark room for interpretation.

- By using IF, it is only possible to see a shadow of the background tissue. In fact, IF cannot be precisely categorized as an *in situ* method.
- Because of the short half-life of fluorophores, it is not possible to see the reactions after few days. This hampers the archiving of the IF-stained slides and assessment of reproducibility of IF examinations.

Immunohistochemistry (IHC)

Principally, thebasis of IHCis very similar to that of IF. InIHCexamination, instead of conjugation with a fluorescent material, the secondary antibody is conjugated with an enzyme. This enzyme changes a chromogene to a chromatic substance, and produces a color signal wherever a specific antigen–antibody reaction takes place on the slide. This means that the final reaction can be seen under an ordinary light microscope as a brown or red color change, depending on the type of chromogenic material and conjugated enzyme. During the past three decades, IHC has gradually become an integral part of routine diagnostic pathology as well as the basis for most researches in the field of biology of neoplastic and non-neoplastic disease processes. In routine practice of clinical pathology, IHC examinations are used to confirm a line of differentiation in undifferentiated tumors (e.g., lymphoma vs small-cell carcinoma vs sarcoma in the so-called small blue round cell tumor), the original tissue of a metastatic carcinoma in metastases of undefined origin (or the so-called carcinoma of undefined primary (CUP)), classification of lymphomas (e.g., B-cell vs T-cell lymphomas as well as subclassification of B- and T-cell lymphomas), assessment of tumor prognostic factors (e.g., hormone receptors in breast carcinoma), and assessment of tumor predictive factors (e.g., Her-2-neu expression in breast and gastric carcinomas). In comparison with IF, IHC has many advantages:

- Most IHC reactions are satisfactory enough to be performed on FFPE tissues. This means they can be carried out on normally processed tissue sections. On the other hand, it can be applied on archived paraffin blocks, irrespective of the age of the blocks.
- The IHC-stained slides can be archived and reassessed any time, because the color signals of IHC reactions do not fade rapidly.
- The IHC reactions can be seen and assessed under normal ordinary bright-field microscopes.
- Using counterstaining for cell nuclei, it is possible for pathologists to localize the reactions (normal vs neoplastic cells; membranous vs cytoplasmic vs nuclear).
- It can be performed by automated IHC stainers.

Fluorescent *In Situ* Hybridization (FISH)

The basis of FISH is the attachment of a fluorescent labeled array of nucleotides (a probe) to its complementary genetic structure of a normal or an abnormal gene. After washing the excess unbound probes, any microscopically detectable fluorescent signal evidences the presence of the investigated target gene or specific arrangement of nucleotides. The main application of FISH in daily practice is the assessment of gene amplification (e.g., Her-2-gene amplification in case of questionable Her2 IHC results). With some modifications, FISH has been used successfully for the assessment of some frequent forms of translocations or fusions in specific types of tumors (e.g., BCR-ABL/t(9;22)(q34;q11) in chronic myelogenous leukemia (CML) or IgH-gene translocations in follicular lymphoma). Another modification of this method is the labeling of the probes with chromogenic substances similar to IHC detection systems, which is called *chromogene in situ hybridization* (*CISH*), or labeling with silver dyes (*silver in situ hybridization* or *SISH*). The main advantages of these two methods are the possibility of interpretation of the results by a conventional bright-field light microscope and the possibility to assess the location of the reaction (i.e., tumoral vs nontumoral tissue).

NON-*IN SITU* METHODS

In many instances, the pathologist might want to know the presence or absence (or sometimes the quantity) of a specific chemical compound or gene in the assessed tissue regardless of the localization of that compound. During the past decades, several methods have been developed that enable the pathologist to carry out such measurements even on small biopsy samples. The list of such methods is already long and still growing rapidly. One of the breakthroughs in such molecular assessments was the introduction of PCR. This method was first introduced by Mullis, an American biochemist, and has found rapid and widespread applications in different fields of science, particularly diagnostic and researchmedicine. The inventor was awarded the Nobel Prize in the year 1993. The basis of this method is cycling thermal melting and enzymatic replication of DNA. By using small known DNA sequences (primers), it is possible to amplify the target gene. The number of amplified genes reaches a sufficient level after a few cycles, allowing qualitative or (semi)quantitative measurements. Other than in research activities, the most frequent applications of PCR in daily pathology practice are the following:

- Detection of the presence and subclassification of infecting microorganisms (viral particles, fungal elements, mycobacterial infections, etc.).
- Detection ofmutations (e.g., KRASmutation inmetastatic colorectal carcinomas, platelet-derived growth factor receptor (PDGFR) mutations in lung adenocarcinomas, and c-kit mutations in gastrointestinal stromal tumors (GISTs)).
- Assessment of the monoclonality of B- or T-lymphocyte proliferations in cases of suspected B- or T-cell lymphomas.

The other more advanced technologies are based partly on the PCR and gene amplification (gene sequencing). Some other methods, such as gene expression profiling, are expensive and time consuming, and are rarely used for diagnostic purposes. Other than genes, the chemical compositions and other cell structure constituents such as proteins are among the attractive targets for specific measurements. Although IHC is a rather inexpensive and readily available method for this purpose, it is not sometimes accurate enough for research purposes. Blotting and proteomics are two examples of fine measurement methods for assessing the protein composition of tissues. A schematic presentation of work flow in a pathology laboratory is illustrated in. Performing autopsies, teaching pathology to medicine and other students and research activities are not displayed in this simplified schema.

MAJOR TERMS IN CLINICAL PATHOLOGY

INJURY AND ADAPTATION

- *Homeostasis*: A steady state in which the cells, a tissue, or an organ is in balance with their microenvironment.
- *Cell injury*: Any external or internal insult that deranges the homeostasis.
- *Injurious (noxious) agent*: Any type of energies, physical stresses, chemical compounds, or invading microorganisms that can affect homeostasis. Examples: Toxins, radiation, burning, trauma, and bacterial infection.
- *Adaptation*: A series of cell changes at the molecular and cellular levels that serve to protect the cells from cell death when they are exposed to a noxious agent. These changes result in a new steady state in which the cell molecular composition,microscopic appearance, ormacroscopic features are different from the original ones.
- *Reversible adaptations*: A couple of changes in the chemical composition and structure of injured cells that enable them to protect themselves against an injurious event. The changes can disappear after the cessation of exposure to the injurious agent. The microscopically andmacroscopically detectable morphologic changes in reversible adaptation are usually of one of the following forms:
  - *Hypertrophy*: Increase in the size of tissue due to an increase in the size or the number of constituting cells. Examples: heart muscle hypertrophy in blood hypertension and hypertrophied muscles in an athlete.
  - *Atrophy*: Decrease in the size of the tissue due to decrease in the size of the constituting cells. Examples: Disuse atrophy of the limb muscle after longterm immobility and endometrial

atrophy in postmenopausal, women. Thus, atrophy is the opposite of hypertrophy and hyperplasia. Sometimes, the term *atrophy* is accompanied by an attribute to differentiate between its two major causes, that is, numerical atrophy (in apposite to hyperplasia) and simple atrophy (in apposite to hypertrophy).

  — *Hyperplasia*: Increase in the size of a tissue or an organ due to increase in the number of constituting cells and reactive cell proliferation. Examples: Endometrial hyperplasia in patients with estrogenic excess and hyperplasia of the parathyroid glands in patients with chronic hypocalcemic states.
  — *Metaplasia*: Substitution of a mature form of tissue with another mature form of tissue that is not normal for that position. Examples: Squamous metaplasia of the columnar epithelial cells of the respiratory tract and columnar metaplasia of the normal squamous epithelium of distal esophagus (Barrett's esophagus).

- *Irreversible injury*: Specific forms of tissue change that happen when the effect of injury is extensive, stark, and long, or the capacity of the injured cell for adaptation is low. It appears in two basic morphologic forms:
  — *Tissue necrosis*: Typical intravital form of cell death (cell death in a fixed tissue or autolytic changes in an unfixed tissue are not categorized as cell necrosis).
  — *Apoptosis*: Specific morphologic form of cell death that happens normally in tissues with high turnover (endometrial tissue and lymph nodes) as well as neoplastic or pathologically changed tissues.

INFLAMMATION AND REPAIR

- *Inflammation*: A series of vascular and cellular changes in response to invading microorganisms or injurious agents, which specifically happen in multicellular and vascularized organisms.
- *Acute inflammation*: An inflammatory response with sudden onset and short (usually 24–48 h) duration. The typical morphologic changes in an acutely inflamed tissue are vascular dilatation, blood congestion, intercellular edema, and acute inflammatory cell (neutrophilic) infiltration.
- *Chronic inflammation*: An inflammatory response of longer duration (on the order of days). The typical morphologic features that differentiate the chronic from acute inflammation are more pronounced tissue destruction, beginning of tissue fibrosis, and infiltration of chronic inflammatory cells (lymphocytes, plasma cells, and macrophages).

- *Granuloma*: A typical structure representative of a typical form of chronic inflammation (e.g., granulomatous inflammation) composed basically of aggregation of epithelioid (epithelial-like) macrophages. Other usually present components are a central area of necrosis (typical for tuberculosis granulomas), multinucleated giant cells (dispersed in between histiocytes), and peripheral layer of lymphoplasmacytic infiltration and fibrosis. Examples: Specific forms of infections (tuberculosis and mycotic infections), reaction to foreign bodies, and autoimmune diseases (sarcoidosis).

NEOPLASTIC DISEASES

- *Neoplasia*: An autonomous and usually uncontrollable proliferation of cells. The autonomy of proliferation is a key point in the definition of a neoplasia. It has to be differentiated from reactive hyperplasia in which the proliferation is usually dependent on a stimulatory factor. A neoplasm usually leads to the formation of a tumor (a mass lesion that can be differentiated from the background organ tissue by its different consistency, appearance, or shape). A neoplasm (or a tumor) can be benign or malignant.
- *Tumor differentiation*: In tumor pathology, the term *differentiation* is usually used to define the "level of differentiation" which signifies the level of morphologic similarity of the constituting tumor cells with the normal cells of counterpart tissue. The higher the similarity, the higher the differentiation. That means that most benign tumors are well differentiated. A similar concept can be expressed in an opposite way. Anaplasia is used to define the level of dissimilarity of tumor cells with presumed normal counterparts. The higher the anaplasia, the lower the differentiation. Morphologically, at the microscopic level most anaplastic tumors, regardless of the tissue of origin, are similar to each other. It is very hard to recognize the tissue of origin of an undifferentiated anaplastic tumor when microscopic examination is the only method of evaluation. In some anaplastic undifferentiated tumors, it is sometimes very hard, if not completely impossible, to determine the "line of differentiation" without the application of ancillary methods such as IHC or electron microscopy. That means that it is hard to define whether this tumor is a carcinoma (a malignant tumor with epithelial differentiation/origin), a sarcoma (amalignant tumor with mesenchymal differentiation/origin), or even a lymphoma (a malignant tumor with lymphoid differentiation/origin).
- *Tumor grade* (*of malignancy*): A concept providing a scale of the level of aggressiveness of a tumor and its potential for lymph node or

distant organ metastasis. One of the most important parameters in defining the grade of malignancy of a tumor is the "level of differentiation." In fact, the grading of malignancy is multifactorial and, other than the level of differentiation, is related also to some other parameters such as the number of mitosis as well as the presence and extent of necrosis. For most malignant tumors, a three-tiered grading system is applicable, for example, G1=low grade of malignancy<"high differentiation; G2=medium grade of malignancy<"moderate differentiation; and G3=high grade of malignancy<"low/poor tumor differentiation. Highly anaplastic and undifferentiated tumors are considered as G4. In these cases, the "level of differentiation" is very low and the line of differentiation during routine microscopic examination will be uncertain.

- *Benign tumors*: They are well-differentiated tumors with little, if any, anaplasia. Benign tumors usually have a very slow growth rate. That in turn let the host tissue to react to this new growth and produce a fibrous wall. The presence of a fibrous capsule is considered by surgeons and pathologists as one of the indicators of a benign tumor. There are exceptions to this general rule. For example, hemangiomas are benign neoplasms of vascular tissue that have no regular boundaries and no fibrous capsule. Most benign tumors are named by addition of the suffix "-oma" at the end of the tissue name. Examples: Lipoma (benign tumors of adipose tissue) or leiomyoma (benign tumors of smooth muscle tissue). Adenoma is the name of benign neoplastic proliferations originating from a glandular tissue or with glandular differentiation. There are also exceptions to this rule of nomenclature. Melanoma is a highly malignant tumor originating from melanocytes (pigment-containing cells in the skin and mucosal surfaces). Lymphoma is a group of usually highly malignant neoplastic proliferations of lymphocytes or lymphoid cells. In the gastrointestinal tract, the term *adenoma* is usually used to describe the polypoid epithelial proliferations with some attributes of malignant proliferations butwithout tissue invasion.
- *Dysplasia or dysplastic changes*: They are defined as morphologically detectable preneoplastic changes. That means that they have the capacity to progress to a (malignant) neoplasm, but in principle, they can also revert to the normal state. The dysplastic changes represent morphological alterations at the cellular microscopic level and in the nuclei of the composing cells. These morphologic features are to a large extent common between malignant neoplastic and preneoplastic (dysplastic) lesions and include nuclear hyperchromasia, nucleomegaly (increase in the size of the nucleus),

irregularity of nuclear border, clumped chromatin pattern, nuclear pleomorphism (different shape and size of the nucleus from one tumor cell to another), loss of polarity, and nuclear pseudostratification. For many of the frequently encountered dysplastic lesions, such as dysplasia of the uterine cervix epithelium or adenomatous polyps of gastrointestinal tract, there is a grading system. Grading a dysplastic lesion provides a basis for their classification according to the probability of development of a neoplasia. For example, the chance of progression to cancer and local recurrence after resection of an adenomatous polyp with low-grade dysplasia is much lower in comparison with a polyp with high-grade dysplasia. It is noteworthy that, according to the latest edition of WHO classification of gastrointestinal tumors, in addition to changes in nuclear features, the architectural changes also play an important role in the grading of dysplastic changes in an adenomatous polyp.

- *Malignant tumors*: An autonomous proliferation of cells with the potential for local invasion of background normal tissue or metastasis to regional lymph nodes or distant organs. In comparison with benign tumors and dysplastic changes, malignant tumors show a substantially low level of differentiation (higher anaplasia) and increased mitotic activity. There are again a few exceptions to this rule. Glioblastoma multiforme (a malignant brain tumor) and basal cell carcinoma (a malignant skin tumor) are locally aggressive tumors that never metastasize. .
- On the other hand, chondroblastoma is generally considered a benign bone tumor. But some cases show well-documented metastasis in the lung tissue. Malignant tumors of epithelial origin or with epithelial differentiation are named by adding the suffix "carcinoma" to the name of the normal tissue cells. Examples: Adenocarcinoma of the lung (malignant epithelial proliferation of lung tissue with the predilection to form glandular elements), renal cell carcinoma (malignant epithelial tumors of the kidney tissue), and colon carcinoma (malignant epithelial tumors of colon). Malignant tumors of mesenchymal origin or with mesenchymal differentiation are named by adding the suffix "sarcoma" to the name of the background or differentiated tissue. Examples: Liposarcoma (malignant tumors of adipose tissue) or osteosarcoma (malignant mesenchymal tissue with the potential to form osteoid or background osseous substance).
- *Tumor metastasis*: A unique capability of malignant tumor cells to detach from parent tumoral mass, invade the lymphatic or blood vessel wall, circulate with lymphatic or blood flow to regional lymph nodes

or distant organs, and finally produce a new tumoral mass in the new location. It has been considered as the most reliable criterion of malignancy of a neoplasm. Two other important characteristics of a malignant tumor are the invasion into and the destruction of local normal tissue.

- *Tumor stage*: The term that defines the extent of tumor expansion in the body of the patient. The staging of almost all carcinomas is performed according to the assessment of three basic parameters: the local extension of the primary tumor (T), lymph node metastasis (N), and distant (hematogenous) tissue metastasis (M). For any kind of carcinoma, there are a set of precisely defined definitions of various levels of the above-mentioned parameters that let the physicians to categorize the tumor stage for each patient. This system of staging is called *TNM staging* and is considered a standard approach in the evaluation of every carcinoma. At the same time, there might be other specific staging systems for a same tumor that can be applied in parallel or independent ofTNMstaging. Some examples for such a specific staging systems are FIGO staging (abbreviation of the French name for International Federation of Gynecology and Obstetrics) and Astler–Coller and Duke staging systems for colon carcinomas. It has been recommended that the TNM system be used for staging soft-tissue and bone sarcomas. As, in general, the lymph node metastasis of sarcomas is a very rare event, in practice, the staging of these tumors depends mainly on two parameters (T and M). Other than a few exceptions, lymphomas are considered generally as a systemic disease and their staging is dependent not on the local manifestations but on the extent of involvement of different areas of the body and possible extranodal manifestations such as bone marrow, spleen, or liver infiltration.

LIMITATIONS OF CLINICAL AND DIAGNOSTIC PATHOLOGY

One of the reasons why diagnostic pathology is sometimes called *surgical pathology* is the fact that the first generations of pathologists were surgeons. They could diagnose different disease processes during the operation only by looking at the organ by the naked eye.

The invention of the microscope and the application of microscopic examination was a great breakthrough. It showed the surgeons and pathologists that the assumptions that are made during gross examination of organs can be completely wrong. Further developments provided important tools that have changed the practice of pathology for ever. Some of these methods (IHC, IF, PCR, and FISH), their applications, and their influence on pathology practice have been comprehensively described previously in this chapter. Although the achievements have been tremendous, they are not enough. In routine practice of diagnostic pathology, it can be assumed that at least 50–60% of specimens can be diagnosed solely on the basis of gross examination and microscopic evaluation.

For a large proportion of remaining cases, it is necessary to apply further supplementary methods. In many of these cases, additional information is needed to provide support to the primary histology-based diagnosis or to exclude possible and frequent differential diagnoses.

Nevertheless, there is always aminor but very important group of cases that, even for experienced pathologists, are very challenging and sometimes cannot be solved. Subspecialization in specific diagnostic fields can help resolve the diagnostic problems of a group of these complicated cases. Even in this situation, the diagnoses of expert pathologists are sometimes rather subjective, difficult to formulate, and somehow inspirational. The following situations exemplify some difficulties and problems encountered in the field of diagnostic pathology.

PREDICTION OF TUMOR BEHAVIOR

The prediction of tumor aggressiveness, velocity of progression, and even sometimes discrimination of benign and malignant neoplastic proliferations from each other are some of the most important tasks of a pathologist. Sometimes, this task cannot be accomplished accurately even with the help of IHC or molecular genetic methods.

For instance, in pheochromocytoma (a sort of tumor of the adrenal medulla), the level of nuclear atypia, nuclear pleomorphism, and abnormal nuclear features (which basically are good microscopic indicators of malignancy in a neoplasm) are very high. These changes can easily impact the diagnosis of a malignant neoplasm. It has been shown that such nuclear changes in endocrine glands, in contrast to other organs, play no essential role in making the diagnosis of malignancy.

A similar situation can happen in the parathyroid gland. Gastrointestinal stromal tumors (GISTs) are a group of mesenchymal tumors of the gastrointestinal tract and the peritoneal cavity. Potentially, all of these tumors can be aggressive.

By definition, there is no "benign" or "malignant" GIST, simply because the pathologists cannot predict the tumor behavior accurately solely on the basis of macroscopic and microscopic features. To predict the behavior of a GIST, a constellation of clinical and pathological findings, including tumor size, tumor location, tumor encapsulation, local aggression, presence of necrosis, the number of mitotic figures, and the evaluation of the proliferation index using IHC evaluation of mitosis associated molecules (Ki67), is used to provide a sort of risk stratification. There is no single marker or a combination of IHCmarkers that can discriminate accurately a benign tumor from a malignant one. Application of clonality analysis in the assessment of T- and B-lymphocyte proliferations is a very helpful tool for the discrimination of neoplastic (predictably monoclonal) and non-neoplastic or reactive (polyclonal) processes. Even such a valuable tool is not always reliable.

Other than false positive (for example, in samples with a few analyzable target cells) or false negative results, there are situations in which a truly monoclonal population of B lymphocytes (e.g., monoclonal B-cell lymphocytosis) or plasma cells (e.g., monoclonal gammopathy of undetermined significance (MGUS)) is present in the bonemarrow, without any further indications of amalignant behavior. There is no need for immediate therapeutic intervention in these types of changes.

DIAGNOSIS OF TUMOR ORIGIN IN A CASE WITH METASTATIC TUMOR DISEASE

Detection of a metastatic carcinoma in a patient with no known primary site (the so-called CUP) is always challenging not only for clinicians but also for pathologists. IHC(for example, application of a set of low and highmolecular weight cytokeratins) can provide helpful information to narrow down the list of differential diagnoses.

In fact, there are some tables in which the metastatic carcinomas are classified according to their cytokeratin expression pattern (CK7+/CK20", CK7"/CK20+, CK7+/CK20+, and CK7"/CK20"). Unfortunately, in many cases, the spectrum of differential diagnoses is too wide. Until now, there is no organ- or tissue-specific IHC marker. Many of the allegedly "specific" markers are not totally specific.

For instance, the expression of prostatic specific antigen (PSA), which is supposed to be restricted to only normal prostatic tissue and the tumors of prostate, is also detected in some salivary gland tumors. Thyroid transcription factor 1 (TTF1) can be expressed other than in thyroid follicular epithelial cells by lung tissue. This is the reason why all these markers need to be evaluated within the context of conventional histology. It may also explain why the comments of pathologists remain speculative in many cases and are sometimes disappointing for the clinician.

INDIVIDUALIZED MEDICINE AND TARGETED THERAPY

Although tumor grading and staging are very helpful tools for the prediction of prognosis and can determine the need for supplementary treatments, they are no longer the only satisfactory pieces of information that a pathologist can and have to report in the evaluation of malignant tumors. Alongside the vast improvement of our knowledge about the pathogenesis and progression of different types of tumors, the treatment of cancer patients has been revolutionized.

Instead of blind application of high doses of strong toxic chemotherapeutic drugs, nowadays the predilection is to provide treatments that can act effectively and specifically on tumor cells and destroy them without affecting normal tissues with as little side effects as possible. These new treatment options are expensive.

It is the job of the pathologist to find the cases that benefit maximally from targeted therapies. For example, all breast cancers are examined immunohistochemically and, if indicated, by FISH for the evaluation of overexpression or amplification of a growth factor receptor, Her2 protein and/or Her2 gene.

Only those with evident overexpression of protein and/or those with evident gene amplification will get the maximum benefit from treatment with herceptin (blockers of Her2 protein on the cell surface). All GISTs, and to some extent other soft tissue tumors, are examined for the overexpression of CD117 (c-kit) to identify those patients who can benefit from targeted treatment against this protein.

The growing number of prognostic and predictive factors in different tumor types is fascinating. By pinpointing the examination at the molecular level, it seems that classification of a tumor under one of the well-characterized diagnostic entities is rather arbitrary. It has been shown that the tumor cells in two different patients with a microscopically similar form of cancer at the same stage can have different genetic and/or chemical characteristics. This difference is sometimes critical and determines the likelihood of response to specific forms of treatment.

Some examples are the KRAS mutation in colon carcinoma, BRAF mutation in malignant melanoma, and epidermal growth factor receptor (EGFR) mutation in lung adenocarcinoma. But these genes and their products are only one of tens or even hundreds of factors whose over- or underactivity results in tumor formation or accentuates its progression. It is imaginable that, in order to achieve the best therapeutic result, it is necessary to have a complete view of the chemical composition and pathogenetic pathways of tumor cells in each individual case.

Use of the contemporary routine methods makes it cumbersome to assess easily and cost and time effectively all the relevant parameters in every case. Such an assessment needs rapid and reliable methods with the integration of a set of assessments for diagnostic, prognostic, and predictive factors in a few steps or, optimally, simultaneously.

Many other situations in diagnostic pathology can be added to the above list (preneoplastic and preinvasive neoplastic conditions, infectious organisms and their possible relation to carcinogenesis, manifestations and complications of nonneoplastic diseases in the elderly, such as atherosclerosis and diabetesmellitus, etc.). The pathologists hope that new breakthrough technologies such as spectroscopic examinations can help them to resolve some of these processes and assist them in providing an explicit and reliable set of clinically relevant information.

3

Laboratory and Clinical Pathology

HEMATOLOGY

Hematology, also spelled haematology is the branch of medicine concerned with the study, diagnosis, treatment, and prevention of diseases related to the blood. Hematology includes the study of etiology. It involves treating diseases that affect the production of blood and its components, such as blood cells, hemoglobin, blood proteins, and the mechanism of coagulation. The laboratory work that goes into the study of blood is frequently performed by a medical technologist or medical laboratory scientist. Hematologists also conduct studies in oncology—the medical treatment of cancer.

Physicians specialized in hematology are known as hematologists or haematologists. Their routine work mainly includes the care and treatment of patients with hematological diseases, although some may also work at the hematology laboratory viewing blood films and bone marrow slides under the microscope, interpreting various hematological test results and blood clotting test results. In some institutions, hematologists also manage the hematology laboratory.

Physicians who work in hematology laboratories, and most commonly manage them, are pathologists specialized in the diagnosis of hematological diseases, referred to as hematopathologists or haematopathologists. Hematologists and hematopathologists generally work in conjunction to formulate a diagnosis and deliver the most appropriate therapy if needed. Hematology is a distinct subspecialty of internal medicine, separate from but overlapping with the subspecialty of medical oncology. Hematologists may specialize further or have special interests, for example, in:

- treating bleeding disorders such as hemophilia and idiopathic thrombocytopenic purpura
- treating hematological malignancies such as lymphoma and leukemia
- treating hemoglobinopathies
- the science of blood transfusion and the work of a blood bank
- bone marrow and stem cell transplantation

SCOPE

- Blood
  - Venous blood
  - Venipuncture
  - Hematopoiesis
  - Blood tests
  - Cord blood
- Red blood cells
  - Erythropoiesis
  - Erythropoietin
  - Iron metabolism
  - Hemoglobin
  - Glycolysis
  - Pentose phosphate pathway
- White blood cells
- Platelets
- Reticuloendothelial system
  - Bone marrow
  - Spleen
  - Liver
- Lymphatic system
- Blood transfusion
  - Blood plasma
  - Blood bank
  - Blood donors
  - Blood groups
- Hemostasis
  - Coagulation
  - Vitamin K
- Complement system
  - Immunoglobulins

(abnormality of the hemoglobin molecule or of the rate of hemoglobin synthesis)

- Anemias (lack of red blood cells or hemoglobin)
- Hematological malignancies
- Coagulopathies (disorders of bleeding and coagulation)
- ...Sickle Cell Anemia
- ...thalassemia

TREATMENTS

Treatments include:

- Diet advice

- Oral medication - tablets or liquid medicines
- Anticoagulation therapy
- Intramuscular injections (for example, Vitamin B12 injections)
- Blood transfusion (for anemia)
- Venesection also known as therepeutic phlebotomy (for iron overload or polycythemia)
- Bone marrow transplant (for example, for leukemia)
- All kinds of anti-cancer chemotherapy
- Radiotherapy (for example, for cancer)

BLOOD COLLECTION

EQUIPMENT REQUIRED FOR BLOOD COLLECTION

- Blood collection system: VACUETTE®
- Swab
- Tourniquet
- Disinfectant
- Disposable gloves
- Plasters

Vein Selection: Priority List

1. Median antecubital veins

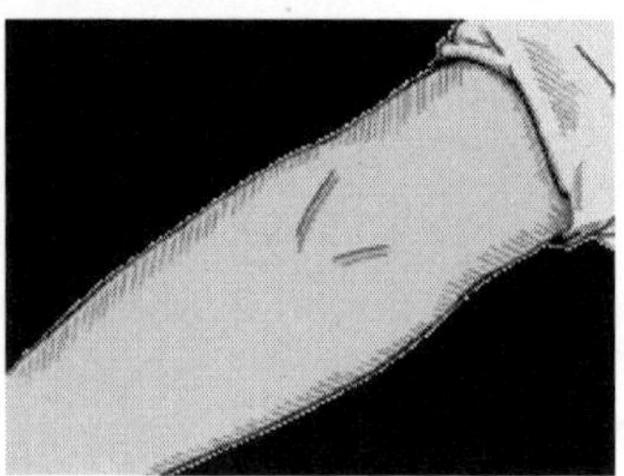

2. Dorsal hand veins

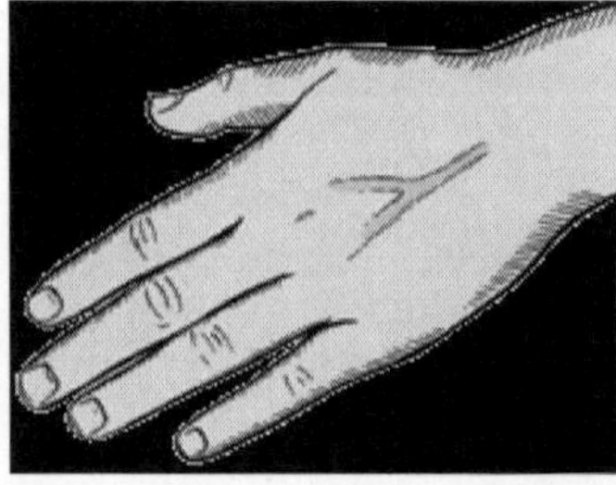

3. Foot veins

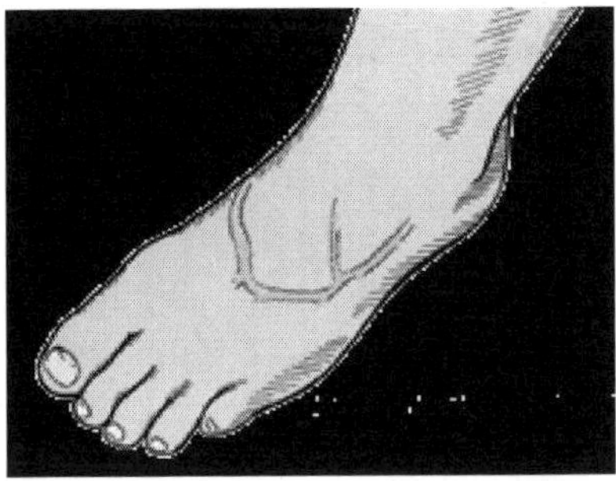

4. Subclavian vein

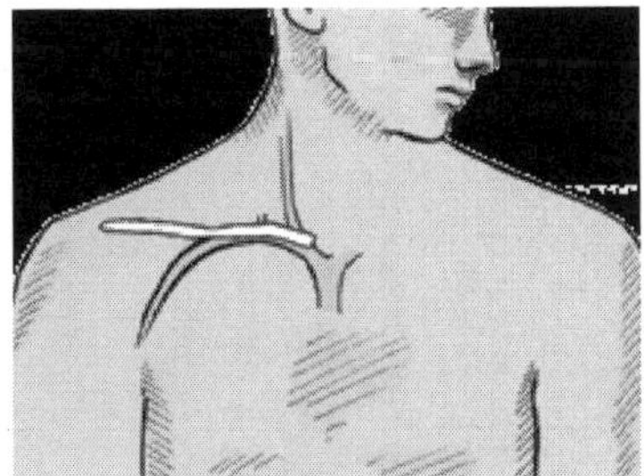

5. Femoral vein or artery

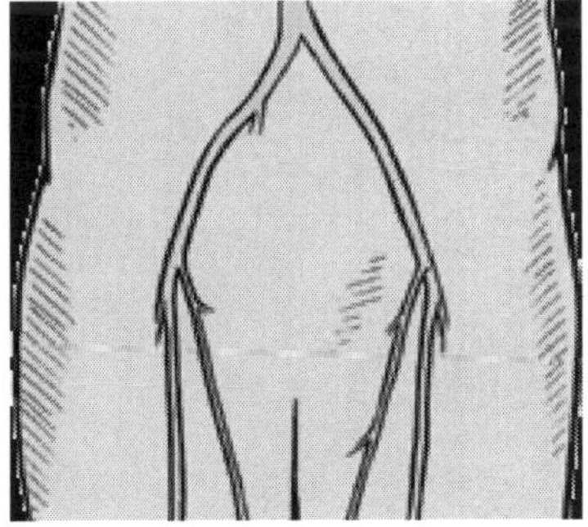

Inspection

Before deciding on a puncture site, an inspection of all possible areas is imperative.

The order of inspection should correspond to the list of priority sites, whereby the first and second sites should be suitable in 95% of the cases. The back of the foot can be quite painful, and is not popular amongst patients. Puncture of the subclavian vein or the femoral vein / artery requires a special blood collection technique, and should only be considered if there is no better alternative, and should only be carried out by experienced personnel.

Measures to Improve Prominence of Vein

1. Incline the arm in a downward position

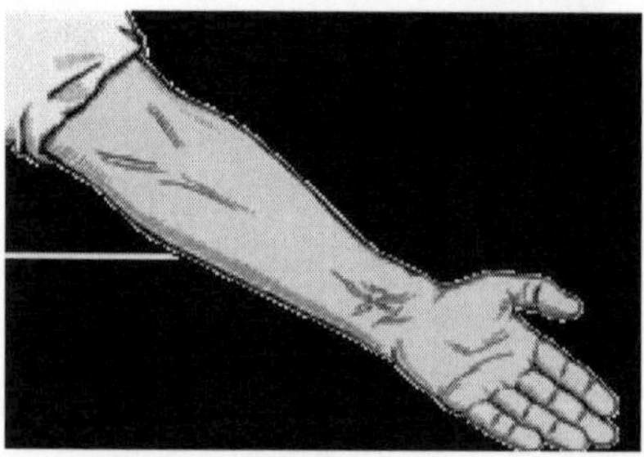

2. Stroke the vein in a distal direction

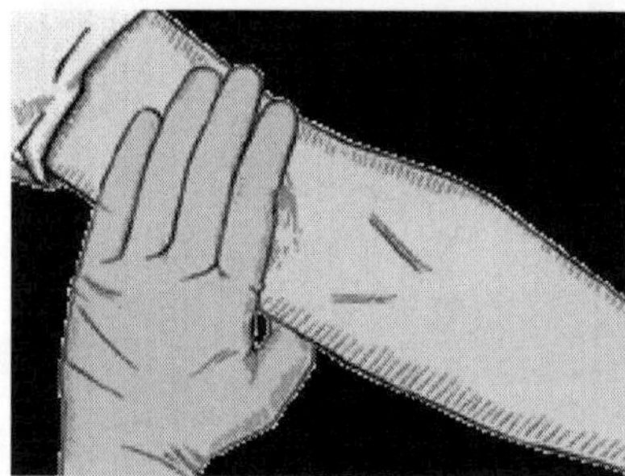

3. Clench the fist

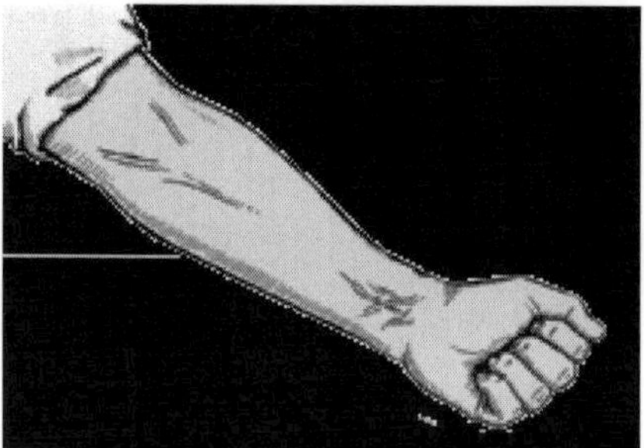

4. Tap the vein

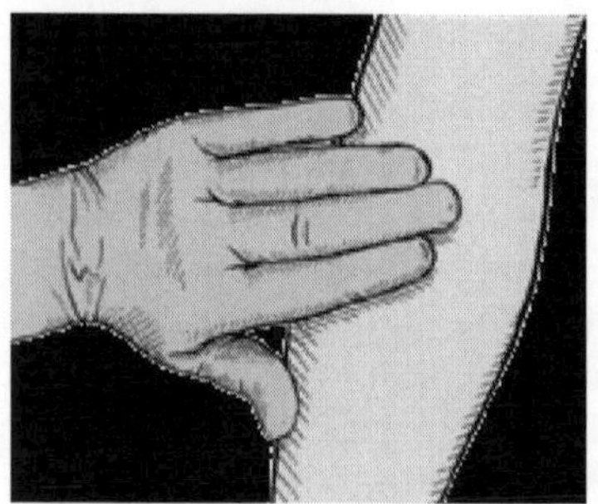

5. Warm the area (bathe arm or use a heating pad)

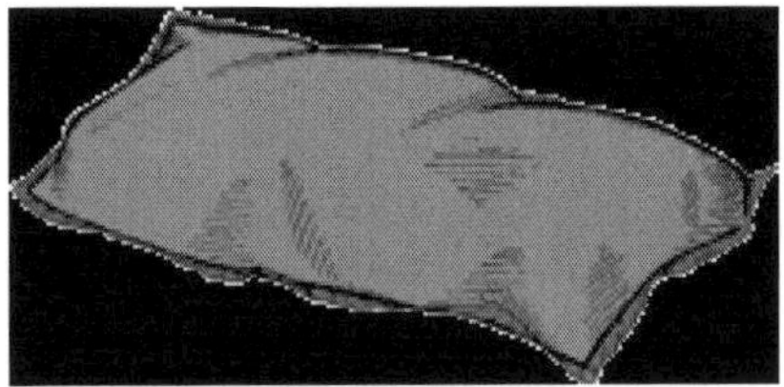

6. Skin patch with local anaesthetic

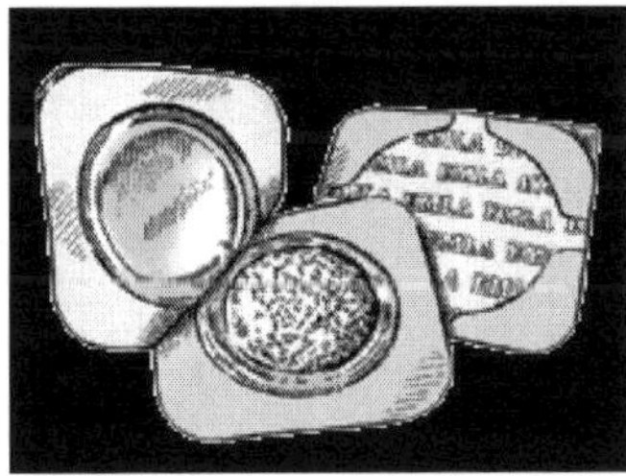

Applying the Tourniquet

A standard tourniquet or blood pressure cuff is applied about one hand breadth above the anticipated puncture site.

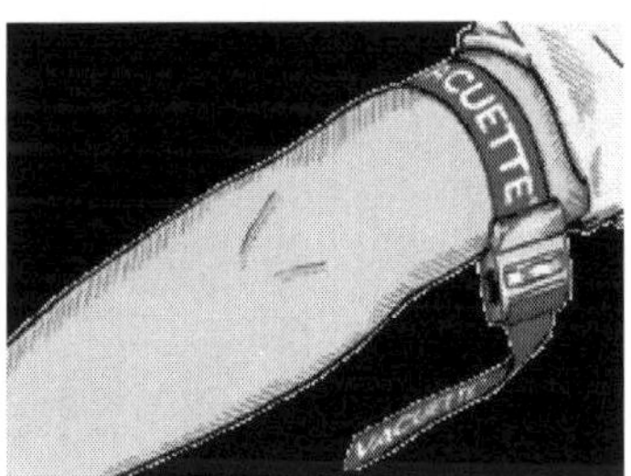

The stasis should not cause the patient any pain, and systolic blood pressure should be reduced by around 20 - 30 mm Hg, so that arterial blood flow remains as normal. For a normal healthy person with a systolic blood pressure of 120 - 130 mm Hg, the pressure from the tourniquet should be around 100 mm Hg, and should not last for longer than one minute (to avoid falsifying laboratory results).

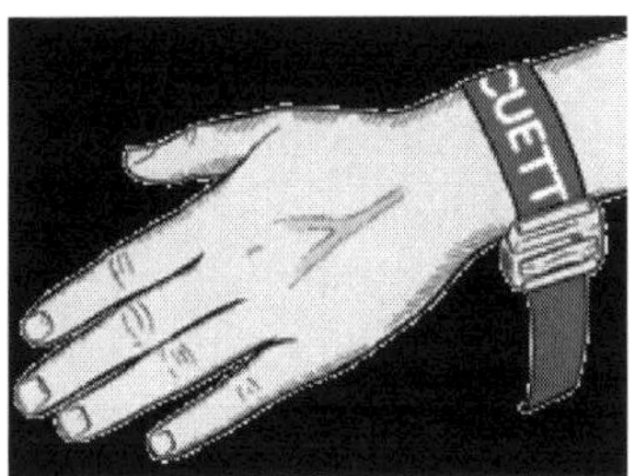

If a longer stasis is required, then the tourniquet should be loosened occasionally, if the skin becomes discoloured. Once the skin around the puncture site has returned to its normal colour, the tourniquet can be reapplied. If the tourniquet has been applied too tightly, the extremities will take on a blue colour, and it should be released immediately until the skin returns to its normal colour. The ideal stasis is as short as possible, and should not last longer than one minute. If the blood flow is insufficient for specimen collection, the tourniquet can be reapplied lightly during the collection procedure.

Disinfecting the Puncture Site

The puncture site should be disinfected thoroughly. It is not enough to wipe over the puncture site with disinfecting solution once, and venipuncture may not be carried out immediately, because some time is necessary for the disinfection to take effect. The skin should be cleansed with a disinfection solution using a circular motion moving outwards. For standard blood collection, reduction of bacteria in skin flora takes place after about 15 - 30 seconds* when an alcoholic solution is used. If puncture is planned with an intravasal catheter, the effect takes place after about 1 minute and furthermore, the puncture site should be covered up with a sterile swab, and mouth protection, cap as well as a sterile laboratory coat must be worn.

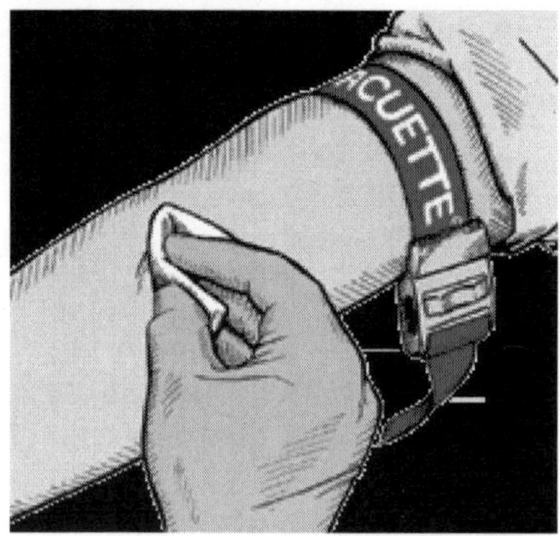

It is obligatory to wear disposable gloves for every venipuncture (NB: risk of infection with hepatitis, HIV).

Routine Puncture Sites

Puncture site: median anticubital veins

This is the most popular site for venipuncture! It is always worth taking time to inspect both arms, to be able to choose the arm with the most prominent veins. If the patient has a particular preference for a puncture site, then this should be heeded whenever possible.

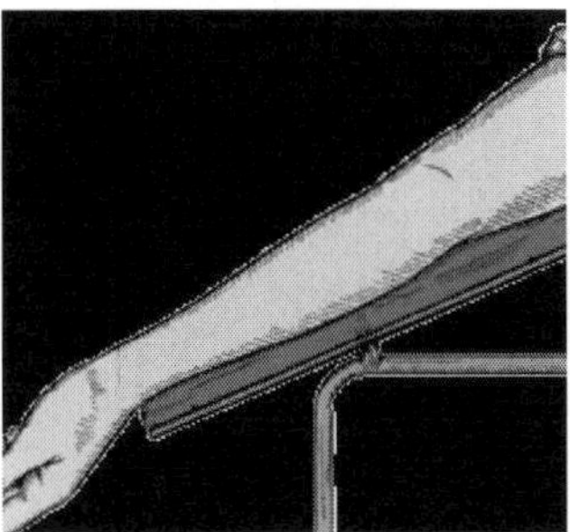

It is of utmost importance, that the patient is relaxed and sitting comfortably (or if convenient lying). The arm should be extended across a suitable padded armrest. The vein calibre of a healthy, relaxed adult varies in diameter from 5 - 10 mm. Light hand pressure on the upper arm should cause the veins to dilate significantly. Palpation of the vein can at this point be carried out without wearing gloves. The arm should be placed on the cushion so that the area for venipuncture is hyperextended.

Puncture site: Dorsal hand veins

A right handed person should use his/her left hand to take the patient's hand intended for venipuncture, pulling the skin in a downward direction until taut.

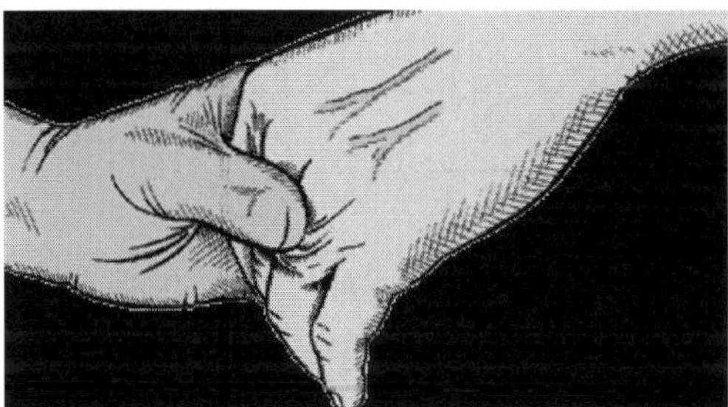

The needle or blood collection set is inserted into the middle of the targeted vein, at an angle of 10 - 20 degrees. As soon as the blood flow starts, the tourniquet can be released. Ideally, a blood pressure cuff can be used to measure the reduction of the systolic blood pressure by 30 mm Hg.

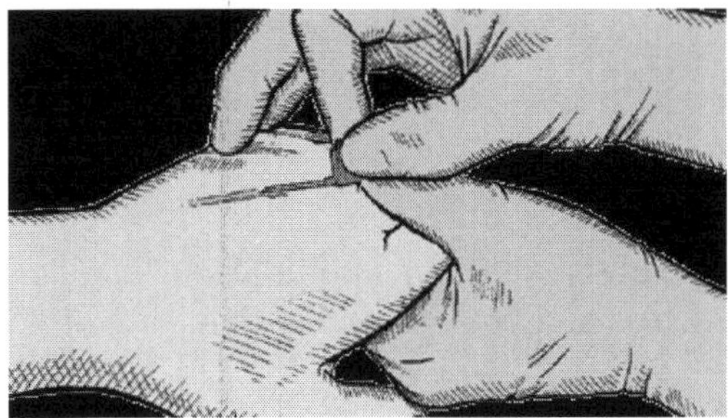

The forefinger should be used to check the prominence of the vein, and to make sure that veins are not under too much pressure (arterial puncture). The area is then thoroughly disinfected.

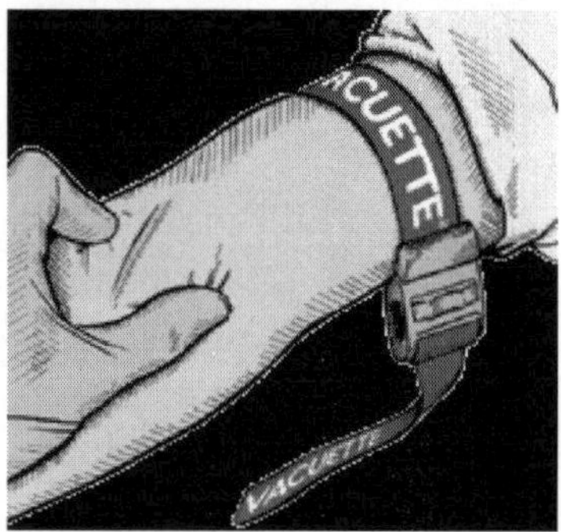

Using the left hand, the skin below the tourniquet is pulled to the sides of the underarm.

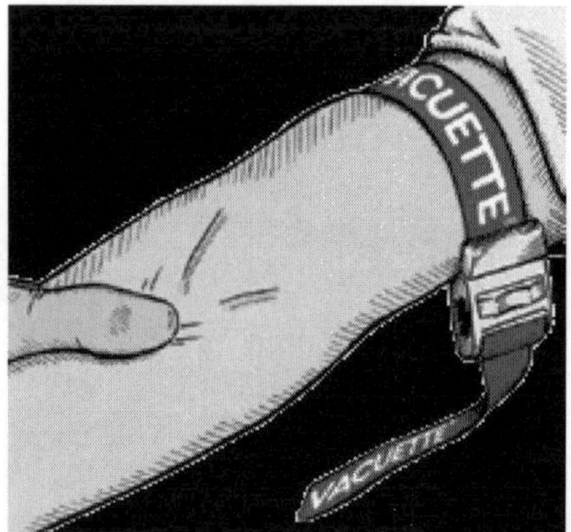

This reduces the chance of veins rolling away from the needle. The puncture is carried out with the right hand, at an angle of 10 to 20 degrees.

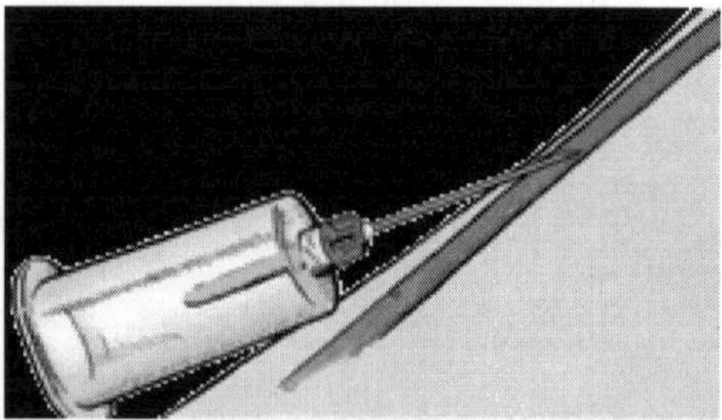

After 10 - 15 mm, the vein lumen should have been reached. If the needle penetrates any further, this would probably mean that the target has been missed.

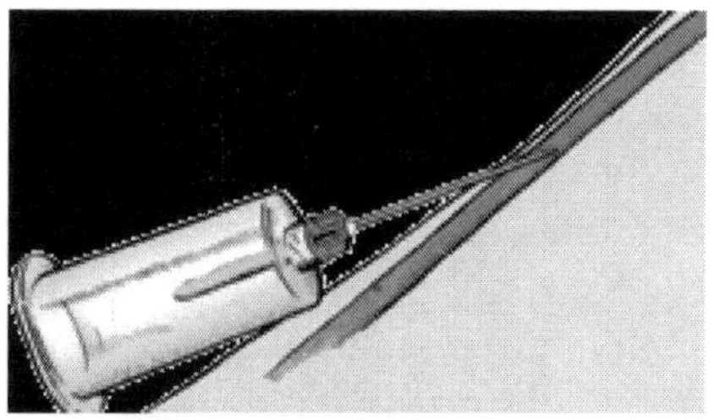

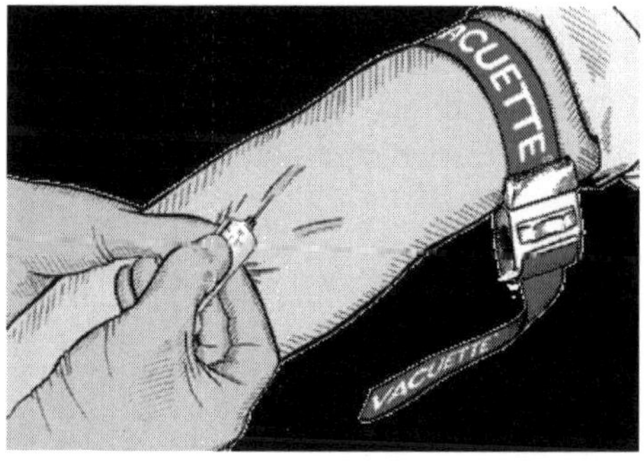

The puncture hand should continue to hold the puncturing device. After some practice, it is possible to sense a "click" when the vein wall has been penetrated. Unnecessary hand changes should be avoided. Any jerky movements with the needle in the vein may cause additional pain. With the left hand an evacuated tube is inserted into the holder. As soon as blood begins to flow, the tourniquet is released. In case the blood flow lightens considerably, the tourniquet can be reapplied briefly.

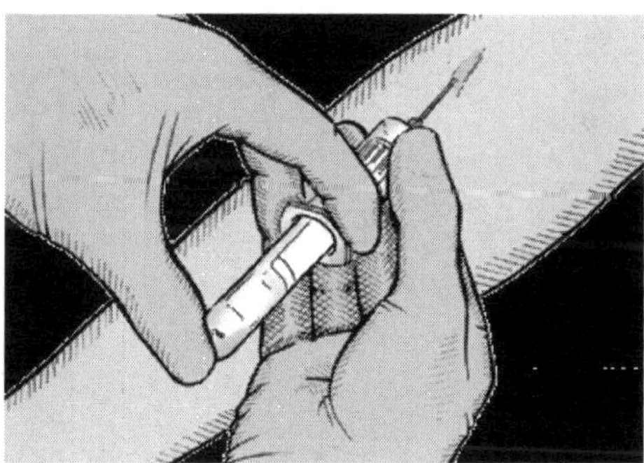

Alternative Puncture Sites

Puncture: Foot veins

The tourniquet is positioned a handbreadth above the site for venipuncture. After tightening the skin, a blood collection set is used to penetrate the vein (at an angle of 10 to 20 degrees). If the blood flows into the thin plastic tubing on the end of the blood collection set, the needle position is correct.

Puncture: Subclavian veins

Puncture of the subclavian vein is almost always in conjunction with the set-up of a central catheter. Puncture of the subclavian vein purely for blood collection reasons is very unusual and is subject to very restricted indications. The range between the sternoclavicular joint and shoulder joint is divided intro three equal areas. The patient is asked to relax as best as possible. The patient's head is then turned slightly to the opposite side, without stretching. An assistant pulls the arm on the venipuncture side towards the caudal, making sure that the patient does not become tense. After applying a little local anaesthetic, the needle is inserted in the transition area between the first to the second directly on the clavicle. The needle must always be in direct contct with the clavicle. The needle should be lowered to skin of the chest immediately up on penetration, with the needle tip pointing towards the jugulum. For a patient of normal weight, the subclavian vein is reached after 2 to 3.5cm (max.). If this is not the case, then the penetration was not directly on the clavicle. The subclavian vein is always open, even when a patient is in shock. As is the case with all punctures of the upper caval vein, depending on skill as well as chance, there is always a risk of pneumothorax. For this reason, the puncture should only be carried out by personnel experienced and competent enough to deal with any complications that could arise (e.g. closed pleural drainage).

Puncture: Femoral artery or vein

Puncture of the femoral artery is simple, if the infrainguinal artery has been palpated. Anchor the artery between the forefinger and middle finger of the left hand. After applying a local anaesthetic solution to the skin, the needle is inserted in the vessel vertically. By lightly moving the needle, it can be determined if the centre of the artery has been reached. If the needle deviates in direction, this can now be corrected, so that the tip is directly on the artery. The needle tip is then tilted towards the cranial (75 degrees), penetrating the vessel wall, so that pulsating light red blood flows. The procedure for puncture of the femoral vein, which is directly next to the artery, is practically identical. However, in this case the blood is not quite so red and does not pulsate in the same way.

FACTORS LEADING TO DIFFICULT VEIN CONDITIONS

- Anxiety
- Delicate veins (children / woman)
- Cold
- Poor hydration
- Vasoconstriction of veins
- Pre-shock or shock
- Thin veins

- Brittle veins
- Repeatedly punctured veins
- Long term treatment with steroids
- Sclerosed veins
- Cachexia
- Rolled veins

The above list of possible unfavourable factors is by no means complete. It is a wellknown fact, that there are a number of adverse situations that can make blood collection difficult. Every step that can lead to vasoconstriction on a patient is a hindrance. Comments such as "You've got bad veins" are not very helpful, and serve more to express helplessness of the blood collector. The first priority is to reduce the patient's anxiety, which is the main cause of vasoconstriction. A calm atmosphere is of prime importance. A hectic mood, a cold room or personnel with cold hands can lead to vasoconstriction. If a patient would prefer to lie down or if a particular venipuncture site is preferred, these wishes should be fulfilled whenever possible. Nevertheless, even if the puncture is carried out correctly, suction of the needle tip to the vein wall may still occur. This can be corrected by rotating the needle slightly in the vein lumen. If this is insufficient, the evacuated tube must be pulled out of the holder until the cap is no longer penetrated by the rear end of the needle.

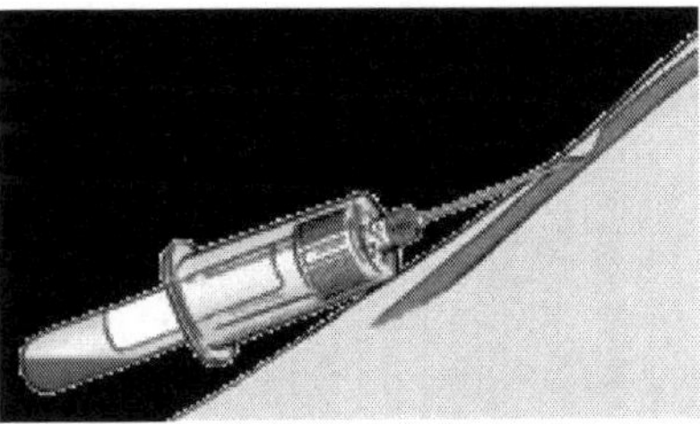

The suction from the vein is then released, and the tip of the needle is freed from the vein wall. The same evacuated tube can now be successfully reapplied. If this still does not work, then use of a blood collection set is to be recommended.

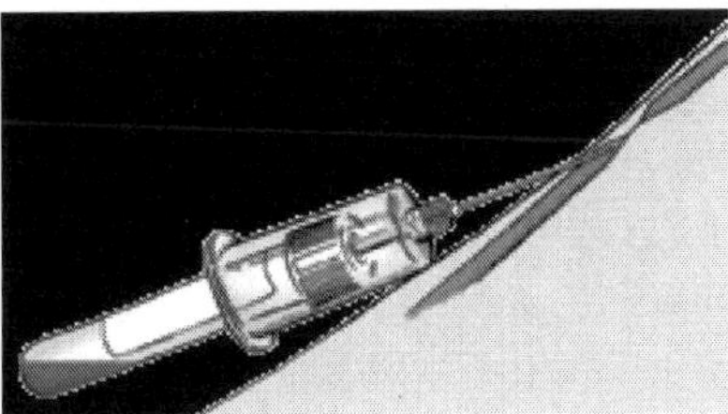

HELPFUL HINTS FOR BLOOD COLLECTION

After removing the rear protective cover, the double-ended blood collection needle is threaded into the holder. The front protective cap is removed before puncture. For hygienic reasons as well as to protect against infection, gloves are required. The blood collection equipment is held between forefinger, middle finger and thumb. The hand carrying out the venipuncture is not to be swapped during the procedure, in order to ensure that the system is securely attached to the patient‘s hand or arm. After penetrating the vein, the free hand is used to push the evacuated tube into the holder. If the needle is in the correct position, blood flows into the tube. If there is no blood flow, a frequent cause is that the needle tip is no longer in the vein lumen. Lightly pulling back the needle and correcting the needle tip can remedy this.

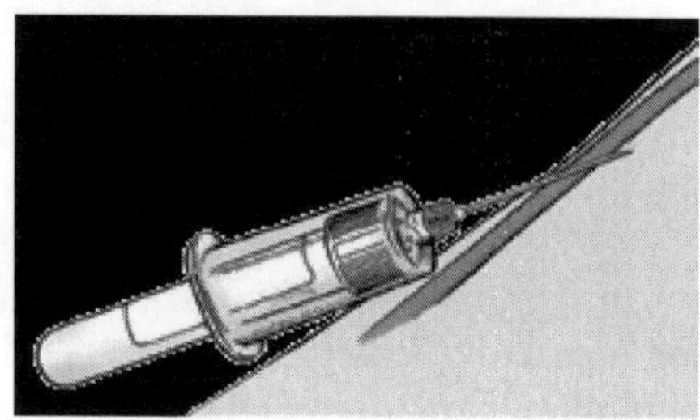

BLOOD COLLECTION FROM A VENOUS OR ARTERIAL CATHETER

Blood collection with a catheter is a possibility, but is only recommended on certain conditions, using a venous catheter. Good patency and optimal care are the essential requirements for this. Depending on the length and type of catheter, 5 - 10ml blood are taken and disposed of either using a syringe or a VACUETTE® Blood Collection Tube (Discard Tube). This ensures that the line is free of flush-out solutions etc. If the manual aspiration using a syringe was without problems, then the following blood collection using an evacuated tube should also be straightforward. The evacuated tube is connected directly to the catheter via a Luer adapter. After collection, the catheter should be rinsed thoroughly using a physiological saline solution (20ml NaCl 0.9%) to prevent any blockages.

Procedure After Blood Collection

Nothing is more unsightly than a bruise after blood collection. The phlebotomist is, to a certain extent, judged on successful penetration, and the extent of any bruising afterwards. This complication can largely be avoided. Before removing the needle from the vein, the tube is removed from the holder. The tourniquet should already have been released completely - this should be made sure of! This is followed by compression using a sterile swab. If the compression is too heavy when the needle is still being pulled out of the vein, the vein wall could be slit, injuring the vein. This can lead to a large haematoma at the puncture site. The compression must be carried out directly after removing the needle.

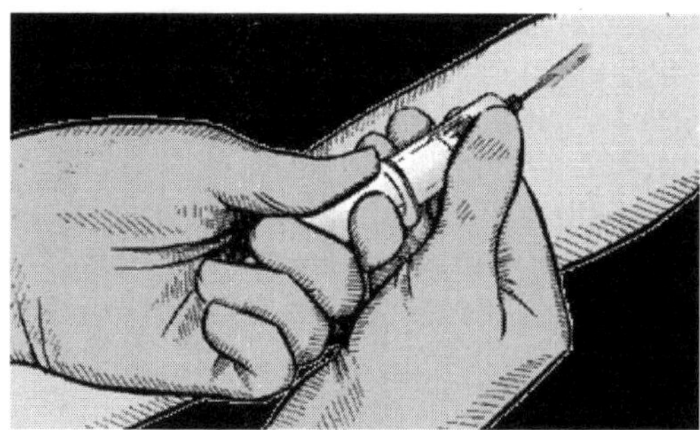

Taking normal coagulation time into account, 2 - 4 minutes time for compression is necessary to prevent a haematoma from forming. This must be explained to the patient, as it is he/she who profits from this measure. If the patient is too weak, the phlebotomist or assistant should make sure that compression is carried out adequately.

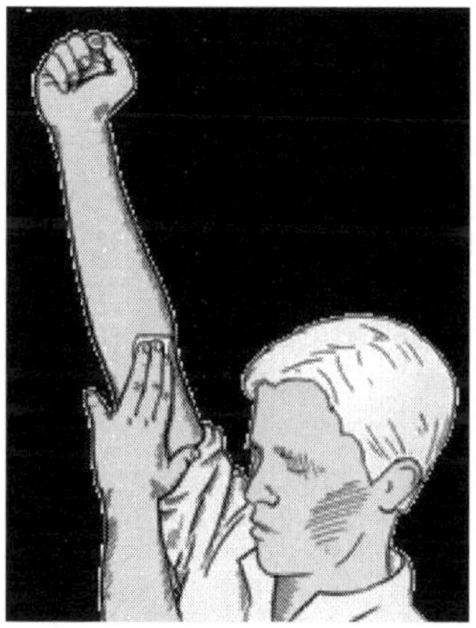

A sterile adhesive plaster should only be applied, when compression is complete. If the antecubital area has been punctured, the arm should be held upwards, without bending. A bent arm could once again cause stasis, and thus lead to formation of a haematoma. For patients undergoing anticoagulation therapy, good manual compression is essential. Rather a minute too long than a minute too short! Physical exertion should not follow blood collection too soon, e.g. sawing, hammering, even climbing stairs. This could lead to formation of a haematoma.

BLOOD COLLECTION WITH SMALL CHILDREN

Technically speaking, blood collection with children from around 2 years and onwards is not that different to blood collection with adults. The collection equipment must be suitable for the smaller dimensions of the vessels. Above all, a calm and friendly atmosphere is extremely important for the young patients. Children are far more cooperative, if the procedure has been explained to them. Application of a local anaesthetic patch on the area intended for venipuncture about an hour beforehand is very important for ensuring that the puncture procedure is as harmonious as possible. The situation can be made easier, if the child is sitting on the mother‘s lap or on the lap of an assistant. Puncture on the back of the hand or in the antecubital area is to be carried out using a small bore vein set. Evcuated tubes with a reduced volume are used. It is very important to hold the arm steady, as reflex movements to escape must be reckoned with.

Puncture in the antecubital area

For venipuncture in the antecubital area, the assistant holds the upper arm of the child, the grip acting at the same time as a tourniquet. If the arm circumference is already too big, a child‘s tourniquet can be used. With the left hand, the phlebotomist pulls the skin in this area taut. With the right hand, the needle of a blood collection set is inserted into the vein at an angle of approx. 15 degrees. The vein area should no longer be sensitive to pain due to the application of a local anaesthetic patch. When the vein has been reached, and blood flow can be seen in the plastic tubing of the collection set, the grip with the left hand can be released. The tube holder can then be connected to the blood collection set, and a VACUETTE® tube with reduced vacuum can be inserted. The assistant or accompanying parent makes sure that the child remains as calm and quiet as possible during the whole procedure.

Dorsal vein puncture

The stasis should be carried out by the assistant, preferably gripping firmly around the arm a handbreadth above the wrist. The fingers are held with the left hand, and pulled downwards, so that the skin on the back of the hand is taut. The needle should be inserted at an angle of 10 to 20 degrees. The limb should be held firmly during the whole venipuncture procedure, in order to avoid jerky movements that could pull the needle out of the vein.

Foot vein puncture

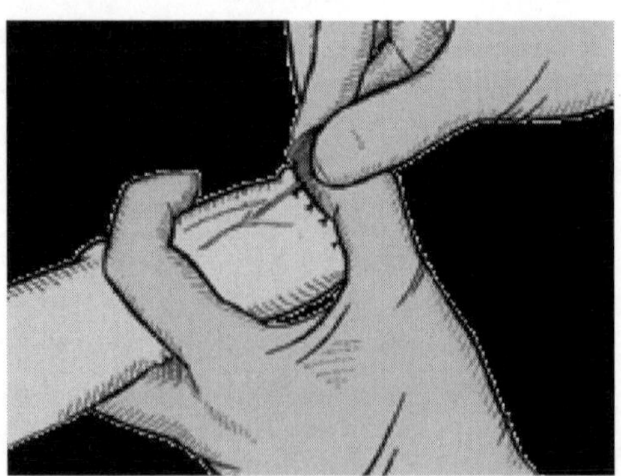

Puncture of a foot vein is carried out after stasis by an assistant‘s hand grip. The toes are pulled downwards, and the skin on the back of the foot is pulled taut. The puncture is carried out very tangentially using a blood collection set. As soon as blood begins to flow, a low-volume VACUETTE® Blood Collection Tube is attached.

BLOOD COLLECTION WITH NEONATES AND INFANTS

Scalp vein puncture

Using a cloth, the infant‘s arms are fastened to his/her body, to prevent defensive movements. By combing through the hair on the scalp, the best suitable vein can be located.

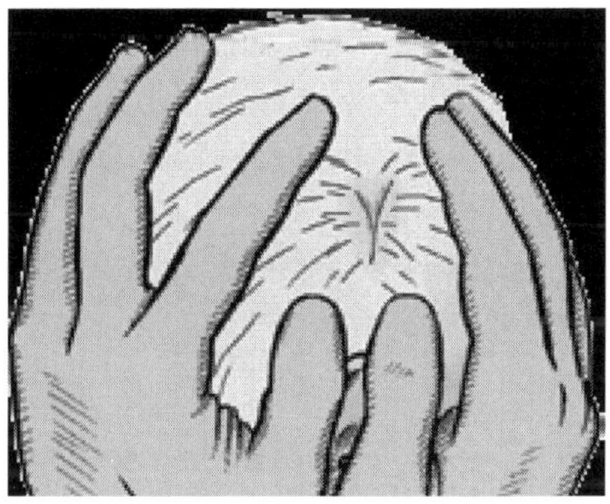

An assistant holds the head firmly but gently, fixing the scalp area where the intended vein for puncture is. Using both hands, the hair is parted, and the skin of the scalp below pulled taut. The vein can then be pressed with the fingers.

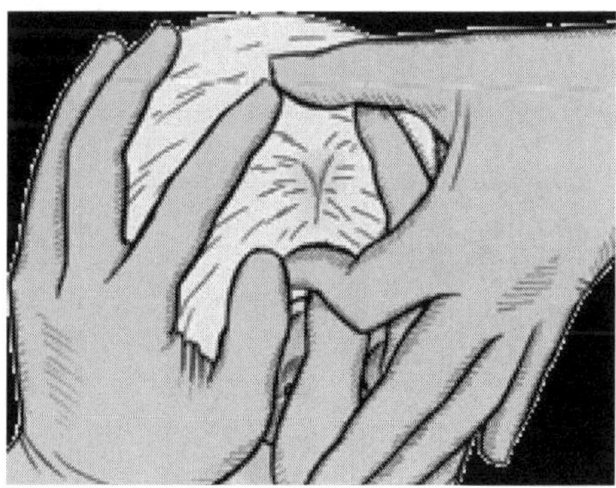

The phlebotomist spreads his fingers of the left hand across the scalp, keeping the skin taut to avoid rolled veins. After disinfection, the vein is punctured very tangentially using a small dimension blood collection set (angle 5 - 10 degrees).

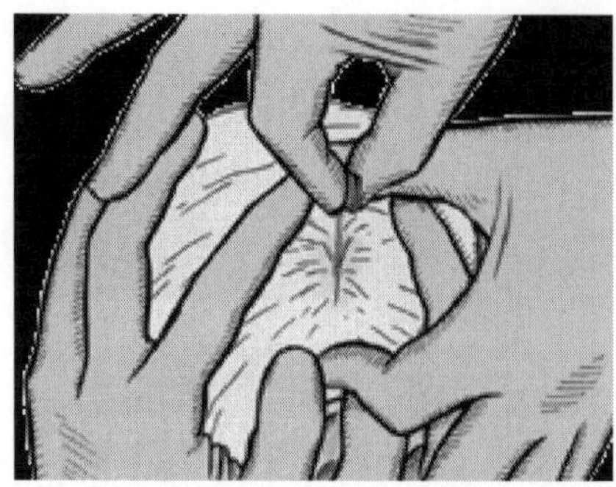

As soon as the blood flows, a VACUETTE® Blood Collection Tube is inserted. When the tube is full, it is first removed from the holder and then the blood collection set can be removed. Using a sterile swab, light pressure is placed on the puncture site for at least 2 minutes, until the blood flow has stopped. The infant is then placed in an upright position and is soothed.

SAFETY ASPECTS DURING BLOOD COLLECTION

Due to the high risk of infection (e.g. HIV, hepatitis), great care should be taken to ensure correct application of materials and equipment, taking particular care to avoid distractions or loss of attention.

Use of thick-walled plastic tubes

By using thick-walled plastic tubes (PET) instead of glass, the risk of tube breakage and thus injury due to glass splinters is virually eliminated.

VACUETTE® QUICKSHIELD Safety Tube Holder

The VACUETTE® QUICKSHIELD Safety Tube Holder is especially suitable for use on isolation wards and for application in making safe diagnoses of HIV, hepatitis etc. When using this holder, blood collection is carried out as usual. When the last tube has been filled, withdraw the needle carefully from the vein.

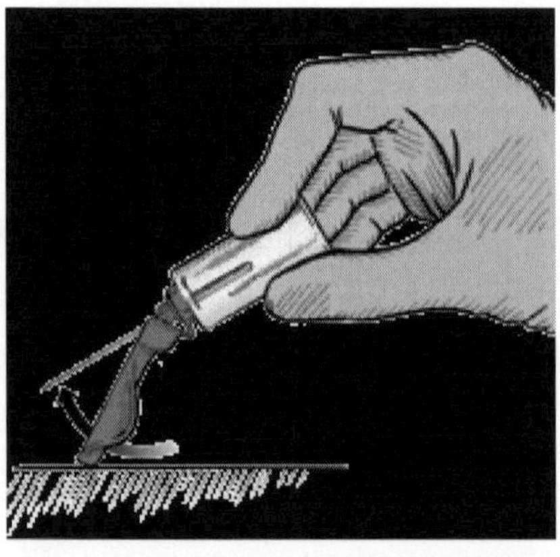

With the aid of a solid support, the needle is enclosed with the protective shield attached to the holder. An audible "click" signifies to the user, that the safety shield has been properly activated.

VACUETTE® Safety Blood Collection Set

After using the safety blood collection set, the safety mechanism is activated in the patient's vein. Whilst removing the tube, a dry, sterile swab and one wing of the set is held by the fingers of one hand.

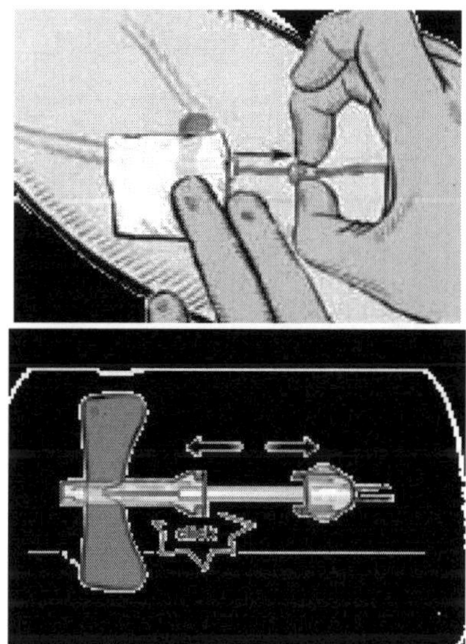

With the other hand, the trigger mechanism is released and locked in place, by pushing together both sides of the stopper. The slide is then pulled back until a click indicates that the safety mechanism has been correctly activated.

VACUETTE® PREMIUM Safety Needle System

The safety mechanism is activated automatically when pressed against the skin. The safety shield can then move freely, enclosing the needle via the spring mechanism as it is withdrawn from the vein. Features of the system are extreme comfort and maximum safety.

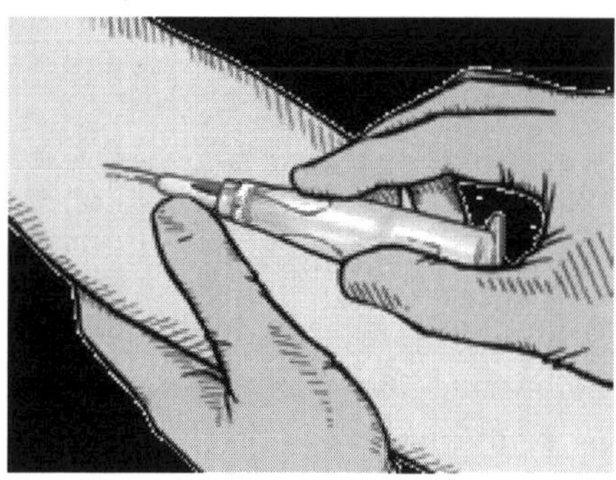

In addition to the „skin-touch" activated product version, there is the „tube-touch" activated version. As soon as the tube is inserted into the holder, the safety mechanism is automatically activated.

VACUETTE® TIPGUARD Safety Tube Holder with automatic needle withdrawal

After completion of blood collection, the last tube is gently removed. Holding the holder with one hand, the safety retractable mechanism is activated by pressing in both sides of the hub. The used needle is then enclosed in the holder and can be disposed of with absolutely no risk of danger.

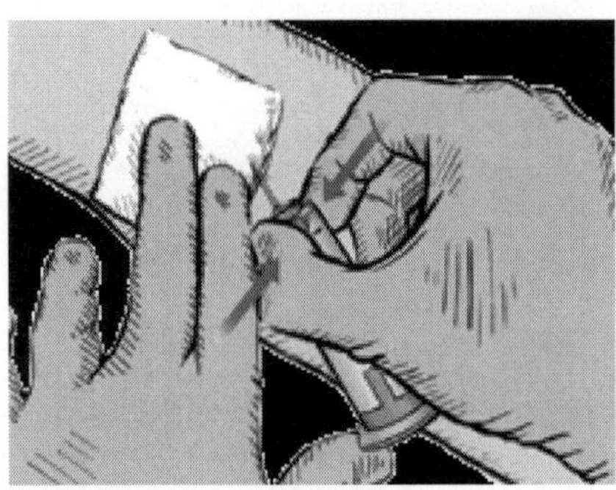

LABORATORY REQUIREMENTS

From the laboratory's point of view, the stasis should always be as short as possible (NB: laboratory values can be falsified, if the stasis is too long). A long stasis can in particular have an effect on the protein values, the cell count, lipids and on other substances bound to protein. Furthermore, excessive application of the tourniquet can lead to haemolysis. To prevent potassium values from increasing, excessive handling of the veins, for example heavily tapping the veins, should not be carried out routinely. This should only be applied in special cases. Tubes containing anticoagulants should be drawn last. This prevents impurities from anticoagulants occuring in other samples.

- Blood culture tubes
- Citrate tubes for coagulation diagnostics
- Serum tubes with and without gel
- Heparin tubes with and without gel
- EDTA tubes
- Glucose tubes
- Others

Coagulation tubes should be fully inverted (180°) 4 times after filling, and all other tubes 8 times. To obtain the full effect of anticoagulants, a thorough mixing is necessary. The air bubble should move from one end to the other, and then back again, for a full inversion.

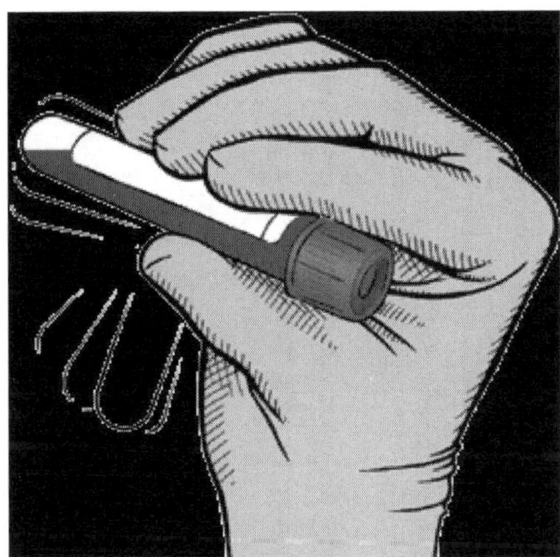

Incorrect collection from venous catheters can lead to contamination from infusion solutions or dilution. Complaints about incorrect laboratory values can usually be led back to the blood collection procedure. Clear labelling of samples with patient data is essential. Any labels attached should not block view of blood as it flows into tube. The tubes should be transferred to the laboratory immediately after blood collection.

HOW TO SAFELY COLLECT BLOOD SAMPLES FROM PERSONS SUSPECTED TO BE INFECTED WITH HIGHLY INFECTIOUS BLOOD-BORNE PATHOGENS (E.G. EBOLA)

Step 1: Before entering patient room, assemble all equipment (1st part)

Step 1a : Assemble equipment for collecting blood

Laboratory sample tubes for blood collection (sterile glass or plastic tubes with rubber caps, vacuum-extraction blood tubes, or glass tubes with screw caps). EDTA tubes are preferred.

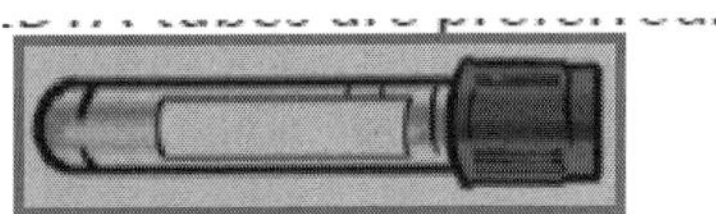

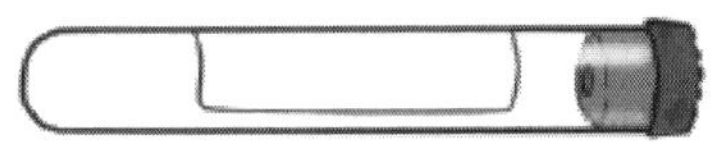

Blood sampling systems (Needle and syringe system, vacuum extraction system with holder, winged butterfly system (vacuum extraction) or winged butterfly system

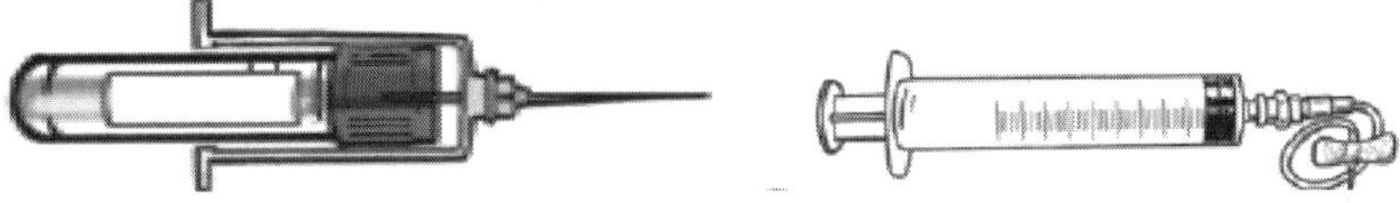

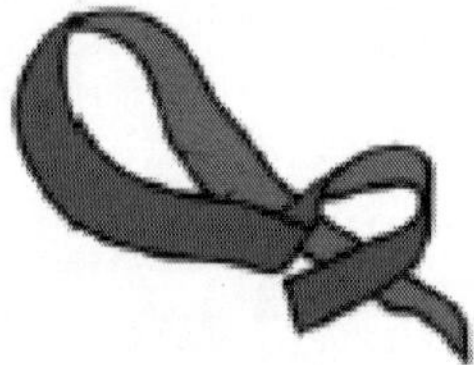

Skin antiseptic solution: 70% isopropyl alcohol

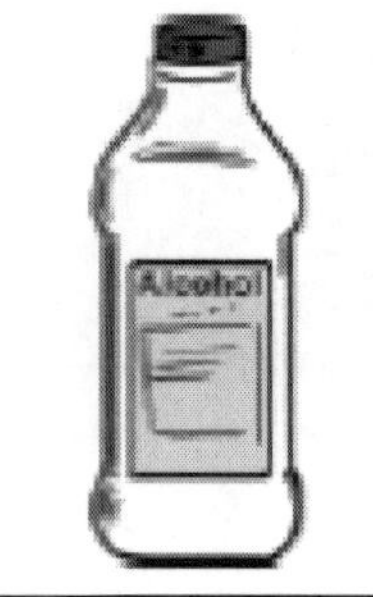

Gauze pads

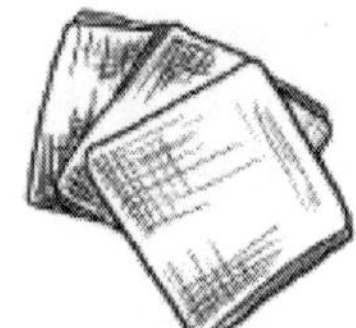

Adhesive bandage

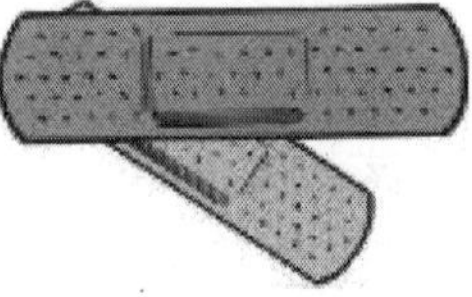

Tray for assembling blood collection tools

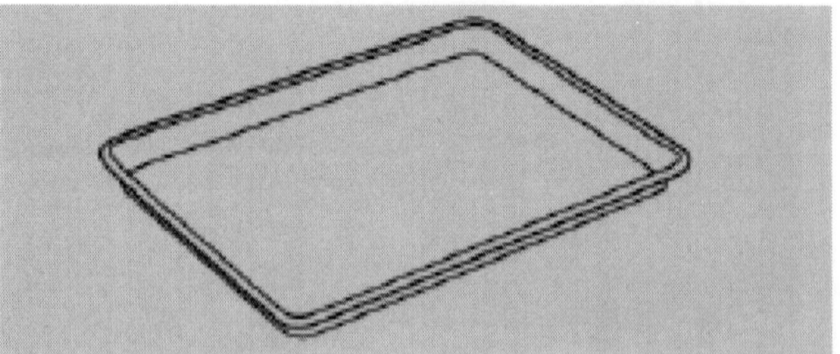

Rack for holding blood tubes

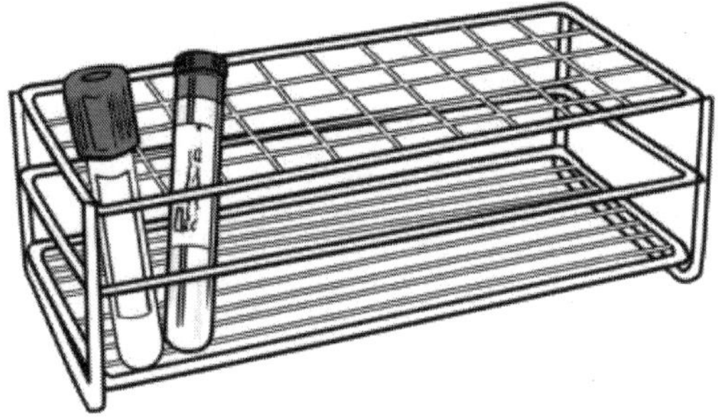

Durable marker for writing on laboratory sample

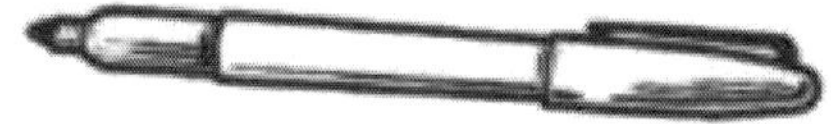

Step 1b : Assemble equipment for preventing infections

For Hand Hygiene: use Alcohol-based handrub OR

- Clean, running water
- Soap
- Disposable (paper) towel

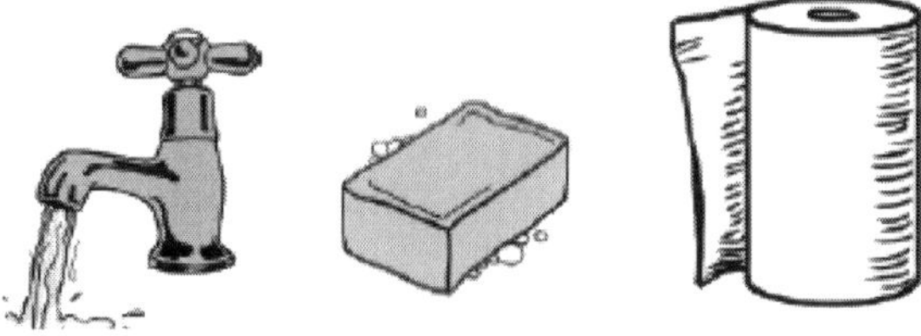

Personal Protective Equipment (PPE):

- Several pairs of disposable gloves (non-sterile, ambidextrous, single layer)
  - — One pair of gloves for blood collection
  - — One additional pair as a replacement if they become damaged or contaminate

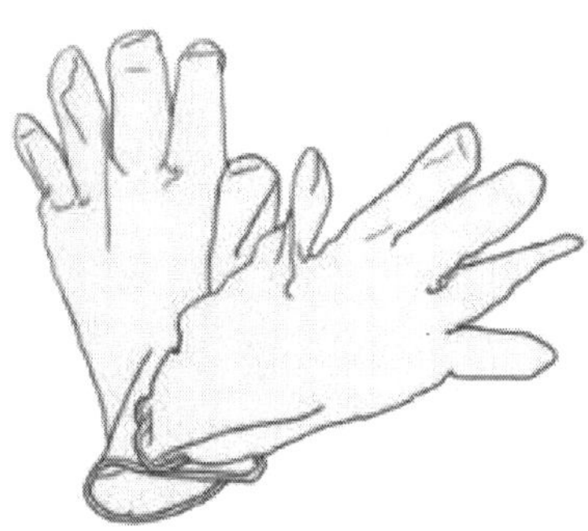

- Footwear: If in hospital: wear shoes with puncture-resistant soles or rubber boots; If in rural setting or patient home wear rubber boots or shoes with puncture-resistant soles with disposable overshoes secured around the shoes to prevent direct contact with ground and infected bodily fluid spills

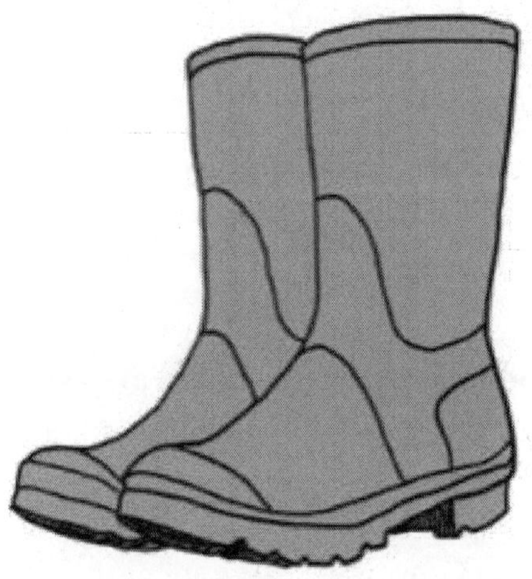

For waste management materials:

- Leak-proof and puncture resistant sharps container
- Two leak-proof infectious waste bags: one for disposable material (destruction) and one for reusable materials (disinfection)

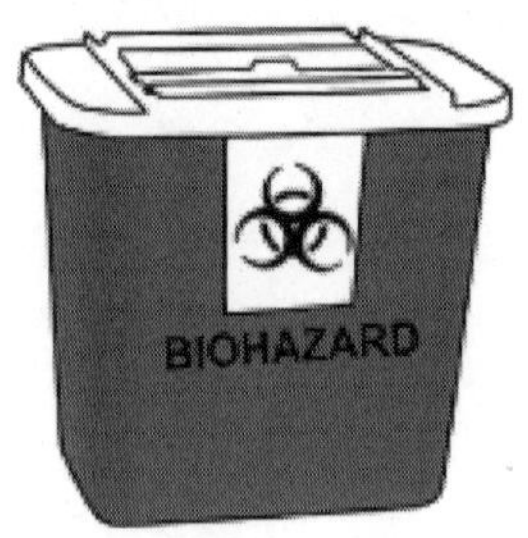

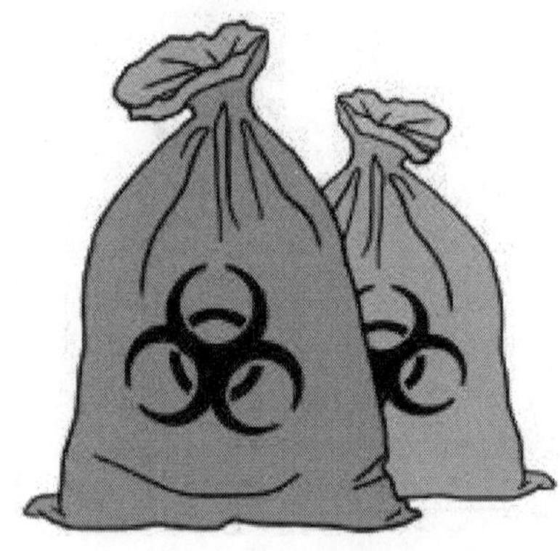

Long-sleeved, cuffed gowns (if in hospital) or disposable coverall suit (if in rural area) Note: Tasks where contact with blood or body fluid could happen, Impermeable gown or a plastic apron over the non impermeable gown are recommended.

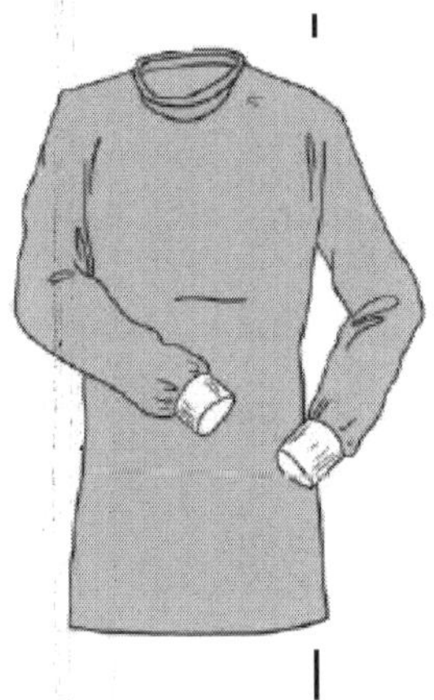

Face protection: Face shield or “goggles and mask

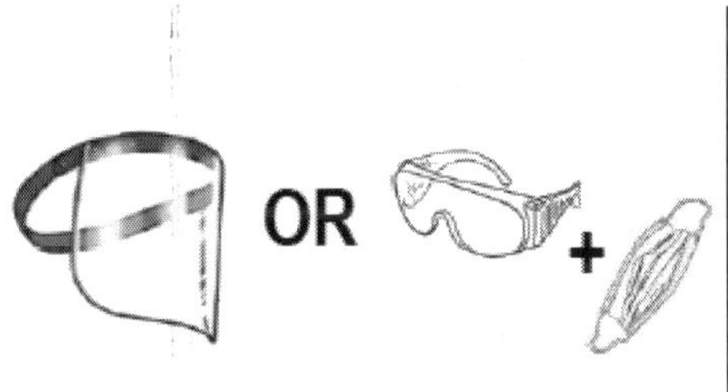

BEFORE ENTERING PATIENT ROOM, ASSEMBLE ALL EQUIPMENT (LAST PART)

Fill out patient documentation:

- Label blood collection tubes with date of collection, patient name, and his/her identifier number.
- Do NOT forget to fill out necessary laboratory form and epidemiological questionnaire.

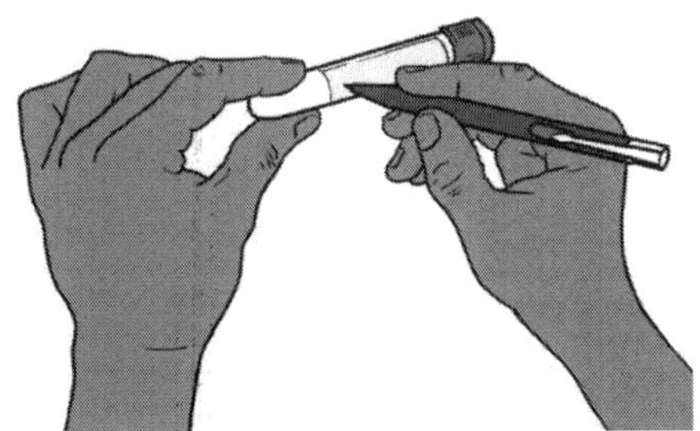

- If several patients have to be sampled in the same place or during the same investigation, create a line list. One patient per line. The list should include: patient name, identifier number, sex, age (birthdate), clinical information: symptoms, date of onset, date specimen was collected, type of sample taken.

Assemble materials for packaging of samples:

- Plastic leak-proof packaging container
- Disposable (paper) towels
- Cooler or cold box, if sample requires refrigeration

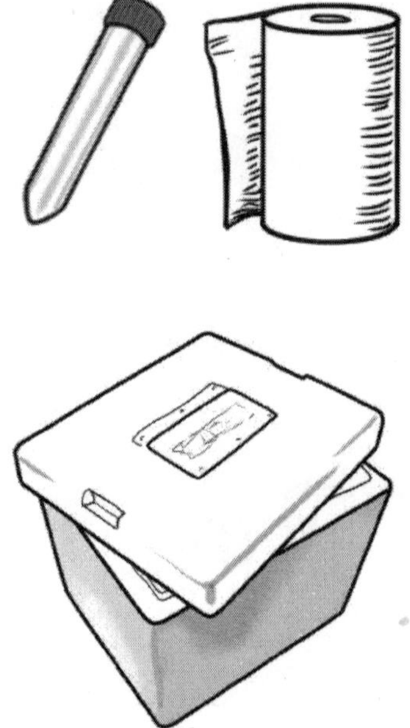

For the shipment of samples to the National Central Laboratory follow Sample Shipment packaging requirements (see document "How to safely ship Emerging and Dangerous Pathogen samples")

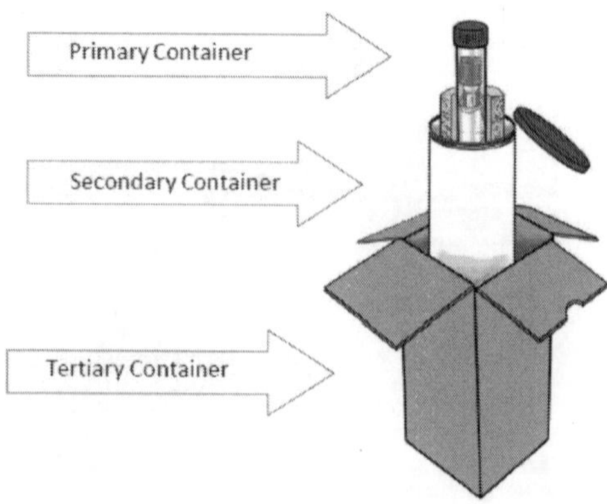

Important: A designated Assistant wearing gloves should be available to help you. This person should stand outside the patient room. He/She will help you prepare the sample for transport, assist you with putting on the personal protective equipment, or provide any additional equipment you may need.

Step 2: Put on all personal protective equipment (PPE)

Step 2a: Perform hand hygiene. Duration of the entire procedure: 40-60 sec.:

- Wet hands with water and enough soap to cover all hand surfaces

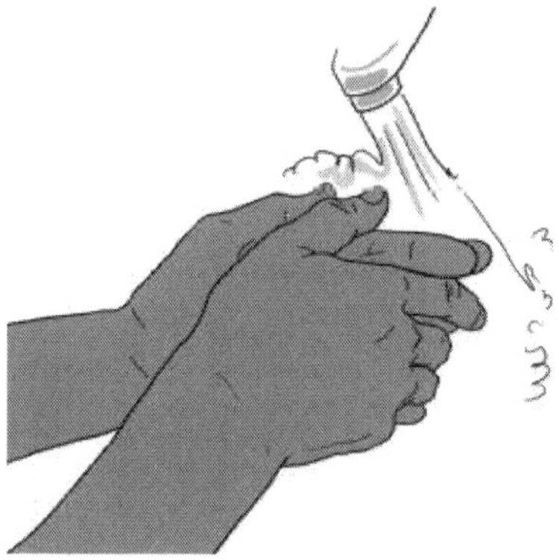

Rub hands, palm to palm,

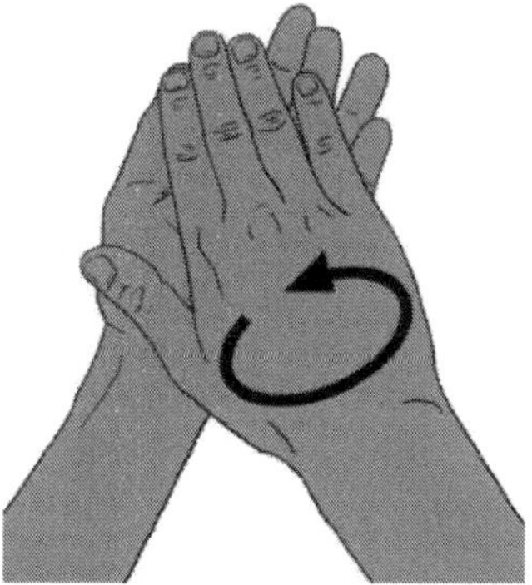

Right palm over left dorsum with interlaced fingers and vice versa,

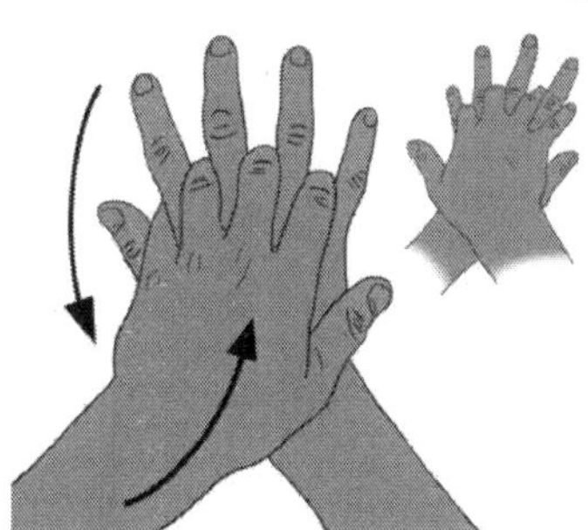

Palm to palm with fingers interlaced

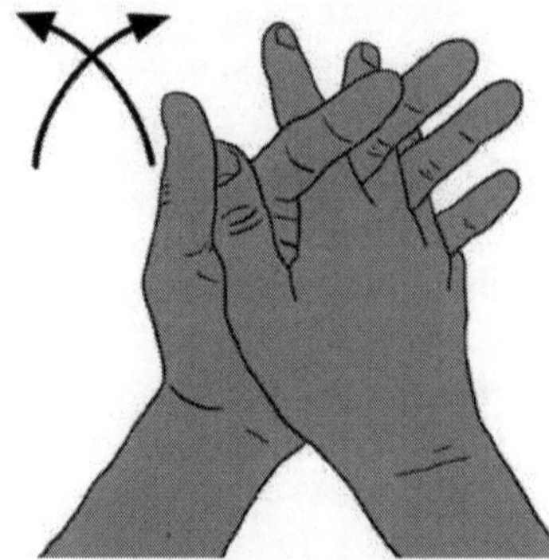

Back of fingers to opposing palms with fingers interlocked

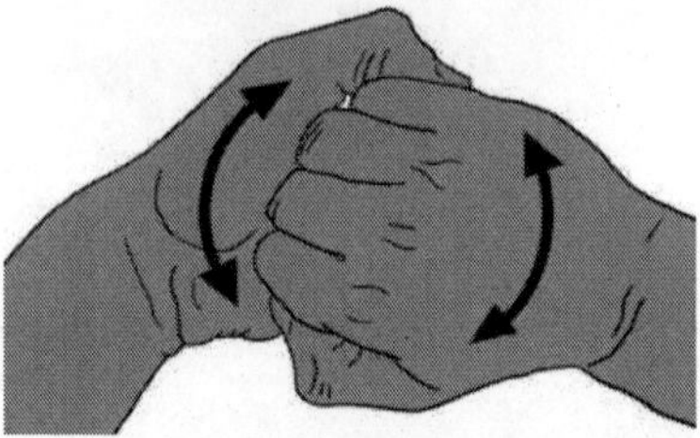

Rotational rubbing of left thumb clasped in right palm and vice versa,

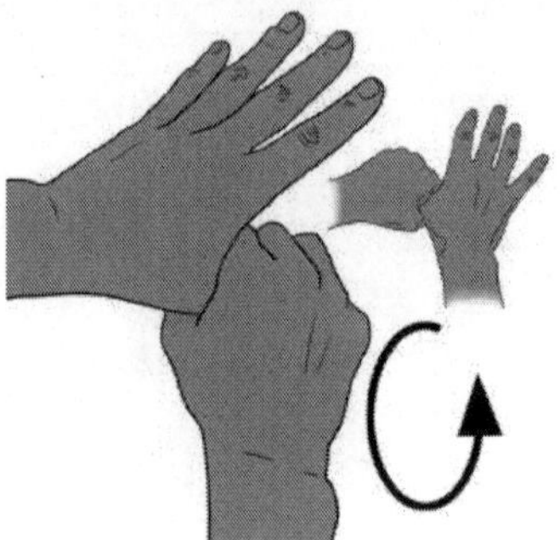

Rinse hands with water.

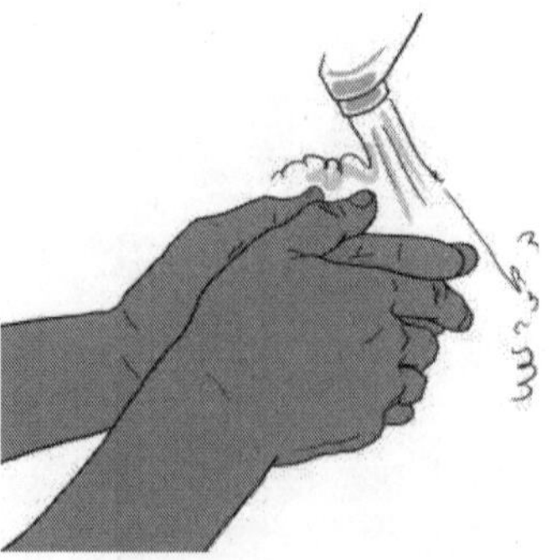

Dry hands thoroughly with single use towel.

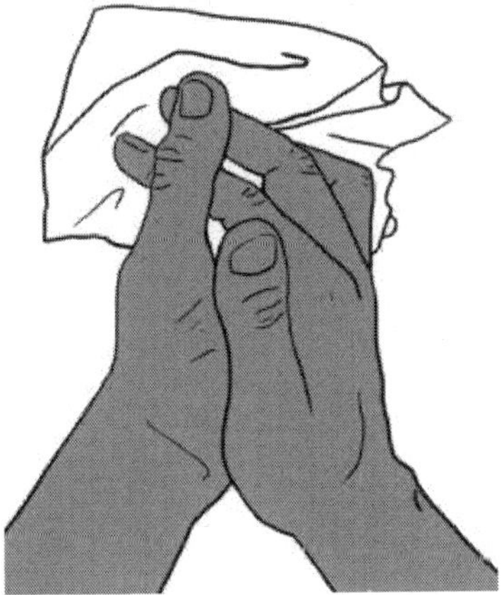

Step 2b: Put on a gown :

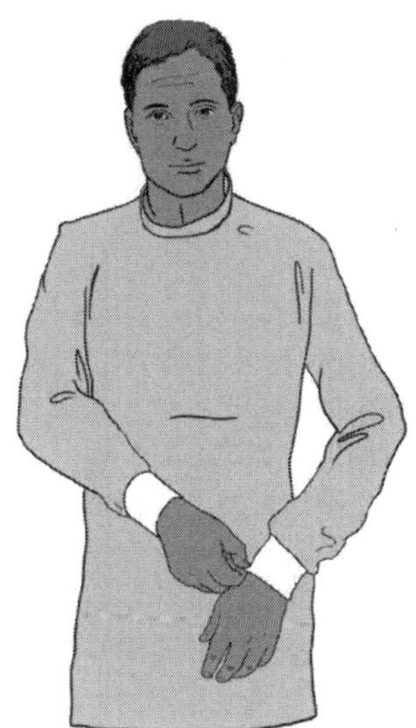

Put on face protection:

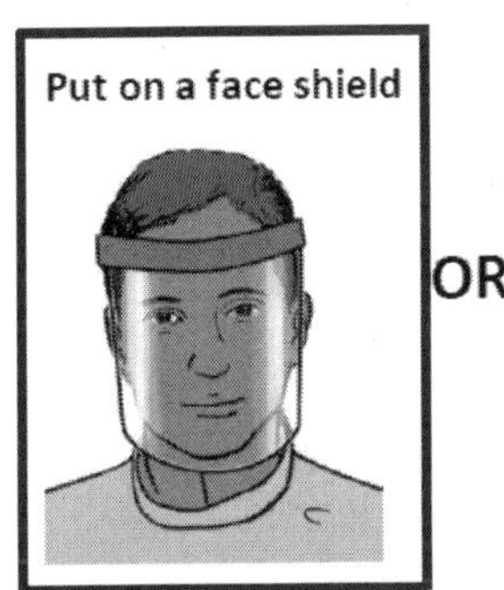

OR

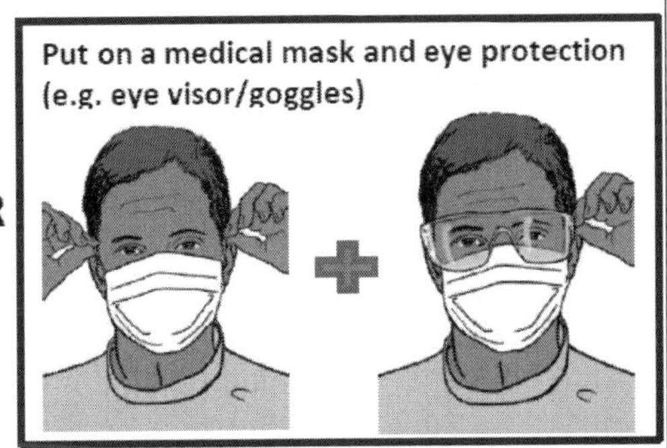

If the patient has respiratory symptoms, wear a medical mask underneath the face shield.

Put on gloves (over gown cuffs).

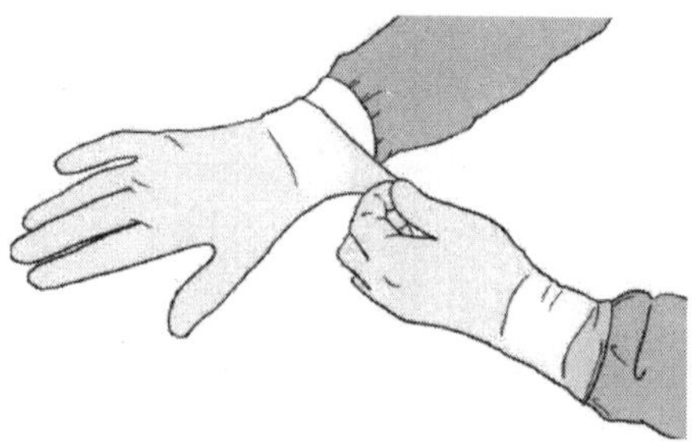

STAINING

Staining is an auxiliary technique used in microscopy to enhance contrast in the microscopic image. Stains and dyes are frequently used in biology and medicine to highlight structures in biological tissues for viewing, often with the aid of different microscopes. Stains may be used to define and examine bulk tissues (highlighting, for example, muscle fibers or connective tissue), cell populations (classifying different blood cells, for instance), or organelles within individual cells.

In biochemistry it involves adding a class-specific (DNA, proteins, lipids, carbohydrates) dye to a substrate to qualify or quantify the presence of a specific compound. Staining and fluorescent tagging can serve similar purposes. Biological staining is also used to mark cells in flow cytometry, and to flag proteins or nucleic acids in gel electrophoresis.

Simple staining is staining with only one stain/dye. There are various kinds of multiple staining, many of which are examples of counterstaining, differential staining, or both, including double staining and triple staining.

Staining is not limited to biological materials, it can also be used to study the morphology of other materials for example the lamellar structures of semi-crystalline polymers or the domain structures of block copolymers.

IN VIVO VS *IN VITRO*

In vivo staining (also called vital staining or intravital staining) is the process of dyeing living tissues—*in vivo* means "in life" (compare with *in vitro* staining). By causing certain cells or structures to take on contrasting colour(s), their form (morphology) or position within a cell or tissue can be readily seen and studied. The usual purpose is to reveal cytological details that might otherwise not be apparent; however, staining can also reveal where certain chemicals or specific chemical reactions are taking place within cells or tissues.

In vitro staining involves colouring cells or structures that have been removed from their biological context. Certain stains are often combined to reveal more details and features than a single stain alone. Combined with specific protocols for fixation and sample preparation, scientists and physicians can use these standard techniques as consistent, repeatable diagnostic tools. A counterstain is stain that makes cells or structures more visible, when not completely visible with the principal stain.

- For example, crystal violet stains only Gram-positive bacteria in Gram staining. A safranin counterstain is applied that stains all cells, allowing identification of Gram-negative bacteria.

While ex vivo, many cells continue to live and metabolize until they are "fixed". Some staining methods are based on this property. Those stains excluded by the living cells but taken up by the already dead cells are called vital stains (e.g. trypan blue or propidium iodide for eukaryotic cells). Those that enter and stain living cells are called supravital stains (e.g. New Methylene Blue and Brilliant Cresyl Blue for reticulocyte staining). However, these stains are eventually toxic to the organism, some more so than others. Partly due to their toxic interaction inside a living cell, when supravital stains enter a living cell, they might produce a characteristic pattern of staining different from the staining of an already fixed cell (e.g. "reticulocyte" look versus diffuse "polychromasia"). To achieve desired effects, the stains are used in very dilute solutions ranging from 1:5000 to 1:500000 (Howey, 2000). Note that many stains may be used in both living and fixed cells.

In vitro methods

Preparation

The preparatory steps involved depend on the type of analysis planned; some or all of the following procedures may be required.

Fixation–which may itself consist of several steps–aims to preserve the shape of the cells or tissue involved as much as possible. Sometimes heat fixation is used to kill, adhere, and alter the specimen so it accepts stains. Most chemical fixatives (chemicals causing fixation) generate chemical bonds between proteins and other substances within the sample, increasing their rigidity. Common fixatives include formaldehyde, ethanol, methanol, and/or picric acid. Pieces of tissue may be embedded in paraffin wax to increase their mechanical strength and stability and to make them easier to cut into thin slices.

Permeabilization involves treatment of cells with (usually) a mild surfactant. This treatment dissolves cell membranes, and allows larger dye molecules into the cell's interior.

Mounting usually involves attaching the samples to a glass microscope slide for observation and analysis. In some cases, cells may be grown directly on a slide. For samples of loose cells (as with a blood smear or a pap smear) the sample can be directly applied to a slide. For larger pieces of tissue, thin sections (slices) are made using a microtome; these slices can then be mounted and inspected.

Staining proper

At its simplest, the actual staining process may involve immersing the sample (before or after fixation and mounting) in dye solution, followed by rinsing and observation. Many dyes, however, require the use of a mordant: a chemical compound that reacts with the stain to form an insoluble, coloured precipitate. When excess dye solution is washed away, the mordanted stain remains. Most of the dyes commonly used in microscopy are available as certified stains. This means that samples of the manufacturer's batch have been tested by an independent body, the Biological Stain Commission, and found to meet or exceed certain standards of purity, dye content and performance in staining techniques. These standards are published in detail in the journal Biotechnic & Histochemistry. Many dyes are inconsistent in composition from one supplier to another. The use of certified stains eliminates a source of unexpected results.

Negative staining

A simple staining method for bacteria that is usually successful, even when the "positive staining" methods detailed below fail, is to use a negative stain. This can be achieved by smearing the sample onto the slide and then applying nigrosin (a black synthetic dye) or India ink (an aqueous suspension of carbon particles). After drying, the microorganisms may be viewed in bright field microscopy as lighter inclusions well-contrasted against the dark environment surrounding them. Note: negative staining is a mild technique that may not destroy the microorganisms, and is therefore unsuitable for studying pathogens.

Specific techniques

Gram staining

Gram staining is used to determine gram status to classify bacteria broadly. It is based on the composition of their cell wall. Gram staining uses crystal violet to stain cell walls, iodine as a mordant, and a fuchsin or safranin counterstain to mark all bacteria. Gram status is important in medicine; the presence or absence of a cell wall changes the bacterium's susceptibility to some antibiotics. Gram-positive bacteria stain dark blue or violet. Their cell wall is typically rich with peptidoglycan and lacks the secondary membrane and lipopolysaccharide layer found in Gram-negative bacteria.

On most Gram-stained preparations, Gram-negative organisms appear red or pink because they are counterstained. Because of presence of higher lipid content, after alcohol-treatment, the porosity of the cell wall increases, hence the CVI complex (crystal violet – iodine) can pass through. Thus, the primary stain is not retained. Also, in contrast to most Gram-positive bacteria, Gram-negative bacteria have only a few layers of peptidoglycan and a secondary cell membrane made primarily of lipopolysaccharide.

Endospore staining

Endospore staining is used to identify the presence or absence of endospores, which make bacteria very difficult to kill. This is particularly useful for identifying endospore-forming bacterial pathogens like *Clostridium difficile*.

Ziehl-Neelsen stain

Ziehl-Neelsen staining is used to stain species of *Mycobacterium tuberculosis* that do not stain with the standard laboratory staining procedures like Gram staining. The stains used are the red coloured Carbol fuchsin that stains the bacteria and a counter stain like Methylene blue

Haematoxylin and eosin (H&E) staining

Haematoxylin and eosin staining protocol is used frequently in histology to examine thin sections of tissue. Haematoxylin stains cell nuclei blue, while eosin stains cytoplasm, connective tissue and other extracellular substances pink or red. Eosin is strongly absorbed by red blood cells, colouring them bright red. In a skilfully made H & E preparation the red blood cells are almost orange, and collagen and cytoplasm (especially muscle) acquire different shades of pink. When the staining is done by a machine, the subtle differences in eosinophilia are often lost. Hematoxylin stains the cell nucleus and other acidic structures (such as RNA-rich portions of the cytoplasm and the matrix of hyaline cartilage) blue. In contrast, eosin stains the cytoplasm and collagen pink.

Papanicolaou staining

Papanicolaou staining, or Pap staining, is a frequently used method for examining cell samples from various bodily secretions. It is frequently used to stain Pap smear specimens. It uses a combination of haematoxylin, Orange G, eosin Y, Light Green SF yellowish, and sometimes Bismarck Brown Y.

PAS staining

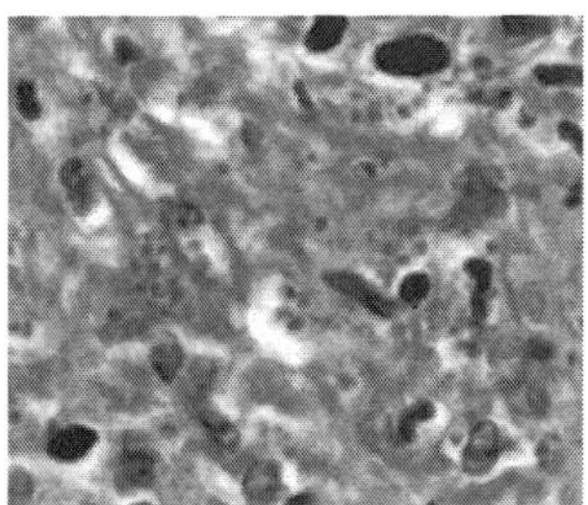

Fig. PAS diastase showing the fungus Histoplasma.

Periodic acid-Schiff staining is used to mark carbohydrates (glycogen, glycoprotein, proteoglycans). It is used to distinguish different types of glycogen storage diseases.

Masson's trichrome

Masson's trichrome is (as the name implies) a three-colour staining protocol. The recipe has evolved from Masson's original technique for different specific applications, but all are well-suited to distinguish cells from surrounding connective tissue. Most recipes produce red keratin and muscle fibers, blue or green staining of collagen and bone, light red or pink staining of cytoplasm, and black cell nuclei.

Romanowsky stains

The Romanowsky stains are all based on a combination of eosinate (chemically reduced eosin) and methylene blue (sometimes with its oxidation products azure A and azure B). Common variants include Wright's stain, Jenner's stain, May-Grunwald stain, Leishman stain and Giemsa stain.

All are used to examine blood or bone marrow samples. They are preferred over H&E for inspection of blood cells because different types of leukocytes (white blood cells) can be readily distinguished. All are also suited to examination of blood to detect blood-borne parasites like malaria.

Silver staining

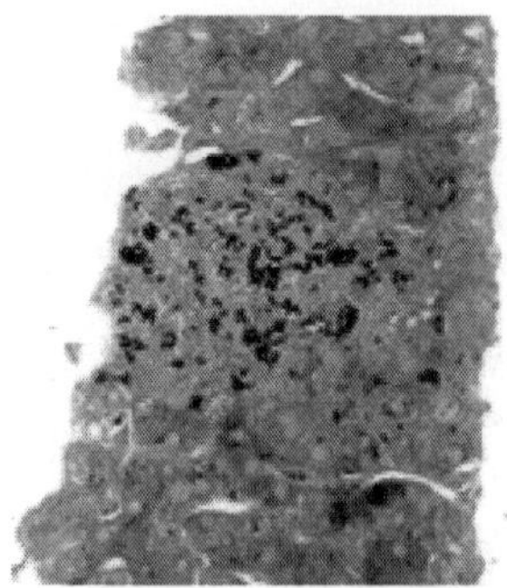

Fig. Gömöri methenamine silver stain demonstrating histoplasma (black round balls).

Silver staining is the use of silver to stain histologic sections. This kind of staining is important especially to show proteins (for example type III collagen) and DNA. It is used to show both substances inside and outside cells. Silver staining is also used in temperature gradient gel electrophoresis.

Some cells are *argentaffin*. These reduce silver solution to metallic silver after formalin fixation. This method was discovered by Italian Camillo Golgi, by using a reaction between silver nitrate and potassium dichromate, thus precipitating silver chromate in some cells (see Golgi's method). Other cells are *argyrophilic*. These reduce silver solution to metallic silver after being exposed to the stain that contains a reductant, for example hydroquinone or formalin.

Sudan staining

Sudan staining is the use of Sudan dyes to stain sudanophilic substances, usually lipids. Sudan III, Sudan IV, Oil Red O, Osmium tetroxide, and Sudan Black B are often used. Sudan staining is often used to determine the level of fecal fat to diagnose steatorrhea.

Conklin's staining

Special technique designed for staining true endospores with the use of malachite green dye, once stained, they do not decolourize.

COMMON BIOLOGICAL STAINS

Different stains react or concentrate in different parts of a cell or tissue, and these properties are used to advantage to reveal specific parts or areas. Some of the most common biological stains are listed below. Unless otherwise marked, all of these dyes may be used with fixed cells and tissues; vital dyes (suitable for use with living organisms) are noted.

- Acridine orange: Acridine orange (AO) is a nucleic acid selective fluorescent cationic dye useful for cell cycle determination. It is cell-permeable, and interacts with DNA and RNA by intercalation or electrostatic attractions. When bound to DNA, it is very similar spectrally to fluorescein. Like fluorescein, it is also useful as a non-specific stain for backlighting conventionally stained cells on the surface of a solid sample of tissue (fluorescence backlighted staining).
- Bismarck brown: Bismarck brown (also Bismarck brown Y or Manchester brown) imparts a yellow colour to acid mucins.
- Carmine: Carmine is an intensely red dye used to stain glycogen, while Carmine alum is a nuclear stain. Carmine stains require the use of a mordant, usually aluminum.

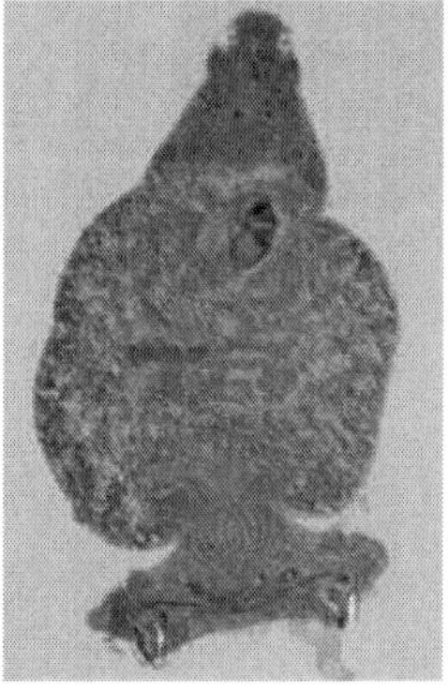

Fig. Carmine staining of a parasitic flatworm.

- Coomassie blue: Coomassie blue (also brilliant blue) nonspecifically stains proteins a strong blue colour. It is often used in gel electrophoresis.
- Cresyl violet: Cresyl violet stains the acidic components of the neuronal cytoplasm a violet colour, specifically nissl bodies. Often used in brain research.

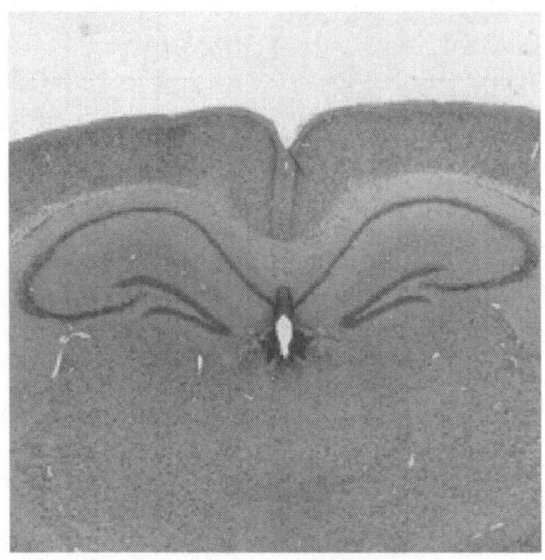

Fig. Cresyl violet staining is commonly used in histology to stain nervous tissues

- Crystal violet: Crystal violet, when combined with a suitable mordant, stains cell walls purple. Crystal violet is the stain used in Gram staining.
- DAPI: DAPI is a fluorescent nuclear stain, excited by ultraviolet light and showing strong blue fluorescence when bound to DNA. DAPI binds with A=T rich repeats of chromosomes. DAPI is also not visible with regular transmission microscopy. It may be used in living or fixed cells. DAPI-stained cells are especially appropriate for cell counting.
- Eosin: Eosin is most often used as a counterstain to haematoxylin, imparting a pink or red colour to cytoplasmic material, cell membranes, and some extracellular structures. It also imparts a strong red colour to red blood cells. Eosin may also be used as a counterstain in some variants of Gram staining, and in many other protocols. There are actually two very closely related compounds commonly referred to as eosin. Most often used is eosin Y (also known as eosin Y ws or eosin yellowish); it has a very slightly yellowish cast. The other eosin compound is eosin B (eosin bluish or imperial red); it has a very faint bluish cast. The two dyes are interchangeable, and the use of one or the other is more a matter of preference and tradition.
- Ethidium bromide: Ethidium bromide intercalates and stains DNA,

providing a fluorescent red-orange stain. Although it will not stain healthy cells, it can be used to identify cells that are in the final stages of apoptosis – such cells have much more permeable membranes. Consequently, ethidium bromide is often used as a marker for apoptosis in cells populations and to locate bands of DNA in gel electrophoresis. The stain may also be used in conjunction with acridine orange (AO) in viable cell counting. This EB/AO combined stain causes live cells to fluoresce green whilst apoptotic cells retain the distinctive red-orange fluorescence.

- Acid fuchsine: Acid fuchsine may be used to stain collagen, smooth muscle, or mitochondria. Acid fuchsine is used as the nuclear and cytoplasmic stain in Mallory's trichrome method. Acid fuchsine stains cytoplasm in some variants of Masson's trichrome. In Van Gieson's picro-fuchsine, acid fuchsine imparts its red colour to collagen fibres. Acid fuchsine is also a traditional stain for mitochondria (Altmann's method).
- Haematoxylin: Haematoxylin (hematoxylin in North America) is a nuclear stain. Used with a mordant, haematoxylin stains nuclei blue-violet or brown. It is most often used with eosin in H&E (haematoxylin and eosin) staining—one of the most common procedures in histology.
- Hoechst stains: Hoechst is a *bis*-benzimidazole derivative compound that binds to the *minor groove* of DNA. Often used in fluorescence microscopy for DNA staining, Hoechst stains appear yellow when dissolved in aqueous solutions and emit blue light under UV excitation. There are two major types of Hoechst: *Hoechst 33258* and *Hoechst 33342*. The two compounds are functionally similar, but with a little difference in structure. Hoechst 33258 contains a terminal hydroxyl group and is thus more soluble in aqueous solution, however this characteristics reduces its ability to penetrate the plasma membrane. Hoechst 33342 contains an ethyl substitution on the terminal hydroxyl group (i.e. an ethylether group) making it more hydrophobic for easier plasma membrane passage
- Iodine: Iodine is used in chemistry as an indicator for starch. When starch is mixed with iodine in solution, an intensely dark blue colour develops, representing a starch/iodine complex. Starch is a substance common to most plant cells and so a weak iodine solution will stain starch present in the cells. Iodine is one component in the staining technique known as Gram staining, used in microbiology. Lugol's solution or Lugol's iodine (IKI) is a brown solution that turns black in the presence of starches and can be used as a cell stain, making the cell nuclei more visible. Iodine is also used as a mordant in Gram's

staining, it enhances dye to enter through the pore present in the cell wall/membrane.

- Malachite green: Malachite green (also known as diamond green B or victoria green B) can be used as a blue-green counterstain to safranin in the Gimenez staining technique for bacteria. It also can be used to directly stain spores.
- Methyl green: Methyl green is used commonly with bright-field microscopes to dye the chromatin of cells so that they are more easily viewed.
- Methylene blue: Methylene blue is used to stain animal cells, such as human cheek cells, to make their nuclei more observable. Also used to stain the blood film and used in cytology.
- Neutral red: Neutral red (or toluylene red) stains Nissl substance red. It is usually used as a counterstain in combination with other dyes.
- Nile blue: Nile blue (or Nile blue A) stains nuclei blue. It may be used with living cells.
- Nile red: Nile red (also known as Nile blue oxazone) is formed by boiling Nile blue with sulfuric acid. This produces a mix of Nile red and Nile blue. Nile red is a lipophilic stain; it will accumulate in lipid globules inside cells, staining them red. Nile red can be used with living cells. It fluoresces strongly when partitioned into lipids, but practically not at all in aqueous solution.
- Osmium tetroxide (formal name: osmium tetraoxide): Osmium tetraoxide is used in optical microscopy to stain lipids. It dissolves in fats, and is reduced by organic materials to elemental osmium, an easily visible black substance.
- Rhodamine: Rhodamine is a protein specific fluorescent stain commonly used in fluorescence microscopy.
- Safranin: Safranin (or Safranin O) is a nuclear stain. It produces red nuclei, and is used primarily as a counterstain. Safranin may also be used to give a yellow colour to collagen.

STAINABILITY OF TISSUES

Tissues which take up stains are called chromatic. Chromosomes were so named because of their ability to absorb a violet stain. Positive affinity for a specific stain may be designated by the suffix *-philic*. For example, tissues that stain with an azure stain may be referred to as azurophilic. This may also be used for more generalized staining properties, such as acidophilic for tissues that stain by acidic stains (most notably eosin), basophilic when staining in basic dyes, and *amphophilic* when staining with either acid or basic dyes. In contrast, chromophobic tissues do not take up coloured dye readily.

ELECTRON MICROSCOPY

As in light microscopy, stains can be used to enhance contrast in transmission electron microscopy. Electron-dense compounds of heavy metals are typically used.

- Phosphotungstic acid: Phosphotungstic acid is a common negative stain for viruses, nerves, polysaccharides, and other biological tissue materials.
- Osmium tetroxide: Osmium tetroxide is used in optical microscopy to stain lipids. It dissolves in fats, and is reduced by organic materials to elemental osmium, an easily visible black substance. Because it is a heavy metal that absorbs electrons, it is perhaps the most common stain used for morphology in biological electron microscopy. It is also used for the staining of various polymers for the study of their morphology by TEM. OsO_4 is very volatile and extremely toxic. It is a strong oxidizing agent as the osmium has an oxidation number of +8. It aggressively oxidizes many materials, leaving behind a deposit of non-volatile osmium in a lower oxidation state.
- Ruthenium tetroxide: Ruthenium tetroxide is equally volatile and even more aggressive than osmium tetraoxide and able to stain even materials that resist the osmium stain, e.g. polyethylene. Other chemicals used in electron microscopy staining include: ammonium molybdate, cadmium iodide, carbohydrazide, ferric chloride, hexamine, indium trichloride, lanthanum nitrate, lead acetate, lead citrate, lead(II) nitrate, periodic acid, phosphomolybdic acid, potassium ferricyanide, potassium ferrocyanide, ruthenium red, silver nitrate, silver proteinate, sodium chloroaurate, thallium nitrate, thiosemicarbazide, uranyl acetate, uranyl nitrate, and vanadyl sulfate.

SMEAR PREPARATION

The preparation of a smear is required for many laboratory procedures, including the Gram-stain. The purpose of making a smear is to fix the bacteria onto the slide and to prevent the sample from being lost during a staining procedure. A smear can be prepared from a solid or broth medium. Below are some guidelines for preparing a smear for a Gram-stain.

1. Place one needle of solid bacterial growth or two loops of liquid bacterial growth in the center of a clean slide.

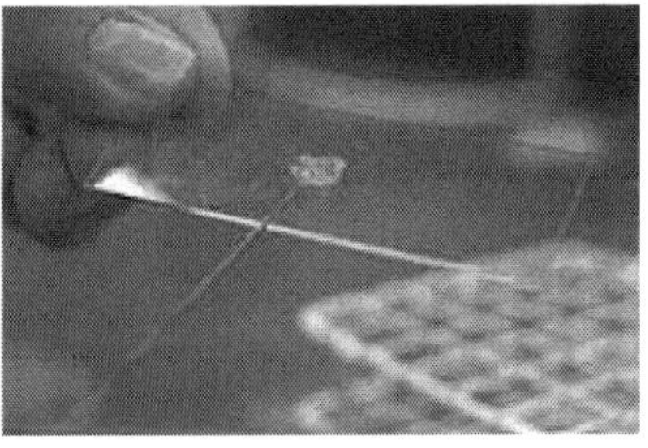

2. If working from a solid medium, add one drop (and only one drop) of water to your specimen with a water bottle. If using a broth medium, do not add the water.

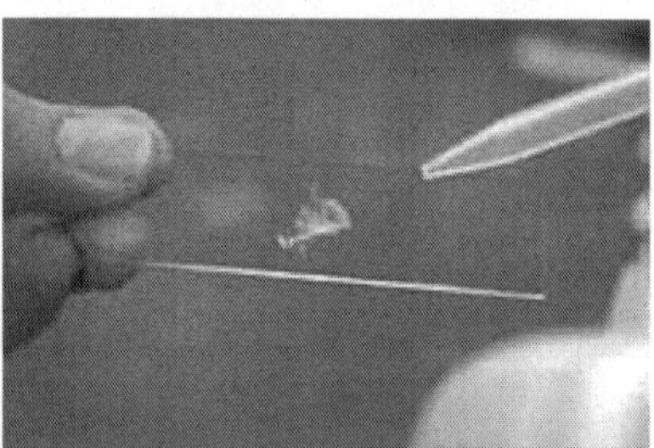

3. Now, with your inoculating loop, mix the specimen with the water completely and spread the mixture out to cover about half of the total slide area.

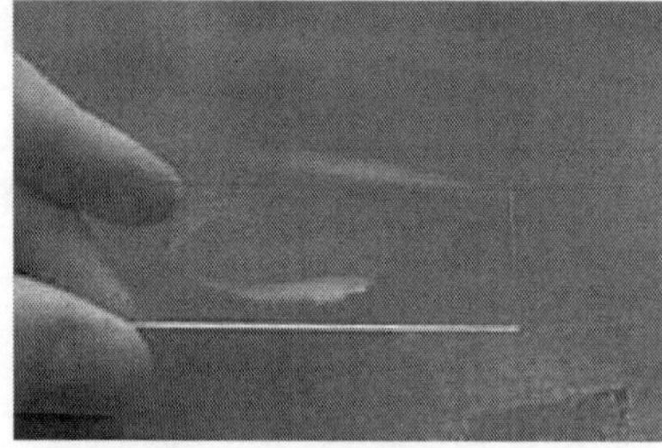

4. Place the slide on a slide warmer and wait for it to dry. The smear is now ready for the staining procedure.

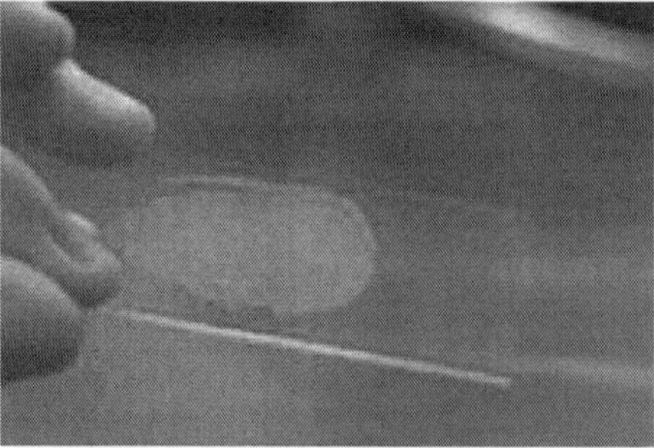

HEMOGLOBIN DETERMINATION

A routine test performed on practically every patient is the hemoglobin determination. Hemoglobin determination, or hemoglobinometry, is the measurement of the concentration of hemoglobin in the blood. Hemoglobin's main function in the body is to carry oxygen from the lungs to the tissues and to assist in transporting carbon dioxide from the tissues to the lungs. The formation of hemoglobin takes place in the developing red cells located in bone marrow.

Hemoglobin values are affected by age, sex, pregnancy, disease, and altitude. During pregnancy, gains in body fluids cause the red cells to become less concentrated, causing the red cell count to fall. Since hemoglobin is contained in red cells, the hemoglobin concentration also falls. Disease may also affect the values of hemoglobin. For example, iron deficiency anemia may drop hemoglobin values from a normal value of 14 grams per 100 milliliters to 7 grams per 100 milliliters. Above-normal hemoglobin values may occur when dehydration develops. Changes in altitude affect the oxygen content of the air and, therefore, also affect hemoglobin values. At higher altitudes there is less oxygen in the air, resulting in an increase in red cell counts and hemoglobin values. At lower altitudes there is more oxygen, resulting in a decrease in red cell counts and hemoglobin values.

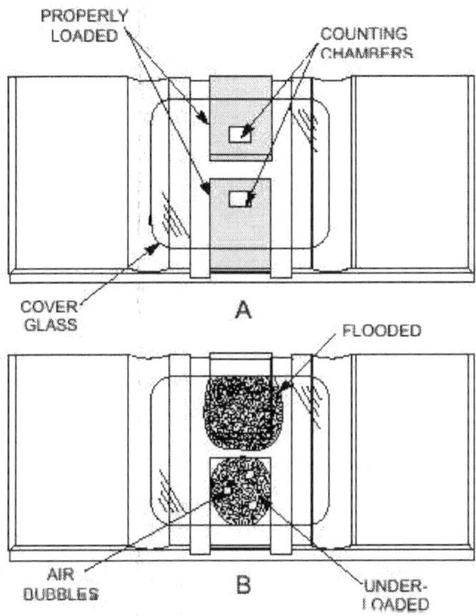

Fig. Loading hemacytometer: A. Hemacytometer properly loaded; B. Hemacytometer improperly loaded.

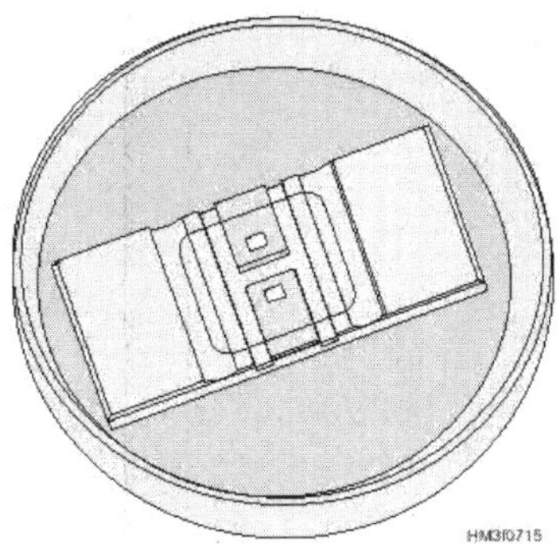

Fig. Loaded hemacytometer placed inside petri dish.

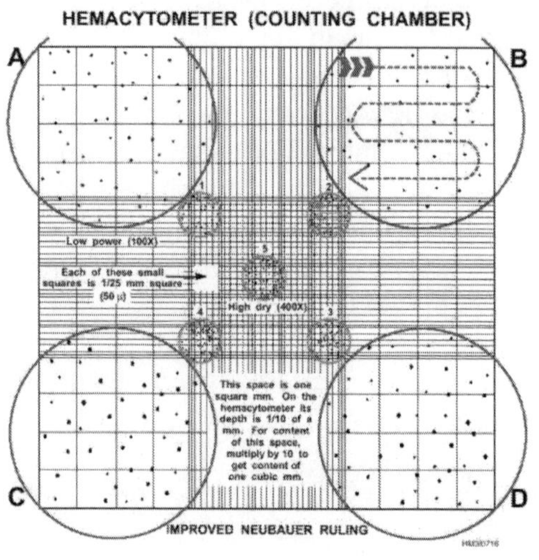

A-B-C-D ARE FIELDS USED IN DOING THE WHITE BLOOD CELL COUNT.

1-2-3-4-5 ARE FIELDS USED IN DOING THE RED BLOOD CELL COUNT.

(Letters, numbers, and arrows are not actually seen in the counting chamber. They are for illustration only. Circles depict areas seen through the microscope.)

Fig.-Hemacytometer counting chamber.

The normal values for hemoglobin determinations are as follows:

	Grams per 100 ml blood	Percent
Woman	12.5 to 15	83 to 110
Men	14 to 17	97 to 124
Newborn infants	17 to 23	97 to 138

Methods for hemoglobin determination are many and varied. The most widely used automated method is the cyanmethemoglobin method. To perform this method, blood is mixed with Drabkin's solution, a solution that contains ferricyanide and cyanide. The ferricyanide oxidizes the iron in the hemoglobin, thereby changing hemoglobin to methemoglobin. Methemoglobin then unites with the cyanide to form cyanmethemoglobin. Cyanmethemoglobin produces a color which is measured in a colorimeter, spectrophotometer, or automated instrument. The color relates to the concentration of hemoglobin in the blood.

Manual methods for determining blood hemoglobin include the Haden-Hausse and Sahli-Hellige methods. In both methods, blood is mixed with dilute hydrochloric acid. This process hemolyzes the red cells, disrupting the integrity of the red cells' membrane and causing the release of hemoglobin, which, in turn, is converted to a brownish-colored solution of acid hematin. The acid hematin solution is then compared with a color standard.

HEMATOCRIT DETERMINATION (PCV)

The hematocrit (Ht or HCT, British English spelling haematocrit), also known as packed cell volume (PCV) or erythrocyte volume fraction (EVF), is the volume percentage (%) of red blood cells in blood. It is normally 45% for men and 40% for women. It is considered an integral part of a person's complete blood count results, along with hemoglobin concentration, white blood cell count, and platelet count. Because the purpose of red blood cells is to transfer oxygen from the lungs to body tissues, a blood sample's hematocrit—the red blood cell volume percentage—can become a point of reference of its capability of delivering oxygen. Additionally, the measure of a subject's blood sample's hematocrit levels may expose possible diseases in the subject. Anemia refers to an abnormally low hematocrit, as opposed to polycythemia, which refers to an abnormally high hematocrit. For a condition such as anemia that goes unnoticed, one way it can be diagnosed is by measuring the hematocrit levels in the blood. Both are potentially life-threatening disorders.

The term *hematocrit* comes from the Ancient Greek words *haima* and *kritçs* . Together, hematocrit means "to separate blood". It was coined by Magnus Blix at Uppsala in 1891 as *haematokrit*, modeled after *lactokrit*, which was used in dairy farming.

MEASUREMENT METHODS

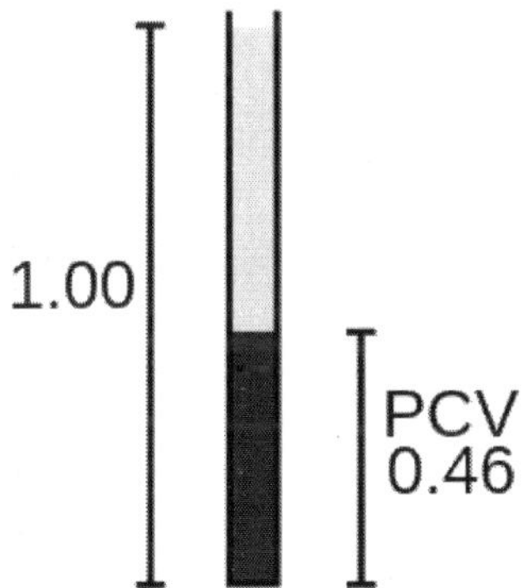

Fig. Packed cell volume diagram

With modern lab equipment, the hematocrit is calculated by an automated analyzer and not directly measured. It is determined by multiplying the red cell count by the mean cell volume. The hematocrit is slightly more accurate as the PCV includes small amounts of blood plasma trapped between the red cells. An estimated hematocrit as a percentage may be derived by tripling the hemoglobin concentration in g/dL and dropping the units.

The packed cell volume (PCV) can be determined by centrifuging heparinized blood in a capillary tube (also known as a microhematocrit tube) at 10,000 RPM for five minutes. This separates the blood into layers. The volume of packed red blood cells divided by the total volume of the blood sample gives the PCV. Since a tube is used, this can be calculated by measuring the lengths of the layers.

Another way of measuring hematocrit levels has been through optical methods such as spectrophotometry has also been developed. Through differential spectrophotometry, the differences in optical densities of a blood sample flowing through small-bore glass tubes at isobestic wavelengths for deoxyhemoglobin and oxyhemoglobin and the product of the luminal diameter and hematocrit create a linear relationship that is used to measure hematocrit levels.

There are some risks and side effects that accompany the tests of hematocrit because blood is being extracted from subjects. Subjects may experience a more than normal amount of hemorrhaging, hematoma, fainting, and possibly infection.

While known hematocrit levels are used in detecting conditions, it may fail at times due to hematocrit being the measure of concentration of red blood cells through volume in a blood sample. It does not account for the mass of the red blood cells, and thus the changes in mass can alter a hematocrit level or go undetected while affecting a subject's condition. Additionally, there have been cases in which the blood for testing was inadvertently drawn proximal to an intravenous line that was infusing packed red cells or fluids. In these situations, the hemoglobin level in the blood sample will not be the true level for the patient because the sample will contain a large amount of the infused material rather than what is diluted into the circulating whole blood. That is, if packed red cells are being supplied, the sample will contain a large amount of those cells and the hematocrit will be artificially very high. On the converse, if saline or other fluids are being supplied, the blood sample would be diluted and the hematocrit will be artificially low.

LEVELS

Hematocrit, the volume percentage of red blood cells, can vary from the determining factors of the number of red blood cells. These factors can be from the age and sex of the subject. Typically, a higher hematocrit level signifies the blood sample's ability to transport oxygen, which has led to reports that an "optimal hematocrit level" possibly exists. Optimal hematocrit levels have been studied through combinations of assays on blood sample's hematocrit itself, viscosity, and hemoglobin level.

Hematocrit levels also serve as an indicator of health conditions. Thus, tests on hematocrit levels are often carried out in the process of diagnosis of such conditions and may be conducted prior to surgery. Additionally, the health conditions associated with certain hematocrit levels are the same as ones associated with certain hemoglobin levels.

As blood flow from the arterioles into the capillaries a change in pressure occurs. In order to maintain pressure, the capillaries branch off to a web of vessels that carry blood into the venules. Through this process blood undergoes micro-circulation. In micro-circulation, the Fahraeus effect will take place, resulting in a large change in hematocrit. As blood flows through the arterioles, red cells will act a feed hematocrit (Hf), while in the capillaries a tube hematocrit (Ht) occurs. In tube hematocrit plasma fills most of the vessel while the red cells travel through in somewhat of a single file line. From this stage, blood will enter a the venules increasing in hematocrit, in other words the discharge hematocrit (Hd).

In large vessels with low hematocrit, viscosity dramatically drops and red cells take in a lot of energy. While in smaller vessels at the micro-circulation scale, viscosity is very high. With the increase in shear stress at the wall, a lot of energy is used to move cells.

SHEAR RATE RELATIONS

Relationships between hematocrit, viscosity, and shear rate are important factors to put into consideration. Since blood is non-Newtonian, the viscosity of the blood is in relation to the hematocrit, and as a function of shear rate. This is important when it comes to determining shear force, since a lower hematocrit level indicates that there is a need for more force to push the red blood cells through the system. This is because shear rate is defined as the rate to which adjacent layers of fluid move in respect to each other. Plasma is a more viscous material than typically red blood cells, since they are able to adjust their size to the radius of a tube; the shear rate is purely dependent on the amount of red blood cells being forced in a vessel.

Elevated

Generally at both sea levels and high altitudes, hematocrit levels rise as children mature. These health-related causes and impacts of elevated hematocrit levels have been reported:

- Fall in plasma levels
- Sleep apnea
- Dehydration
- In cases of dengue fever, a high hematocrit is a danger sign of an increased risk of dengue shock syndrome. Hemoconcentration can be detected by an escalation of over 20% in hematocrit levels that will come before shock. For early detection of dengue hemorrhagic fever, it is suggested for hematocrit levels to be kept under observations at minimum every 24 hours, however for in the case of dengue shock syndrome or critical cases of dengue hemorrhagic fever, every 3–4 hours.

- Polycythemia vera (PV), a myeloproliferative disorder in which the bone marrow produces excessive numbers of red cells, is associated with elevated hematocrit.
- Chronic obstructive pulmonary disease (COPD) and other pulmonary conditions associated with hypoxia may elicit an increased production of red blood cells. This increase is mediated by the increased levels of erythropoietin by the kidneys in response to hypoxia.
- Professional athletes' hematocrit levels are measured as part of tests for blood doping or erythropoietin (EPO) use; the level of hematocrit in a blood sample is compared with the long-term level for that athlete (to allow for individual variations in hematocrit level), and against an absolute permitted maximum (which is based on maximum expected levels within the population, and the hematocrit level that causes increased risk of blood clots resulting in strokes or heart attacks).
- Anabolic androgenic steroid (AAS) use can also increase the amount of RBCs and, therefore, impact the hematocrit, in particular the compounds boldenone and oxymetholone.
- Capillary leak syndrome also leads to abnormally high hematocrit counts, because of the episodic leakage of plasma out of the circulatory system.

Hematocrit levels were also reported to be influenced by social factors that influence subjects. In the 1966-80 Health Examination Survey, there was a small rise in mean hematocrit levels in female and male adolescents that reflected a rise in annual family income. Additionally, a higher education in a parent has been put into account for a rise in mean hematocrit levels of the child.

Lowered

Lowered hematocrit levels also pose health impacts. These causes and impacts have been reported:

- A low hematocrit level is a sign of a low red blood cell count. One way to increase the ability of oxygen transport in red blood cells is through blood transfusion, which is carried out typically when the red blood cell count is low. Prior to the blood transfusion, hematocrit levels are measured to help ensure the transfusion is necessary and safe.
- At higher altitudes, there is a lower oxygen supply in the air and thus hematocrit levels may increase over time.
- A low hematocrit with a low mean corpuscular volume (MCV) with a high RDW suggests a chronic iron-deficient anemia resulting in abnormal hemoglobin synthesis during erythropoiesis. The MCV and the red cell distribution width (RDW) can be quite helpful in evaluating

a lower-than-normal hematocrit, because they can help the clinician determine whether blood loss is chronic or acute, although acute blood loss typically does not manifest as a change in hematocrit, since hematocrit is simply a measure of how much of the blood volume is made up of red blood cells. The MCV is the size of the red cells and the RDW is a relative measure of the variation in size of the red cell population.

- Decreased hematocrit levels could indicate life-threatening diseases such as leukemia. When the bone marrow no longer produces normal red blood cells, hematocrit levels deviate from normal as well and thus can possibly be used in detecting acute myeloid leukemia. It can also be related to other conditions, such as malnutrition, water intoxication, anemia, and bleeding.
- Pregnancy may lead to women having additional fluid in blood. This could potentially lead to a small drop in hematocrit levels.

4

Generlised Techniques in Clinical Pathology

ENDOCRINOLOGY

Endocrinology is a practice of medicine that is highly dependent on accurate laboratory measurements because small changes in hormone levels often may be more specific and more sensitive for early disease than the classic physical signs and symptoms. Because most endocrinologists currently do not have facilities to develop and validate laboratory assays, they rely on commercial analytic assays or send a patient's specimen to specialized laboratories. Even most hospital and commercial laboratories have minimal expertise for developing analytic assays.

This critical dependence on quality laboratory measurements, combined with minimal information about the performance of these tests, places endocrinologists in a potentially vulnerable position.

This chapter provides an overview of the strengths and weaknesses of the analytic techniques typically used for endocrine measurements in blood and urine. Concentrations of most hormones are much lower than those of general chemistry analytes, and specialized techniques are necessary to measure these low concentrations.

Four major types of assays for measuring hormones are described: immunoassays (both competitive and sandwich), chromatography, mass spectrometry, and nucleic acid–based assays for evaluation of genetic alterations.

The analytic performance validation required by the Federal Government for laboratories testing specimens of Medicare patients is outlined, along with explanations of these performance parameters. This information should help endocrinologists better assess the performance of the analytic systems that they are using. Techniques to investigate discordant laboratory test values also are presented to help clinicians work with their laboratories to reconcile test values that do not match clinical presentations.

Hormone concentrations are reported in molar units, mass units, or standardized units, such as World Health Organization (WHO) International Units (IU). When these measurements are expressed in molar units, most hormones in blood and urine are present in concentrations of 10^{-6} to 10^{-12} M/L. The terms used to describe these concentrations are micromolar (10^{-6} M/L), nanomolar (10^{-9} M/L), and picomolar (10^{-12} M/L). The range—from the lowest to the highest concentrations—is more than a million-fold difference. Therefore, laboratory techniques must be targeted to the levels of each given hormone.

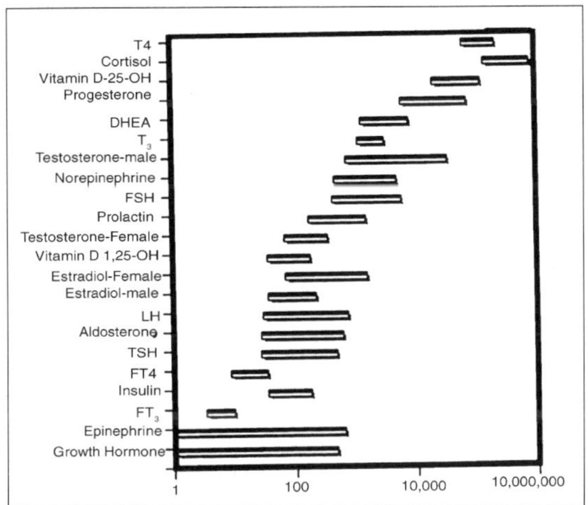

Fig. Six-logarithm range of normal Concentrations for the Plasma Concentrations of EndocrineTests. *DHEA,* Dehydroepiandrosterone. *FSH,* Follicle-Stimulating Hormone. *FT_4,* freeThyroxine. *FT_3,* free Triiodothyronine. *LH,* luteinizing hormone. *T_3,*Triiodothyronine. *T_4,* Thyroxine. *TSH,* Thyrotropin

The major techniques for measuring the lower picomolar concentrations are immunoassay and mass spectrometry, whereas the higher nanomolar and micromolar concentrations can be measured by these methods as well as chromatography and chemical detection systems. Some hormones, such as thyrotropin (TSH), have very low concentrations in the femtomolar (10^{-15} M/L) range in patients with diseases such as thyrotoxicosis. Exquisitely sensitive immunometric assays are usually used to measure these very low concentrations.

TECHNIQUES USED IN ENDOCRINE MEASUREMENTS

The four major techniques used for endocrine measurements are as follows:

1. Antibody-based immunologic assays, of which there are two subcategories: competitive immunoassays andimmunometric(sandwich)assays
3. Chromatographic assays,
3. Mass spectrometry, and
4. Nucleic acid–based assays.

COMPETITIVE IMMUNOASSAYS

The term *competitive radioimmunoassay* refers to a measurement method in which an antigen (*e.g.*, a hormone) in a specimen competes with radiolabeled reagent antigen for a limited number of binding sites on a reagent antibody.

The three basic components of a competitive immunoassay are:

1. Antiserum specific for a unique epitope on a hormone or antigen,
2. labeled antigen that binds to this antiserum,
3. Unlabeled antigen in the specimen or standard that is to be measured.

The antiserum is diluted to a concentration in which the number of binding sites available on the antibodies is fewer than the number of antigen molecules (labeled and unlabeled) in the reaction mixture.

The labeled and unlabeled antigens compete for this limited number of binding sites on the antiserum. The competition is not always equal because the labeled antigen *(tracer)* may react differently with the antibody compared with the native antigen.

This disparity in reactivity may be caused by alteration of the antigen due to the chemical attachment of the label or by differences in the endogenous antigen versus the form of the antigen used in the reagents. As long as the reactions are reproducible, these differences in reactivity are not important because the reaction can be *calibrated* with standard reference materials having known concentrations.

Figure illustrates the concepts of a competitive immunoassay. In the schematic diagram, 8 units of antibody react with 16 units of labeled antigen and 4 units of native antigen. At equilibrium (assuming equal reactivity), 6 units of label and 2 units of native antigen are bound to the limited supply of antibody. The antigen bound to the antibody is separated from the liquid antigen by any of several methods, and the amount of labeled antigen in the bound portion is quantitated. The assay is calibrated by measuring standards with known concentrations and cross-plotting the signal (*i.e.*, counts of the gamma rays emitted from the radioactive label) versus the concentration of the standards to generate a dose-response curve. As the concentration increases, the signal decreases exponentially.

Generally, the antiserum used in a competitive assay is diluted to a titer that binds between 40% and 50% of the labeled antigen when no unlabeled antigen is present. Further dilution of the antiserum increases the analytic sensitivity but decreases both the signal and the range of the assay.

The precision of competitive immunoassays is related to the rate of change of the signal compared with the rate of change of concentration (*i.e.*, the slope of the dose-response curve). In Fig. B, the slope is much lower at higher concentrations, causing the assay precision to be less at higher concentrations. Most competitive immunoassays also have a relatively flat dose-response curve at very low concentrations, causing poor precision at the low end of the assay.

Consequently, the precision profile for most immunoassays is U-shaped, having the best coefficients of variation in the center of the dose-response curve.

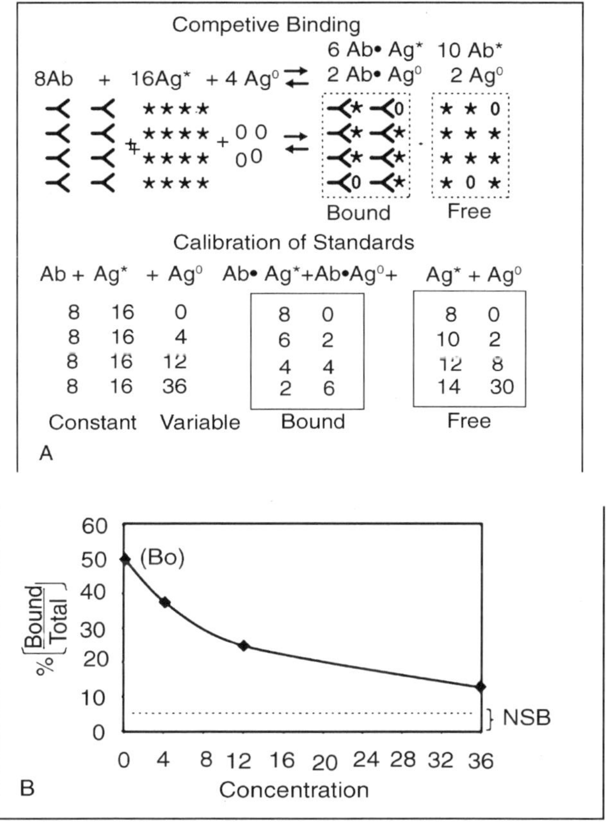

Fig. A, Principles of Competitive Binding assays. B, Typical dose-Response curve

As shown in Fig. the higher the concentration of the unlabeled antigen, the lower the amount of radiolabeled antigen that binds to the limited amount of antiserum. The signal decreases exponentially from the approximately half-maximum at zero concentration to a minimum value at high concentrations. This minimal binding, or *nonspecific binding* (NSB), is a valuable control parameter. Elevations in NSB usually signify impurities in the label that bind to the sides of the tubes and are not competitively displaced. Most assays add surfactants and proteins to minimize the NSB. Monitoring of changes in the NSB provides an early warning of potential assay problems.

Statistical data processing techniques are needed to translate the assay signals into concentrations. As illustrated, these dose-response curves generally are not linear, and numerous curve-fitting algorithms have been developed. Before the introduction of microprocessors, tedious error-prone, manual calculations were required to mathematically transform the data into linear models. A commonly used model was to cross-plot the logit of the normalized signal versus the logarithm of the concentration and to use linear regression lines to establish the dose-response curve.[5] Fortunately, today this procedure of curve fitting usually is accomplished electronically by using programmes that automatically test the robustness of fit of multiparameter curves after statistically eliminating discordant data points.[6] However, users of these systems must understand the limitations and should pay attention to any warnings presented by the programmes during processing of the data.

In radioimmunoassays, radioactive iodine (^{125}I) is usually used to label the antigen. The immune complexes are separated from the unbound molecules by precipitation with centrifugation after reaction with secondary antisera and precipitating reagents (*e.g.*, polyethylene glycol). These radioimmunoassays are labour intensive and may require special handling and licensure to ensure safety of the radioisotopes.

The statistical counting errors associated with the relatively low radioactive counts and the poor reproducibility associated with the multiple manual steps generally necessitate that most laboratories perform the measurements in duplicate. Even when the averages of duplicate measurements are used, many manual radioimmunoassays have coefficients of variation between 10% and 15%.

It is important that key quality control parameters for radioimmunoassays be carefully monitored. In addition to NSB, another key quality control parameter is the percentage binding of the radiolabel when zero antigen (Bo) is present. As the label deteriorates, because of aging, the binding often decreases, resulting in a less reliable assay.

Another important quality control parameter is the slope of the dose-response curve. This parameter can be tracked by monitoring the concentration corresponding to half-maximum binding (50% of B/Bo). If this concentration increases significantly, the slope of the response curve decreases and the assay may not be capable of reliably measuring patient specimens at clinically important concentrations.

Many commercial kits and automated immunoassays use nonisotopic signal systems to measure hormone concentrations. These assays often use colourimetric, fluorometric, or chemiluminescent signals rather than radioactivity to quantitate the response. The advantages of these alternate signals are biosafety, longer reagent shelf-life, and ease of automation. On the other hand, these signals are more subject to matrix interferences than radioactive iodine.

Radioactivity is not affected by changes in protein concentration, hemolysis, colour, or drugs (except for other radioactive compounds), whereas many of the current signal systems may yield spurious results when such interferences are present. In addition, many automated immunoassays are read kinetically before the reactions reach equilibrium. This step accentuates the effects of matrix differences between the reference standards and patient specimens.

Later in this chapter potential troubleshooting steps are outlined to help clinicians evaluate the integrity of test measurements when spurious results are suspected.

Solid-phase reactions often are used in current immunoassays to facilitate the separation of the bound antibody-antigen complexes from the free reactants.

Three frequently used solid-phase materials are:

1. Microtiter plates,
2. Polystyrene beads, and
3. Paramagnetic particles.

Typically, the antibody is attached to the solid phase, and the separation of the immune complexes from the unbound moieties is accomplished by plate washers, bead washers, or magnetic wash stations, eliminating the need for centrifugation. Another novel way of accomplishing this separation is to attach high-affinity linkers to antiserum, which then can be coupled to a complementary linker on the solid phase.

An excellent pair of linkers are biotin and streptavidin. These compounds bind with affinity constants of approximately 10^{15} L/M.

Biotin is a relatively small molecule that can be easily covalently attached to antiserum and used with streptavidin (a 70-kd tetrameric nonglycosylated protein) conjugated to microtiter plates, beads, or paramagnetic particles to facilitate separation. This technique allows the antibody-antigen reaction to proceed faster with less stearic hindrance than when the antibody is directly coupled to the solid phase.

The antiserum used in these assays is a crucial component. Most earlier immunoassays used *polyclonal* antiserum produced in animals. The process of generating these antisera is a combination of art, science, and luck. Generally, a relatively pure form of the antigen is conjugated to a carrier protein (especially if the antigen is less than 10,000 d), mixed with adjuvant (*e.g.*, Freud's complete adjuvant), and injected intradermally into the host animal. After several boosts with conjugated protein plus Freud's incomplete adjuvant, the host animal recognizes the material as foreign and develops immune responses. The antiserum then is harvested from the animal's blood. Under optimal conditions, moderate quantities of high-affinity antisera, which react only with the specific target antigen, are developed.

The analytic sensitivity of a competitive immunoassay is approximately inversely related to the affinity of the antiserum, such that an antiserum with an affinity constant of 10^9 L/M can be used to measure analytes in the nanomolar concentration range.

The polyclonal antiserum developed by immunizing animals represents a composite of many immunologic clones, with each clone having a different affinity and different immunologic specificity. Most clones have affinities in the 10^7 to 10^8 L/M range, with only rare clones having affinities above 10^{12} L/M.

Various techniques are used to develop a specific antiserum, including:

- Altering the form of the antigen by blocking cross-reacting epitopes and
- Purifying the antiserum using affinity chromatography to select antibodies directed towards the epitope of interest. Affinity-column purification also can be used for immunoextraction of higher affinity antisera by selectively eluting antiserum from the column by means of a series of buffers with increasing acidity.

The major disadvantage of a polyclonal antiserum is the limited quantity. The large quantities needed by commercial suppliers of immunoassay reagents often require them to use multiple sources of antisera. These changes in antisera can cause significant changes in assay performance. In many instances, laboratories and clinicians are not informed about these changes, which may cause problems in medical decisions.

Monoclonal antisera are used in many current immunoassays. These antisera are made by immunizing animals (usually mice) using techniques similar to those used for polyclonal antisera. instead of harvesting the antisera from the blood, however, the animal is killed and the spleen is removed. The lymphocytes in the spleen are fused with myeloma cells to make cells that will grow in culture and produce antisera.

These fused cells are separated into clones by means of serial plating techniques similar to those used in subculturing bacteria. The supernatant of these monoclonal cell lines (or ascites fluid if the cells are transplanted into carrier mice) contains monoclonal antisera. The selection processes used to separate the initial clones can be targeted to identify specific clones producing antisera with high affinities and low cross-reactivity to related compounds.

The high specificity of monoclonal antisera can cause problems for some endocrine assays. Many hormones circulate in the blood as heterogeneous mixtures of multiple forms. Some of these forms are caused by genetic differences in patients, whereas other forms are related to metabolic precursors and degradation products of the hormone. Genetic differences cause some patients to produce variant forms of a hormone such as luteinizing hormone (LH). These genetic differences can cause marked variations in measurements made using assays with specific monoclonal antisera compared with more uniform measurements made using assays with polyclonal antisera that cross-react with the multiple forms. Well-characterized monoclonal antisera can be mixed together to make an "engineered polyclonal antiserum" with improved sensitivity and specificity.

Cross-reactivity with precursor forms of the analytes and with metabolic degradation products can cause major differences in assays. For example, cross-reactivity with six molecular forms of human chorionic gonadotropin (hCG) causes differences in hCG assays, and cross-reactivity with metabolic fragments causes differences in parathyroid hormone (PTH) assays. Cortisol is another analyte wherein major cross-reactivity with other steroids such as corticosterone, 11-deoxycortisol, cortisone, and numerous synthetic steroids causes significant immunoassay interferences. Extraction of hormones from serum and urine specimens before measurement is a technique that can enhance both sensitivity and specificity of immunoassays.

Numerous extraction systems have been developed, including:

- Organic-aqueous partitioning to remove water-soluble interferences seen with steroids,
- Solid-phase extraction with absorption and selective elution from resins such as silica gels, and
- Immunoaffinity chromatography. Unfortunately, extraction and purification before immunoassay are seldom used in clinical assays.

These techniques are difficult to automate and require skills and equipment not available in many clinical laboratories. Although commercial assays generally use reagents having adequate sensitivity and specificity to measure *most* patient specimens, some patient specimens may give spurious results and some disease states may require more analytic sensitivity to ensure sound clinical decisions. In these cases, extraction of specimens before measurement may provide more reliable information. Immunoassays measure concentrations rather than biologic activity. For most hormones, there is a strong correlation between the concentration of the protein or steroid being measured and the biologic activity, but this is not universally true. The reactive site for most antibodies is relatively small, about 5 to 10 amino acids for linear peptides. Some antiserum reactions are specific for the tertiary structure that corresponds to unique molecular configurations, but immunoassays seldom react with the exact antigenic structure that confers biologic activity.

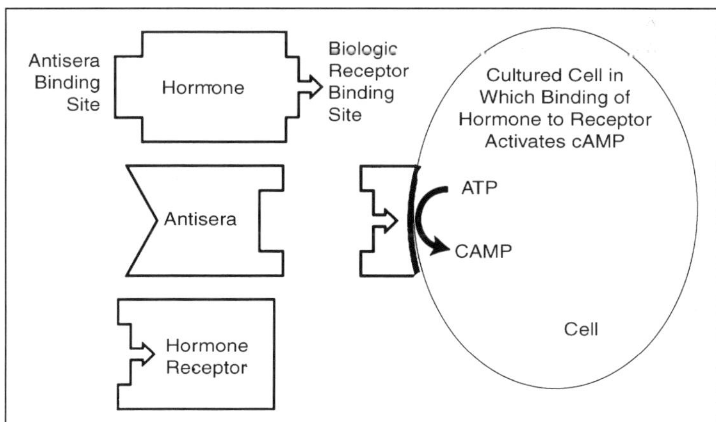

Fig. Comparison of an Immunologic Technique for MeasuringHormone Concentration Versus a ReceptorTechnique for Measuring Hormone Activity. *ATP,* Adenosine Triphosphate. *cAMP,* Cyclic Adenosine Monophosphate

Figure presents a schematic illustration of the difference between immunologic binding site and biologic receptor binding site on a hormone. Indirect immunoassays have been developed using cultured cells that synthesize second messengers such as cyclic adenosine monophosphate (cAMP) at rates proportional to the concentration of hormone in the specimen. An example of this technique is the immunoassay measurement of cAMP produced by osteosarcoma cells to quantitate PTH bioactivity in serum. Unfortunately, these assays are tedious and generally are not reproducible. Techniques using recombinant receptors as immunoassay binders may provide improved specificity with good reliability.

IMMUNOMETRIC (SANDWICH) ASSAYS

A second immunologic technique used to measure hormones is the immunometric (sandwich) assay.

The three basic components of a sandwich assay are:

1. An antigen large enough to allow two antibodies to bind concurrently on different binding sites,
2. A *capture* antiserum directed to one of the antigenic sites on the antigen—this antiserum is attached to a solid phase to permit immunologic extraction of the immune complexes, and
3. A *signal* antiserum directed to a second antigenic site on the antigen—this antiserum is attached to an assay signal system.

In contrast to competitive immunoassays, these assays use a large excess of antiserum-binding sites compared with the concentration of antigen. The capture antibody immunoextracts the antigen from the sample and the signal antibody binds to the capture-antibody-antigen complex to form a tertiary complex. As the antigen concentration increases, the signal increases progressively. Figure schematically illustrates these concepts. The capture antiserum (ATB1) is attached to biotin. The signal antiserum (ATB2) is labeled with a detection system.

The ATB1-antigen-ATB2 complexes are immunologically extracted using a streptavidin solid phase. After the complex is bound to the solid phase, most of the unbound signal antibody is washed away. As shown in Fig. the signal increases progressively with the concentration. For lower concentrations, the signal generally increases proportionally to the assay concentrations (after the offset caused by the NSB). At higher concentrations, the signal generally is less than proportional, so that nonlinear curve-fitting techniques are used to generate the dose-response curves. Again, the relative imprecision, expressed as a coefficient of variation, depends on the slope of the dose-response curve. consequently, the relative precision is less at higher concentrations.

In immunometric assays, the background level of signal is associated with very low concentrations. This background signal is caused by the NSB. The analytic sensitivity of immunometric assays is related to the ratio of the true signal to the NSB signal. Therefore, assays can be made more sensitive either by increasing the response signal or by decreasing NSB. Inadvertent increases in NSB caused by specimen interference or reagent deterioration can significantly alter the assay performance.

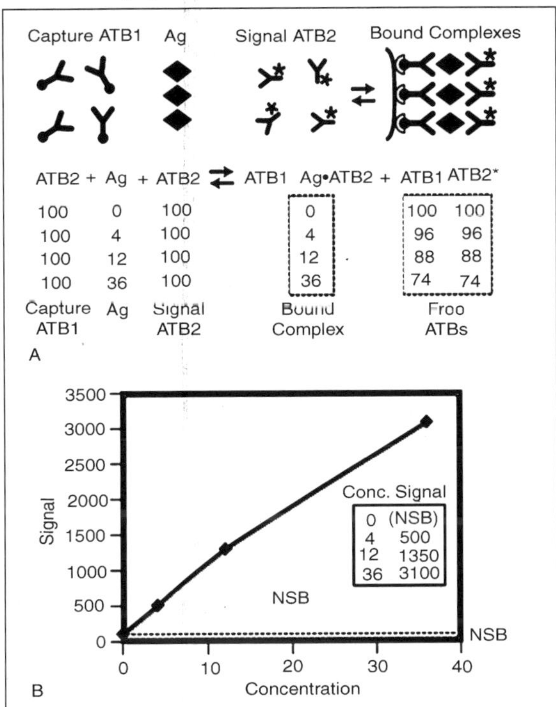

Fig. A, Principles of Immunometric Assays. *Ag,* Antigen. *ATB1,* Capture Antiserum. *ATB2,* Signal Antiserum. B, Typical Dose-response curve. *NSB,* Nonspecific binding

In immunometric assays, it is also important that a large excess of capture antibody be used. When the antigen concentration approaches the effective binding capacity of the capture antibody system, the signal no longer increases. If the antigen concentration exceeds the binding capacity of the capture antibody, the signal may actually decrease.

Figure illustrates this *high-dose hook effect* for immunometric assays caused by insufficient amounts of capture or signal antiserum. The signal increases progressively until the hormone concentration exceeds the binding capacity. the signal then decreases, apparently as a result of the removal of some of the weaker binding antigen-antibody complexes during the wash cycle on the assay. This is a potentially dangerous phenomenon because very high concentrations can give the same "answer" as lower concentrations. If this artifact is suspected, the specimen can be diluted and reanalysed. If the answer for the diluted specimen is higher than the original answer, a high-dose hook effect probably is present.

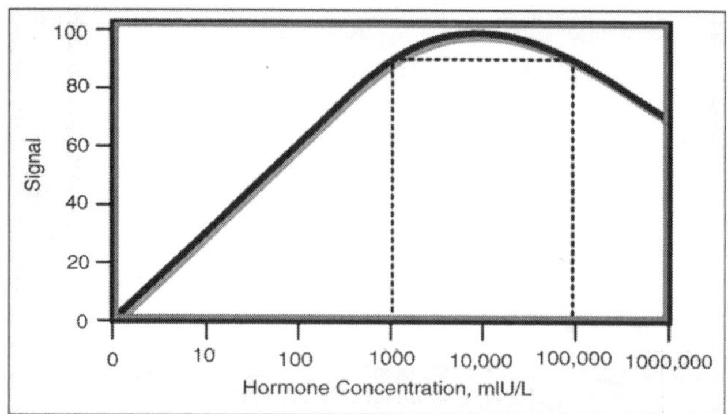

Fig. Immunometric "High-Dose Hook Effect." The Response Signal Reaches a Maximum and then Decreases when the Antigen Concentration Exceeds the limit of the assay

Most manufacturers are aware of this potential problem and configure assays with relatively large amounts of capture antibody. however, some patients produce high concentrations of hormones or antigens that may exceed assay limits. Laboratories are able to detect this phenomenon by analysing specimens at two dilutions, but this practice generally is not cost-effective. Therefore, feedback to the laboratory about results that are inconsistent with clinical findings is essential.

Another potential problem for immunometric assays consists of endogenous heterophile antibodies that cross-react with reagent antiserum. Normally, the signal antibody does not form a "sandwich" with the capture antibody unless the specific antigen is present. however, divalent heterophile antibodies may mimic the antigen by simultaneously binding to the signal and capture reagent antibodies, thereby causing "falsely" elevated results.

Figure schematically illustrates this situation. The problem is most common with monoclonal antibodies but may also occur with polyclonal antibodies. Immunoglobulins contain both a *constant* (Fc) region and a *variable* (Fab) region. As implied in the name, the Fc region is constant, or similar, for all immunoglobulins from that species. Therefore, if a patient receives immunotherapy or imaging reagents containing mouse immunoglobulin, he or she is likely to develop human antimouse antibodies (HAMAs) directed to the Fc fragment. Some patients may develop heterophile antibodies after exposure to foreign proteins from domestic pets or food contaminants. When these endogenous antibodies are present in a patient's specimen, they may bridge across the reagent antibodies used in immunometric assays and may cause falsely high values. These antibodies also may bind to sites on the reagent antibodies, which sterically block the binding of the specific antigen and give falsely low test values. Most manufacturers include nonimmune immunoglobulin in the assays to help block these interferences. as with the high-dose hook effect, however, the amounts added are not always adequate and some patients with high titer antibodies thus may still show in vitro assay interference.

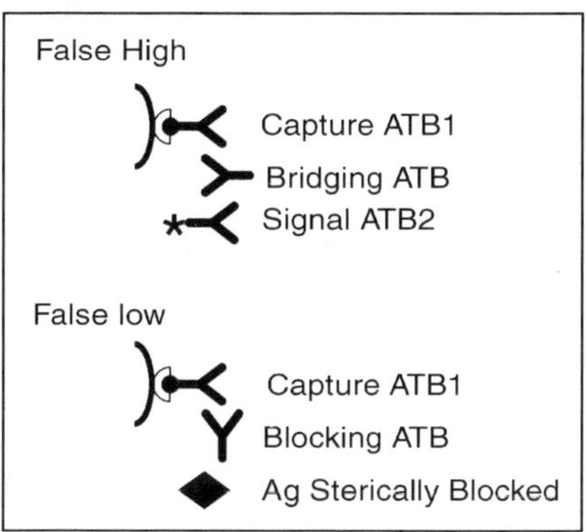

Fig. Assay Interferences Caused by Heterophile Antibodies, which Result in Either False High or False low Results. *Ag,* Antigen. *ATB1,* Capture Antiserum. *ATB2,* Signal Antiserum

The combined specificity of the two antibodies used in an immunometric assay can produce exquisitely sensitive and specific immunoassays. In the past, a common problem with early competitive immunoassays was cross-reactivity among the structurally similar gonadotropins: LH, follicle-stimulating hormone (FSH), TSH, and hCG.

The á subunits of each of these hormones are almost identical, and the â subunits have considerable structural homology. Many individual antisera (especially polyclonal antisera) used for measuring one of these hormones may have cross-reactivity for the other gonadotropins. The cross-reactivity of a pair of antibodies is less than the cross-reactivity of each of the individual antibodies because any cross-reacting substance must contain both of the binding epitopes in order to simultaneously bind to both antibodies.

For example, consider two antibodies for LH, each having 1% cross-reactivity with hCG. The cross-reactivity of the pair is less than the product of the two cross-reactivities or, in this case, less than 0.01%. Most current immunoassays for LH have a cross-reactivity of less than 0.01%. This low cross reactivity is important because pregnant patients and patients with choriocarcinoma may have very high hCG concentrations that could interfere with measurements of the other gonadotropin hormones.

Multiple forms of most hormones circulate in the blood. Some hormones (*e.g.*, prolactin, growth hormone) circulate with macro forms, which can cause difficulty in their analysis if specimens are not pretreated. For hormones composed of subunits (*e.g.*, the gonadotropins), both the intact and the free subunits circulate in blood. Immunometric assays can be made specific for intact molecules by pairing an antibody specific for the á-â bridge site of the subunits with a second antibody specific for the â subunit. Assays using these antibody pairs retain the two-antibody, low cross-reactivity needed for measuring gonadotropins and do not react with the free subunit forms of the hormones.

The heterogeneous forms of circulating hormones and differences in specificity characteristics of immunoassays for these forms make calibration and harmonization difficult. Two immunoassays calibrated with the same reference preparation can give widely varying measurements on patient specimens. Consider the example of hCG in Table. The three assays are calibrated with a pure preparation of intact hCG, such as the WHO Third International Reference Preparation. The three assays differ in their cross-reactivity with free β-hCG (0, 100%, and 200%, respectively). These assays give identical measurements for a specimen containing only intact hCG but progressively disparate values as the percentage of free β-hCG in the specimen increases. In reality, the standardization issue is much more complex because multiple forms of hormones (*i.e.*, intact, free subunits, nicked forms, glycosylated forms, degradation products) circulate in patients and each assay has different cross-reactivities for these forms.

Table. Effect of Immunoassay Specificity on Calibration of Human Chorionic Gonadotropin (Hcg) Assay

	Assay 1	Assay 2	Assay 3
Specificity for intact hCG standard	100%	100%	100%
Cross-reactivity with free β-hCG	0%	100%	200%
Value of specimen with no free β-hCG, IU/L	10.0	10.0	10.0
Value of specimen with 10% free β-hCG, IU/L	9.0	10.0	11.0
Value specimen with 50% free β-hCG, IU/L	5.0	10.0	15.0

FREE (UNBOUND) HORMONE ASSAYS

Many hormones are tightly bound to specific plasma-binding proteins and loosely bound to albumin. The unbound (free) forms as well as some of the loosely bound forms are biologically active.

Multiple methods are available to measure these free, unbound forms of a hormone. Theoretically, the best procedure is direct measurement of the free hormone concentration after physical separation of free-form bound hormone by equilibrium dialysis, ultrafiltration, or gel filtration. Unfortunately, this method is difficult to perform, is thus not readily available, and is subject to technical errors. The two major clinical applications for free hormone measurements are for thyroid hormones (thyroxine [FT_4] and triiodothyronine [FT_3]) and steroids (testosterone and estradiol). Four techniques are commonly used to estimate free thyroid hormone concentrations: indirect index methods, two-step labeled hormone methods, one-step labeled hormone analogue methods, and labeled antibody methods.

Indirect Index Methods

The *indirect indices* involve two measurements: one for total hormone concentration and another for the thyroxine-binding globulin (TBG), followed by calculation of the ratio or a normalized index (FT4I or FT3I). The availability of test results for both the total T_4 and the T_4 binding capacity has the advantage of assessing these two different quantities, but has the disadvantage that ratios and indices are subject to the combined error of both measurements. These methods correct for routine changes in TBG associated with estrogen levels, but they may produce inappropriately abnormal values in patients with extreme variations in TBG levels found in patients with congenital disorders of the TBG gene, familial dysalbuminemic hyperthyroxinemia, thyroid hormone autoantibodies, and nonthyroidal illnesses. Because of the necessity for two measurements and the sensitivity of these methods to interference with drugs, these indirect methods are being used less frequently.

TWO-STEP LABELED HORMONE METHODS

These methods immunologically bind the free and loosely bound thyroid hormone to a solid phase. The other serum components are washed away, and the residual binding sites are back-titrated with labeled hormone. When calibrated with appropriate serum standards, these methods are thought to pose fewer problems with binding protein abnormalities.

One-Step Labeled Hormone Analogue Methods

These methods use synthetic analogues of T_4 and T_3 that bind to the measurement antibody but do not bind to normal TBG. These methods are seldom used because performance has been poor in patients with abnormal albumin concentrations, abnormal free fatty acid concentrations, and all conditions that interfere with the indirect indices.

LABELED ANTIBODY METHODS

These methods use kinetic reactions of antibodies with selected affinities that bind preferentially with the free form of the hormone. These methods work best for automated testing instruments and have become popular.

Complexities in Testing

Each of these methods works well for correcting for minor changes in TBG levels, but each has problems with some patient sera, especially those containing interfering substances such as inhibitors and heterophilic antibodies. Unfortunately, most manufacturers have not fully validated their methods in patients with these abnormalities.

Multiple methods are also available for measuring both the free and the biologically active forms of steroid hormones. The preferred method for measurement of free hormones consists of direct physical separation and high-sensitivity assays similar to those recommended for the thyroid hormones. One-step labeled hormone-analogue methods also have been developed, but these are associated with interference problems similar to the problems with free thyroid hormone assays. The measurement of free testosterone has been problematic. Most immunoassays are unreliable at low concentrations and the concentration of free testosterone is much lower than total testosterone.

Another complexity in regard to steroid hormones is that in addition to the free hormones, testosterone and estrogen bound to albumin also are biologically active. The concentration of the biologically active forms can be estimated using indirect indices calculated from measurements of the total hormones and sex hormone–binding globulin (SHBG) or by measurement of the residual free and albumin-bound steroids after separation of the SHBG-bound forms after differential precipitation with ammonium sulfate. Recent work with tandem mass spectrometry shows promise as a more reliable test method.

CHROMATOGRAPHIC ASSAYS

Another major method of measuring hormone concentrations involves chromatographically separating the various biochemical forms and quantitating specific characteristics of the molecules. High-performance liquid chromatography (HPLC) systems utilize multiple forms of detection, including light absorption, fluorescence, electrochemical properties, and mass spectrometry.

There are two major advantages of these techniques:

1. They can be used to simultaneously measure multiple forms of an analyte.
2. They are not dependent on unique immunologic reagents. Therefore, harmonization of measurements made with different assays is more feasible. The major disadvantages of these methods are their complexity and their limited availability.

Many chemical separation techniques are based on chromatography, but the two most commonly used for liquid chromatography are:

1. *Normal-phase* HPLC and
2. *Reverse-phase* HPLC. In both systems, a bonded solid-phase column is made that interacts with the analytes as they flow past in a liquid solvent.

In normal-phase HPLC, the functional groups of the stationary phase are polar (*e.g.*, amino or nitrile ions) relative to the nonpolar stationary phase (*e.g.*, hexane). in reverse-phase HPLC, a nonpolar stationary phase (*e.g.*, C-18 octadecylsilane molecules bonded to silica) is used.

More recently, polymeric packings made of mixed copolymers have been made with C4, C8, and C18 functional groups directly incorporated so that they are more stable over a wide pH range. The mobile and stationary phases are selected to optimize adherence of the analytes to the stationary phase. The adhered molecules can be eluted differentially from the solid phase after washing to separate specific forms of the analyte from interfering substances as follows: When the composition of the mobile phase remains constant throughout the run, the process is called an *isocratic elution*. If the mobile-phase composition is abruptly changed, a *step elution* occurs. If the composition is gradually changed throughout the run, a *gradient elution* occurs.

The efficiency of separation in a chromatography system is a function of the flow rates of the different substances.[40] *The resolution of the system is a measure of the separation of the two solute bands in terms of their relative retention volumes (V_r) and their bandwidths (ù). Resolution (R_s) of solutes A and B is shown as:*

$$R_s = \frac{2[V_r(B) - V_r(A)]}{\omega(A) + \omega(B)}$$

Values of R_s less than 0.8 result in inadequate separation, and values greater than 1.25 correspond to baseline separation. The resolution of a chromatography column is a function of flow rates and thermodynamic factors.

The simultaneous measurement of the three catecholamines (epinephrine, norepinephrine, and dopamine) can be performed with reverse-phase HPLC with a C-18 column and electrochemical detection system or fluorometric detection. Prior extraction by absorption on activated alumina and acid elution helps improve specificity. Dihydroxybenzylamine, a molecule similar to endogenous catecholamines, can be used as an internal standard.

Mass Spectrometry

The technique of mass spectrometry involves fragmentation of target molecules, followed by separation and measurement of the mass to charge ratio of the components. When coupled with liquid chromatography, a mass spectrometer can function as a unique detector to provide structural information about the composition of individual solutes. Inclusion of internal standards in the specimens, which are molecularly similar to the measured compounds, allows precise quantitation of the concentration of the eluting analytes. The measurement of specific mass fragments makes possible the quantitation of multiple specific analytes in complex mixtures.

The basic components of a quadrupole mass spectrometer are an ionizer, an ion analyser, and a detector (Fig.). The initial step in mass spectrometry is the fragmentation of the target compound into charged ions. Multiple techniques are used to generate these charged ions, including *chemical ionization* and *electron-impact ionization.*

Chemical ionization uses reagent gas molecules, such as methane, ammonia, water, and isobutane, to transfer protons. This process produces less fragmentation than other techniques because the process is not highly excited.

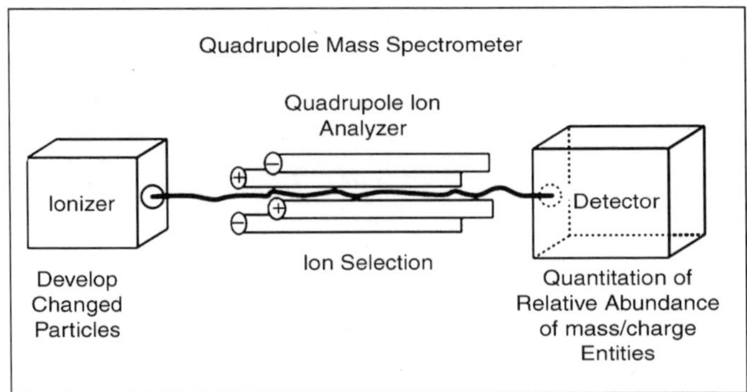

Fig. Basic Components of Quadrupole Mass Spectrometer

The electron impact bombards gas molecules from the sample, with electrons emitted from a heated filament. The process occurs in a vacuum to prevent the filament from burning out. *Electron-spray ionization* is a process in which a solution containing the analyte is introduced into a gas phase and is sprayed across an ionizing potential. The charged droplets are desolvinated and analysed in a mass spectrometer.

The ion analyser uses four charged rods to systematically set up a charged field that selects only certain ions with particular mass-to-charge ratios and facilitates their movement along a path to the detector. Regular calibration is necessary to ensure accuracy of the instrument.

A *mass spectrum* is a bar graph in which the heights of the bars correspond to the relative abundance of a particular ion plotted as a function of the mass-to-charge ratio. Modern mass spectrometers can measure molecular masses so accurately and precisely that the elemental composition of a compound can be predicted by comparison with stored spectral libraries. When these systems are used to measure only a few select compounds having known spectrums, the mass spectrometer can be programmed to focus only on these selected ions. Stable isotopes of the compounds of interest can be used as internal standards through a technique called *isotope dilution mass spectrometry.* Stable isotopes generally perform the same as the native compounds in terms of extraction, chromatography, and mass spectrometry and are thus ideal internal standards. However, they must have a sufficient number of isotopic atoms to ensure that their mass is different from naturally occurring substances that may be in the specimen.

Tandem mass spectrometry (MS/MS) is a powerful new tool consisting of two mass analysers separated by an ion-activation device. The first analyser is used to isolate and dissociate the ion of interest by activation, and the second mass analyser is used to analyse its dissociation products. This technique can be used to provide rapid, definitive measurements of multiple endocrine analytes. For example, liquid chromatography and tandem mass spectrometry can be used to simultaneously quantitate multiple steroid compounds. In Fig.

the chromatograph shows peaks for nine steroids in a standard solution. The nine steroids investigated in positive-ion mode and their respective deuterated internal standards were separated well in 18 minutes. These chromatograms were run on a SCIEX (Applied Biosystems/MDS SCIEX, Foster City, CA/Concord, Ontario, Canada) API-3000 triple quadrupole tandem MS equipped with an APPI (Applied Biosystems/MDS SCIEX) source.

The column eluate was fed directly into an electro-spray ionization device in a triple-quadrupole mass spectrometer (API 3000, Perkin-Elmer SCIEX, Foster City, CA). The stable isotopes were from Cambridge Isotope Laboratories (Andover, MA). A 10-minute analysis provided quantitation of the 10 compounds: cortisone, cortisol, 21-deoxycortisol, corticosterone, 11-deoxycortisol, andro-stenedione, deoxycorticosterone (DOC), 17-hydroxyprogesterone, progesterone, and pregnenolone. The sensitivity for cortisol using d_4 cortisol calibration was 0.1cg/dL.

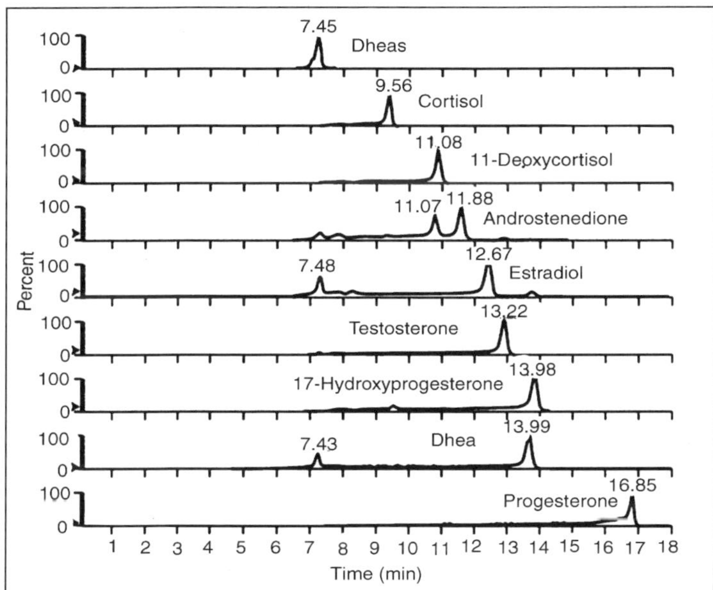

Fig. Liquid Chromatography-Tandem Mass Spectroscopy Profiles of nine Steroids. *DHEAS,* Dehydroepiandrosterone 3-sulfate.*DHEA,* Dehydroe-piandrosterone. (Reproduced with Permission from Archives of Pathology of Laboratory Medicine)

NUCLEIC ACID–BASED ASSAYS

The decoding of the human genome has set the stage for an enormous increase in nucleic acid–based gene assays. The basic principles of nucleic acid–based assays have been known for several decades, but the identification of specific genes and the mapping of gene defects to clinical disease states have now made these measurements clinically useful.

Four concepts important for nucleic acid measurements are:

1. Hybridization,
2. Amplification,
3. Restriction fragment length polymorphisms (RFLPs), and
4. Electrophoretic separation.

Hybridization

Nucleic acid molecules have a unique ability to fuse with complementary base-pair sequences. When a fragment of a known sequence (probe) is mixed under specific conditions with a specimen containing a complementary sequence, hybridization occurs. This feature is analogous to the antibody-antigen binding used in immunoassays. Many of the formats used for immunoassay have been adopted to nucleic acid assays, including some of the same signal systems (*e.g.*, radioactivity, fluorescence, chemiluminescence) and the same solid-phase capture systems (*e.g.*, magnetic beads, biotin-streptavidin binding). In situ hybridization, which involves the binding of probes to intact tissue and cells, provides information about morphologic localization analogous to immunohisto-chemistry.

AMPLIFICATION

Nucleic acid assays have an advantage that low concentrations can be amplified in vitro before quantitation. The best known amplification procedure is the polymerase chain reaction (PCR), first reported by Mullis and Faloona. The three steps in the process (denaturation, annealing, and elongation) occur rapidly at different temperatures. Each "cycle" of amplification can occur in less than 90 seconds by cycling the temperature. The target double-stranded DNA is denatured at high temperature to make two single-stranded DNA fragments. Oligonucleotide primers, which are specific for target region, are annealed to the DNA when the temperature is lowered. Addition of DNA polymerase allows the primer DNA to extend across the amplification region, thus doubling the number of DNA copies.

At 85% to 90% efficiency, this process can amplify the DNA by about 250,000-fold in 20 cycles. This huge amplification is subject to major problems with contamination if special precautions are not taken. In one control technique, a psoralen derivative is used to prevent subsequent copying by polymerase during exposure to ultraviolet light.

RESTRICTION FRAGMENT LENGTH POLYMORPHISMS

Some diseases (*e.g.*, sickle cell anemia) are associated with a specific gene mutation. generally, however, a series of deletions and additions of DNA are involved with the disease. A number of restriction enzymes that cleave DNA at specific locations have been identified. Changes in the sequence of DNA result in different fragment lengths. This technique, or RFLP, is particularly helpful in family studies for disorders that have a unique *genetic fingerprint.*

ELECTROPHORETIC SEPARATION

E. M. Southern invented an electrophoretic separation technique known as *Southern blotting.* Restriction enzymes are used to digest a sample of DNA into fragments, and the product is subjected to electrophoresis. The separated bands of DNA are then transferred to a solid support and hybridized. *Northern blotting* is a similar technique, in which RNA is used as the starting material. *Western blotting* refers to electrophoresis and transfer of proteins.

ANALYTIC VALIDATION

Clinicians generally assume that laboratory methods have been validated and that they function correctly. Although this assumption is generally true, it is helpful to understand the level of assay validation performed and the appropriateness of the validation criteria for each clinical application of a test.

In the United States, the Federal Government regulates all laboratories performing complex tests for patients receiving Medicare. These regulations, published in the Federal Register, outline the validation requirements for both Food and Drug Administration (FDA)-approved instruments, kits, and test systems as well as methods developed in-house. Laboratories must document analytic accuracy, precision, reportable ranges, and reference ranges for all procedures.

The regulations for in-house procedures and modifications of approved commercial procedures are more extensive and require laboratories to further document:

- Analytic sensitivity.
- Analytic specificity, including interfering substances. and
- Other performance characteristics required for testing patient specimens.

Although the details of method validation may be unique to a specific procedure, the following analytic validation studies have proved valuable for most procedures:

- Method comparison,
- Precision,
- Linearity,
- Recovery,
- Detection limit,
- Reportable range,
- Analytic interference,
- Carryover,
- Reference interval,
- Specimen stability, and
- Specimen type. Laboratories should have documentation for each of these performance characteristics, either from the diagnostics manufacturer or from direct studies.

METHOD COMPARISON

Ideally, the system should be compared with an established reference method. however, many endocrine tests do not have reference methods and many laboratories do not have the facilities to perform reference methods when they exist. As a minimum, the assay should be compared with an analytic system that has been clinically validated with specimens from healthy subjects and specimens from patients with the diseases being investigated. The system should be traceable to established reference standards, such as those from the WHO and the National Institute of Standards and Technology (NIST). Between 100 and 200 different specimens distributed over the assay range are recommended for method comparisons.

A cross-plot displaying the new method on the vertical axis versus the established method on the horizontal axis, along with the identity line, reference value lines, and regression statistics, is a useful way of displaying these comparisons. An alternative display method is the Bland-Altman difference plot, in which the difference between the test method and the reference method is plotted against the reference method values.

Although acceptable performance criteria for method comparisons are not well established, some important characteristics to examine are as follows:

- Any grossly discordant test values.
- The degree of scatter about the regression curve
- The size of the regression offset on the vertical axis

The number of points crossing between the low, normal, and high reference intervals for the two methods.

The European Union (EU) has enacted the In Vitro Diagnostics Directive, which requires manufacturers marketing in the European Union after the year 2003 to establish that their products are "traceable to reference standards and reference procedures of a higher order" when these references exist. Hopefully, medically relevant performance characteristics that define the allowable ranges for differences between a specific assay's test values and the traceable standards will be linked with this traceability requirement. This combination of traceability and allow-able error requirements could serve to harmonize many test methods worldwide because most diagnostic companies market internationally.

Precision

Precision is a measure of the replication of repeated measurements of the same specimen. it is a function of the time between repeats and the concentration of the analyte. Both short-term precision (within a run or within a day) and long-term precision (across calibrations and across batches of reagents) should be documented at clinically appropriate concentration levels.

In general, normal range, abnormally low range, and abnormally high range targets are chosen for precision studies. however, targets focused on critical medical decision limits may be more appropriate for some analytes. Twenty measurements are recommended at each level for both short-term and long-term precision validations. Precision generally is expressed as the coefficient of variation, calculated as 100 times the standard deviation divided by the average of the replicate measurements.

There is no universal agreement on the performance criteria for analytic precision, although numerous recommendations have been put forth.

Two major approaches to defining these criteria have been:

1. Comparison with biologic variation and
2. Expert opinion of clinicians based on their perceived impact of laboratory variation on clinical decisions.

The total variation clinically observed in test measurements is a combination of the analytic and biologic variations, for instance: If the analytic standard deviation (SD) is less than one fourth of the biologic SD, the analytic component increases the SD of the total error by less than 3%. If the analytic precision is less than one half of the biologic SD, the total error increases by only 12%.

These observations have led to recommendations for maintaining precision of less than one fourth or one-half of the biologic variation. The expert opinion precision recommendations are based on estimates of the magnitude of change of a test value that would cause clinicians to alter their clinical decisions. Table lists some precision recommendations for selected endocrine tests.

Table. Recommended Analytic Performance Limits[*]

Analyte	Biologic CVi (%)	Precision (%)	Accuracy (%)
Calcium	1.8	0.9[†]	0.7
Glucose	4.4	2.2[†]	1.9
Thyroxine	7.6	3.4[†]	4.1
Potassium	4.4	2.4[†]	1.6
Triiodothyronine	8.7[†]	4.0[‡]	5.5[‡]
Thyrotropin	20.2[†]	8.1[‡]	8.9[‡]
Cortisol	15.2[†]	(7.6)[*]	
Estradiol	21.7[†]	(10.9)[*]	
Follicle-stimulating hormone	30.8[†]	(15.4)[*]	
Luteinizing hormone	14.5[†]	(7.2)[*]	
Prolactin	40.5[†]	(20.2)[*]	
Testosterone	8.3[†]	(4.1)[*]	
Insulin	15.2[†]	(7.6)[*]	
Dehydroepiandrosterone	5.6[†]	(2.8)[*]	
11-deoxycortisol	21.3[†]	(10.6)[*]	

Linearity

Patient specimens commonly contain several different forms of the hormones to be measured compared with the pure form contained in the reference standards and calibrators used to establish the assay dose-response curve. When a patient specimen is diluted, the measured value for these dilutions should parallel the dose-response curve and give results proportional to the dilution. Linearity can be evaluated by measuring serial dilutions of patient specimens with high concentrations diluted in the appropriate assay diluent. The product of the measured value multiplied by the dilution factor should be approximately constant. There are no performance standards for linearity, but a reasonable expectation for most hormones is that dilutions are comparable within 10% of the undiluted value.

Recovery

Two methods of assessing the recovery of assays are:

1. Measuring the increase in test values after the reference analyte is added.
2. Mmeasuring the proportional changes caused by mixing high-concentration and low-concentration specimens.

Some analytes circulate in the blood in multiple forms, and some of these forms may be bound to carrier proteins. The recovery rate of pure substances added to a specimen may be low if the assay does not measure some of the bound forms. Mixtures of patient specimens may not be measured correctly if one of the specimens contains cross-reacting substances such as autoantibodies. A thorough understanding of the chemical forms of the analyte and their cross-reactivities in the assay is important during assessment of recovery data.

Detection Limit

The minimal analytic detection limit is the smallest concentration that can be statistically differentiated from zero. This concentration is mathematically determined as the upper 95% limit of replicate measurements of the *zero standard,* calculated from the average signal plus 2.0 SD. This minimal detection limit is valid *only* for the average of multiple replicate measurements. When individual determinations are performed on a specimen having a true concentration exactly at the minimal detection limit, the probability that the measurement is above the noise level of the assay is only about 50%.

A second term for the lowest level of reliable measurement for an assay is the *functional detection limit,* or the *limit of quantitation.* For this parameter to be measured, multiple pools with low concentrations are made and analysed in the replicate. A cross-plot of the coefficient of variation of the measurements versus the concentration allows one to generate a precision profile. The concentration corresponding to a coefficient of variation of 20% is the functional detection limit. This term generally applies to across-assay variation, but it also can be calculated using within-assay variation if one uses the tests to evaluate results measured within one run (*e.g.*, provocative and suppression tests).

Reportable Range

The reportable range of an assay generally spans from the functional detection limit to the concentration of the highest standard. Values above the highest standard may be reported if they are diluted and the measured value is multiplied by the dilution factor.

The validity of the analytic range is documented by the linearity and recovery studies. Some laboratories erroneously report the exact values displayed by the test systems even if they are outside of the analytic range. Therefore, it is important for clinicians to understand the limitations of valid measurements and not inappropriately use meaningless numbers that may be reported.

Another potential source of error is failure of the technologist to multiply the measured value of diluted specimens by the dilution factor to correct for the dilution. In addition, care should be taken to define the number of significant figures used for reporting test values and to establish an appropriate algorithm for rounding test values to the significant number of digits.

ANALYTIC INTERFERENCE

The cross-reactivity and potential interference of other analytes that may react in a test system should be documented. The choice of potential interfering substances that must be evaluated requires an understanding of both the analytic system and the pathophysiology of the analyte being evaluated. In immunoassays, for example, compounds with similar structures as well as precursor forms and degradation products should be tested. Drugs commonly prescribed for the diseases under evaluation should be assessed for interference both by addition of the drug to a specimen and by analysis of specimens from patients before and after receiving the drug. Most assays also are evaluated for the effects of hemolysis, lipemia, and icterus.

CARRYOVER STUDIES

Many diagnostic systems use automated sample-handling devices. If a specimen to be tested is preceded by a specimen with a very high concentration, a trace amount of the first specimen may significantly increase the reported concentration of the second specimen. The choice of the concentration that should be tested for carryover depends on the pathophysiology of the disease, but high values may need to be tested because some endocrine disorders may produce these high values.

A prudent procedure would be to retest all specimens following a specimen with an extraordinarily high value. One also should document that carryover from the sampling probe has not inadvertently contaminated subsequent specimen vials, there by invalidating subsequently repeated measurements.

REFERENCE INTERVALS

The development and validation of reference intervals for endocrine tests can be a very complex task. The normal reference interval for most laboratory tests is based on estimates of the central 95 percentile limits of measurements in healthy subjects. A minimum of 120 subjects is needed to reliably define the 2.5 and 97.5 percentiles. The reference intervals for many endocrine tests depend on gender, age, developmental status, and other test values. Formal statistical consultation is recommended to determine the appropriate number of subjects to test and to develop statistical models for defining multivariate reference ranges.

Full evaluation of the adrenal, gonadal, and thyroid axes requires simultaneous measurement of the trophic and target hormones. Bivariate displays of these hormone concentrations along with their multivariate reference intervals facilitate the interpretation. Preanalytic conditions should be well defined and controlled during evaluation of both healthy reference subjects and patients.

SPECIMEN STABILITY

Analyte stability is a function of storage conditions and specimen type. Although most hormones are relatively stable in serum or urine if they are rapidly frozen and stored in hermetically sealed vials at -70 °C, multiple freeze/thaw cycles may damage analytes, and storage in frost-free freezers that repeatedly cycle through thawing temperatures can adversely affect stability. Blood specimens collected in edetate (EDTA) often are more stable than serum or heparinized specimens because edetate chelates calcium and magnesium ions, which function as coenzymes for some proteases. The addition of protease inhibitors (*e.g.*, aprotinin) to blood specimens may also improve specimen stability.

Types of Specimens

Most hormones are measured in blood or urine, but alternative testing sources, such as saliva and transdermal membrane monitors, are also used.

Urine Specimens

The 24-hour urine specimen is used for many endocrine tests. Urine specimens represent a time average that integrates over the multiple pulsatile spikes of hormone secretion occurring throughout the day. The 24-hour urine specimen also has the advantage of better analytic sensitivity for some hormones. Urine often contains not only the original hormone but also key metabolites that may or may not have biologic activity.

Drawbacks include the inconvenience of and delays in collecting the 24-hour specimen. Another limitation of urine specimens is the uncertainty of the completeness of the collection. Measurement of urinary creatinine concentrations helps in monitoring collection completeness, especially when it is compared with the patient's muscle mass. Many urinary hormones are conjugated to carrier proteins before excretion. Therefore, both hepatic function and, to a lesser degree, renal function may alter urinary hormone values.

Blood Specimens

Blood specimens have both the advantage and the limitation of time dependency. The ability to direct rapid changes to a provocative stimulus is a strong advantage, whereas the unsuspected changes due to pulsatile secretions may be a major limitation. Most hormones undergo significant biologic variations, including ultradian, diurnal, menstrual, and seasonal changes. Many hormones have short half-lives and are thus rapidly cleared from the blood. The half-life is particularly important when one is attempting to measure the response to a provocative drug, such as the effect of gonadotropin-releasing hormone (GnRH). The development of rapid intraoperative methods for measuring PTH and growth hormone has highlighted the importance of plasma specimens, which do not require extra waiting time for the blood to clot to make serum.

Saliva Specimens

Saliva is becoming an alternative specimen for measuring non–protein-bound hormones and small molecules. Small analytes in blood pass into oral fluid by crossing capillary walls and basement membranes and by passage through lipophilic membranes of epithelial cells. This transport involves passive diffusion, ultrafiltration, and/or active transport. The concentration in saliva depends on the concentration of the non–protein-bound analyte in blood as well as salivary pH, the pKa of the analyte, and the size of the analyte. Analytes entering saliva by passive diffusion generally are less than 500 d, non–protein-bound, and nonionized. Saliva measurements correlate with blood measurements in some hormones like cortisol, progesterone, estradiol, and testosterone, but they do not correlate well for others (*e.g.*, thyroid and pituitary hormones).

Multiple preanalytic variables can affect the salivary measurement. Stimulation of oral fluid production by chewing or the use of candy or drops containing stimulants like citric acid can increase oral fluid volume and stabilize pH, but this stimulation may alter some analyte concentrations. Several commercial devices are available for collection of oral fluid. however, these devices need to be validated for each analyte and each assay system to ensure they adequately recover each of the analytes.

Blood Drops

Blood drops collected on filter paper from punctures of a finger or heel are a convenient system for collecting, transporting, and measuring hormones. If standardized collection conditions and extraction techniques are used, these measurements correlate well with serum measurements. Integration of immunochemistry with computer chip technology has also led to immunochips that can measure multiple analytes using a single drop of blood.

Noninvasive Measurements

Noninvasive transcutaneous measurements also have been developed for some endocrine tests. Transcutaneous glucose measurements using near-infrared spectroscopy correlate well with blood measurements. The GlucoWatch device is also being marketed for noninvasive monitoring of glucose.

QUALITY CONTROL SYSTEMS

Laboratory quality control programmes are intended to ensure that the test procedures are being performed within defined limits. A critical component of control systems is the definition of acceptable performance criteria. Unfortunately, these criteria often are not well defined and many laboratories use floating criteria that change when assays change. Control limits are often set at the mean ± *2 or 3 Standard Deviations (SDs),* where the mean and SD are arbitrarily assigned based on measurements made in that laboratory. When reagents or equipment change, new limits are assigned. These types of control systems provide some assurance that the laboratory is functioning at a level of performance similar to that of the recent past, but they provide little assurance that measurements are adequate for clinical decisions.

Statistically, there are two major forms of analytic errors: random and systematic. *Random error* relates to reproducibility. *systematic error* relates to the offset or bias of the test values from the target or reference value. Performance criteria can be defined for each of these parameters, and quality control systems can be programmed to monitor compliance with these criteria. Control systems must have low false-positive rates as well as high statistical power to detect assay deviations. The multirule algorithms developed by Westgard and colleagues use combinations of control rules, such as two consecutive controls outside of *warning limits,* one control outside of *action limits,* or moving average trend analysers outside of limits to achieve good statistical error detection characteristics.

Traditionally, quality control programmes have focused primarily on precision. however, analytic bias also can cause major clinical problems. When fixed decision levels are used to trigger clinical actions, such as therapy and additional investigations, changes in the analytic set-point of an assay can cause major changes in the number of follow-up cases. This concept is illustrated in Fig. for TSH measurements.

Under stable laboratory testing conditions, approximately 122 per 1000 patients tested have TSH values above 5.0 mIU/L. If the test shifts upward by 20%, the number of patients with TSH values above 5.0 mIU/L increases to

189, which equates to more than a 50% increase in the number of patients flagged as abnormal. These changes in test value distributions often can be sensed by clinicians who encounter multiple patients with unexpected elevated test values, causing them to call the laboratory and enquire whether the "test is running high today." Some modern quality control systems use moving averages of patient test values to help monitor changes in analytic bias.

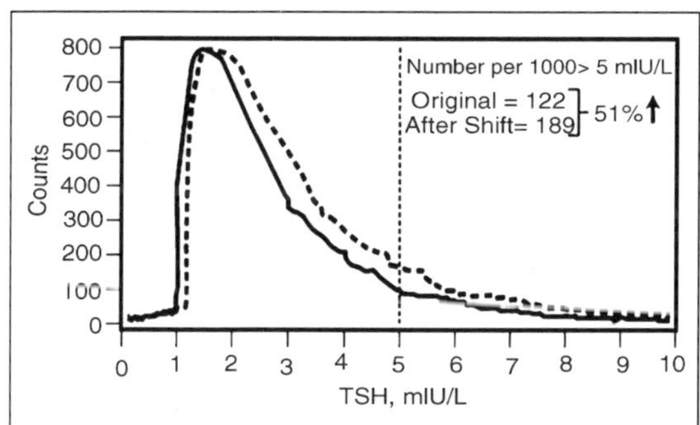

Fig. Effect of Analytic Bias, or Shift, on the Number of Patients with Elevated Levels of Thyrotropin (TSH)

Some medical facilities are linking together into networks to provide more integrated patient care. This crossover of both physicians and patients is increasing the importance of *harmonized* testing systems. For endocrine tests, harmonization is best achieved when all the laboratories in the network use the same test systems. Differences in analytic specificity may cause across-method differences in patient test distributions even when the methods use the same reference standard. Full harmonization of testing requires not only standardization of equipment but also standardization of reagents (including using the same lot numbers) and standardization of laboratory protocols. Real-time quality control monitors with peer group comparisons across the laboratories in the health care network are necessary to ensure uniformity of testing.

Investigation of Discordant Test Values

The practice of modern endocrinology depends extensively on reliable and accurate test values. even in the best laboratories, however, erroneous results sometimes are reported. Careful correlation of pathophysiology with test values can help to identify values that are "discordant." Some of these discordant test values may be analytically correct, but others may be erroneous. Clinicians can help investigate these suspicious test values by requesting laboratories to perform a few simple validation procedures.

Repeated testing of the same specimen is a valuable first step. If the specimen has been stored under stable conditions, the absolute value of the difference between the initial and the repeated measurements should be less than *3 analytic SDs* 95% of the time. Normally, the 95% confidence range is associated with the mean ±2 *SDs.* with repeated laboratory tests, however, errors are associated with the first as well as the second measurement. The confidence interval for the uncertainty of the difference between two measurements can be calculated using the statistical rules for propagation of errors.

To better understand this propagation of error, consider:

$$D = X_1 - X_2$$

where X_1 is the first measurement, X_2 is the repeated measurement, and D is the difference.

$$\text{Variance(D)} = \text{Variance}(X_1) + \text{Variance}(X_2)$$

$$\text{Variance(D)} = 2\text{Varince(X)}$$

$$\text{SD(D)} = \sqrt{2\text{Variance(X)}}$$

$$\text{SD(D)} = \sqrt{2}\text{SD(X)}$$

The variance of D is the *sum* of the variance of X_1 and the variance of X_2. The SD of D is the square root of the variance of D, or the square root of twice the variance of X_1. The SD of D equates to square root of 2 multiplied by the SD of S. Therefore, 95% of the absolute values for D should be within 2 times $\sqrt{2}\text{SD(X)}$ SD(X), or approximately 3 SD(X). If a repeat measurement exceeds this 3 SD(X) limit, the initial (or reagent)measurement is probably in error.

Linearity and recovery are valuable techniques for evaluating test validity. If the initial test value is elevated, serially diluting the specimen in the assay diluent and reassaying should be considered. If the specimen dilutes nonproportionately (Fig.), no meaningful value can be reported with that assay.

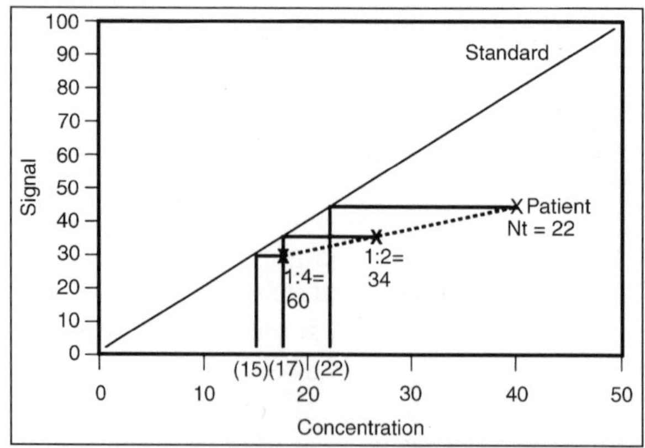

Fig. Nonproportional Dilutions. Discordant Values are Produced when Samples do not Dilute linearly. (Nt = undiluted [neat])

In the example, the undiluted specimen reads 22, the two fold dilution multiplies back to 34 (2×17), and the four fold dilution multiplies back to 60 (4×15). Therefore, the result depends on the dilution factor, so that no reliable answer can be reported. If the initial value is low, one may consider adding known quantities of the analyte to part of the specimen. Analysing these spiked or diluted specimens with the original specimen allows one to evaluate both reproducibility and recovery. It may be helpful to analyse the linearity or recovery of the assay standards at the same time to provide internal controls of the dilution or spiking procedures and the appropriateness of the diluent and spiking material.

If the replication, dilution, or recovery experiment appears successful, further analytic troubleshooting will vary according to the method used. Immunoassays may be affected by interference caused by heterophile antibodies. Addition of nonimmune mouse serum or heterophile antibody-blocking solutions may neutralize these effects. Chromatographic assays are usually more robust than immunoassays. Specimens with suspected interference on one type of assay can be reanalysed by means of an alternative methodology.

Water-soluble interferences have been reported for some direct assays for steroid measurements. Extraction of the hormones into organic solvents, followed by drying down and reconstitution in the assay zero standard, removes these interferences. Similarly, interferences with cross-reacting drugs and metabolic products can be minimized with selective extraction.

The analytic methods of assessing endocrine problems in patients are continually expanding. The newer systems are often based on analytic techniques similar to those outlined in this chapter, but the configurations are generally more user-friendly. These advances make the systems more convenient, but they also become more of a "black box" that conceals most of the details of the system. The performance validation steps outlined in this chapter become important procedures for ensuring that these systems continue to provide the reliable measurements needed for quality medical care.

5

Computed Tomography

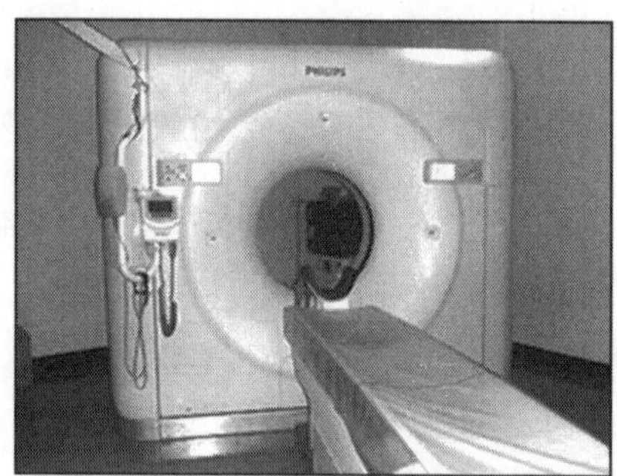

Fig. A Multislice CT Scanner.

Computed tomography (CT), was originally known as "EMI scan" as it was developed at a research branch of EMI, a company best known today for its music and recording business. It was later known as *computed axial tomography* (CAT or CT scan) and *body section roentgenography*.

Computed tomography is a medical imaging method employing tomography where digital geometry processing is used to generate a three-dimensional image of the internals of an object from a large series of two-dimensional X-ray images taken around a single axis of rotation. The word "tomography" is derived from the Greek *tomos* (slice) and *graphein* (to write).

CT produces a volume of data which can be manipulated, through a process known as *windowing*, in order to demonstrate various structures based on their ability to block the X-ray beam.

Although historically the images generated were in the axial or transverse plane (orthogonal to the long axis of the body), modern scanners allow this volume of data to be reformatted in various planes or even as volumetric (3D) representations of structures.

Although most common in healthcare, CT is also used in other fields, for example nondestructive materials testing. Another example is the DigiMorph project at the University of Texas at Austin which uses a CT scanner to study biological and paleontological specimens.

HISTORY

In the early 1930s the Italian radiologist Alessandro Vallebona proposed a method to represent a single slice of the body on the radiographic film. his exam was known as tomography.

The idea is based on simple principles of projective geometry: moving synchronously and in opposite directions the X-ray tube and the film, which are connected together by a rod whose pivot point is the focus; the image created by the points on the focal plane appears sharper, while the images of the other points annihilate as noise.

This is only marginally effective, as blurring occurs only in the "x" plane. There are also more complex devices which can move in more than one plane and perform more effective blurring.Tomography has been one of the pillars of radiologic diagnostics until the late 1970s, when the availability of minicomputers and of the transverse axial scanning method, this last due to Godfrey Newbold Hounsfield and Allan McLeod Cormack, gradually supplanted it as the modality of CT. The first commercially viable CT scanner was invented by Sir Godfrey Newbold Hounsfield in Hayes, United Kingdom at EMI Central Research Laboratories using X-rays. Hounsfield conceived his idea in 1967, and it was publicly announced in 1972.

Allan McLeod Cormack of Tufts University, Massachusetts, USA independently invented a similar process, and both Hounsfield and Cormack shared the 1979 Nobel Prize in Medicine.The original 1971 prototype took 160 parallel readings through 180 angles, each 1° apart, with each scan taking a little over five minutes. The images from these scans took 2.5 hours to be processed by algebraic reconstruction techniques on a large computer. The scanner had a single photomultiplier detector and operated on the Translate/ Rotate principle.

The CT scanner was "the greatest legacy" of The Beatles, with the massive profits resulting from their record sales enabling EMI to fund scientific research, including into computerised tomography.

The first production X-ray CT machine (in fact called the "EMI-Scanner") was limited to making tomographic sections of the brain, but acquired the image data in about 4 minutes (scanning two adjacent slices) and the computation time (using a Data General Nova minicomputer) was about 7 minutes per picture. This scanner required the use of a water-filled Perspex tank with a pre-shaped rubber "head-cap" at the front, which enclosed the patient's head.

The water-tank was used to reduce the dynamic range of the radiation reaching the detectors (between scanning outside the head compared with scanning through the bone of the skull). The images were relatively low resolution, being composed of a matrix of only 80 x 80 pixels.

The first EMI-Scanner was installed in Atkinson Morley's Hospital in Wimbledon, England, and the first patient brain-scan was made with it in 1972.In the U.S., the first installation was at the Mayo Clinic. As a tribute to the impact of this system on medical imaging the Mayo Clinic has an EMI scanner on display in the Radiology Department.

The first CT system that could make images of any part of the body, and did not require the "water tank" was the ACTA (Automatic Computerized Transverse Axial) scanner designed by Robert S. Ledley, DDS at Georgetown University.

This machine had 30 photomultiplier tubes as detectors and completed a scan in only 9 translate/rotate cycles, much faster than the EMI-scanner. It used a DEC PDP11/34 minicomputer both to operate the servo-mechanisms and to acquire and process the images. The Pfizer drug company acquired the prototype from the university, along with rights to manufacture it. Pfizer then began making copies of the prototype, calling it the "200FS" (FS meaning Fast Scan), which were selling as fast as they could make them. This unit produced images in a 256x256 matrix, with much better definition than the EMI-Scanner's 80x80.

Previous Studies

Tomography

CT's primary benefit is the ability to separate anatomical structures at different depths within the body. A form of tomography can be performed by moving the X-ray source and detector during an exposure. Anatomy at the target level remains sharp, while structures at different levels are blurred.

By varying the extent and path of motion, a variety of effects can be obtained, with variable depth of field and different degrees of blurring of 'out of plane' structures.Although largely obsolete, conventional tomography is still used in specific situations such as dental imaging (orthopantomography) or in intravenous urography.

Tomosynthesis

Digital tomosynthesis combines digital image capture and processing with simple tube/detector motion as used in conventional radiographic tomography - although there are some similarities to CT, it is a separate technique. In CT, the source/detector makes a complete 360 degree rotation about the subject obtaining a complete set of data from which images may be reconstructed. In digital tomosynthesis, only a small rotation angle (e.g. 40 degrees) with a small number of discrete exposures (e.g. 10) are used.

This incomplete set of data can be digitally processed to yield images similar to conventional tomography with a limited depth of field. However, because the image processing is digital, a series of slices at different depths and with different thicknesses can be reconstructed from the same acquisition, saving both time and radiation exposure. Because the data acquired is incomplete, tomosynthesis is unable to offer the extremely narrow slice widths that CT offers. However, higher resolution detectors can be used, allowing very-high in-plane resolution, even if the Z-axis resolution is poor. The primary interest in tomosynthesis is in breast imaging, as an extension to mammography, where it may offer better detection rates, with little extra increase in radiation exposure.

Reconstruction algorithms for tomosynthesis are significantly different from conventional CT, as the conventional filtered back projection algorithm requires a complete set of data. Iterative algorithms based upon expectation maximization are most commonly used, but are extremely computationally intensive. Some manufacturers have produced practical systems using commercial GPUs to perform the reconstruction.

TYPES OF MODERN CT ACQUISITION

Scout/Pilot/Topogram

A Scout image is used in planning the exam and to establish where the target organs are located. The beginning and end of the scan are set by the target region and the location of the patient on the table.

Once the Scout image is created it is used to determine the extent of the desired Axial/Helical scan. During the Scout scan the gantry is rotated to a fixed position and the table is translated as x-ray is delivered. The image appears similar to a radiograph.

Axial

In axial "step and shoot" acquisitions each slice/volume is taken and then the table is incremented to the next location. In multislice scanners each location is multiple slices and represents a volume of the patient anatomy. Tomographic reconstruction is used to generate Axial images.

Cine

A cine acquisition is used when the temporal nature is important. This is used in Perfusion applications to evaluate blood flow, blood volume and mean transit time. Cine is a time sequence of axial images. In a Cine acquisition the cradle is stationary and the gantry rotates continuously. Xray is delivered at a specified interval and duration.

Helical/Spiral

Helical is a very fast way to examine the target anatomy. The volume is scanned very quickly because the table is in constant motion as the gantry rotates continuously. There is no interscan delay between slices as in a Axial acquisition.

DRR

A Digitally Reconstructed Radiograph is a simulation of a conventional 2D x-ray image, created from computed tomography (CT) data. A radiograph, or conventional x-ray image, is a single 2D view of total x-ray absorption through the body along a given axis. Two objects (say, bones) in front of one another will overlap in the image. By contrast, a 3D CT image gives a volumetric representation. (Earlier CT data sets were better thought of as a set of 2D cross sectional images.) Sometimes one must compare CT data to a classical radiograph, and this can be done by comparing a DRR based on the CT data.

An early example of their use is the beam's eye view (BEV) as used in radiotherapy planning. In this application, a BEV is created for a specific patient and is used to help plan the treatment.DRRs are created by summing CT intensities along a ray from each pixel to the simulated x-ray source.Since 1993, the Visible Human Project (VHP) has made full body CT data available to researchers. This has allowed several universities and commercial companies to try and create DRR's.

These have been suggested as useful for training simulations in Radiology and Diagnostic Radiography. It takes a significant number of calculations to create a summative 2D image from a large amount of 3D data.

This is an area of medical science and education that has benefited from the advancing of graphics card technology, driven by the computer games industry.Another novel use of DRR's is in identification of the dead from old radiographic records, by comparing them to DRR's created from CT data.

Electron Beam CT

Electron beam tomography (EBCT) was introduced in the early 1980s, by medical physicist Andrew Castagnini, as a method of improving the temporal resolution of CT scanners. Because the X-ray source has to rotate by over 180 degrees in order to capture an image the technique is inherently unable to capture dynamic events or movements that are quicker than the rotation time.

Instead of rotating a conventional X-ray tube around the patient, the EBCT machine houses a huge vacuum tube in which an electron beam is electro-magnetically steered towards an array of tungsten X-ray anodes arranged circularly around the patient. Each anode is hit in turn by the electron beam and emits X-rays that are collimated and detected as in conventional CT.

The lack of moving parts allows very quick scanning, with single slice acquisition in 50-100 ms, making the technique ideal for capturing images of the heart. EBCT has found particular use for assessment of coronary artery calcium, a means of predicting risk of coronary artery disease.

The very high cost of EBCT equipment, and its poor flexibility (EBCT scanners are essentially single-purpose cardiac scanners), has led to poor uptake; fewer than 150 of these scanners have been installed worldwide. EBCT's role in cardiac imaging is rapidly being supplanted by high-speed multi-detector CT, which can achieve near-equivalent temporal resolution with much faster z-axis coverage.

Helical or Spiral CT

Helical, also called spiral, CT was introduced in the early 1990s, with much of the development led by Willi Kalender and Kazuhiro Katada. In older CT scanners, the X-ray source would move in a circular fashion to acquire a single 'slice', once the slice had been completed, the scanner table would move to position the patient for the next slice; meanwhile the X-ray source/detectors would reverse direction to avoid tangling their cables.

In helical CT the X-ray source (and detectors in 3rd generation designs) are attached to a freely rotating gantry. During a scan, the table moves the patient smoothly through the scanner; the name derives from the helical path traced out by the X-ray beam.

It was the development of two technologies that made helical CT practical: slip rings to transfer power and data on and off the rotating gantry, and the switched mode power supply powerful enough to supply the X-ray tube, but small enough to be installed on the gantry.

The major advantage of helical scanning compared to the traditional shoot-and-step approach, is speed; a large volume can be covered in 20-60 seconds. This is advantageous for a number or reasons:

- Often the patient can hold their breath for the entire study, reducing motion artifacts,
- It allows for more optimal use of intravenous contrast enhancement,
- The study is quicker than the equivalent conventional CT permitting the use of higher resolution acquisitions in the same study time.

The data obtained from spiral CT is often well-suited for 3D imaging because of the lack of motion mis registration and the increased out of plane resolution. These major advantages led to the rapid rise of helical CT as the most popular type of CT technology.

Despite the advantages of helical scanning, there are a few circumstances where it may not be desirable - there is, of course, no difficulty in configuring a helical capable scanner for scanning in shoot-and-step mode. All other factors being equal, helical CT has slightly lower z-axis resolution than step-and-shoot (due to the continual movement of the patient).

Where z-resolution is critical but where it is undesirable to scan at a higher resolution setting (due to the higher radiation exposure required) e.g. brain imaging, step-and-shoot may still be the preferred method.

Multislice CT

Multislice CT scanners are similar in concept to the helical or spiral CT but there are more than one detector ring. It began with two rings in mid nineties, with a 2 solid state ring model designed and built by Elscint (Haifa) called CT TWIN, with one second rotation (1993): It was followed by other manufacturers.

Later, it was presented 4, 8, 16, 32, 40 and 64 detector rings, with increasing rotation speeds. Current models (2007) have up to 3 rotations per second, and isotropic resolution of 0.35mm voxels with z-axis scan speed of up to 18 cm/s.This resolution exceeds that of High Resolution CT techniques with single-slice scanners, yet it is practical to scan adjacent, or overlapping, slices - however, image noise and radiation exposure significantly limit the use of such resolutions.

The major benefit of multi-slice CT is the increased speed of volume coverage. This allows large volumes to be scanned at the optimal time following intravenous contrast administration; this has particularly benefitted CT angiography techniques - which rely heavily on precise timing to ensure good demonstration of arteries.

Computer power permits increasing the postprocessing capabilities on workstations. Bone suppression, volume rendering in real time, with a natural visualization of internal organs and structures, and automated volume reconstruction really change the way diagnostic is performed on CT studies and this models become true volumetric scanners.

The ability of multi-slice scanners to achieve isotropic resolution even on routine studies means that maximum image quality is not restricted to images in the axial plane - and studies can be freely viewed in any desired plane.

Dual Source CT

Siemens introduced a CT model with dual X-ray tube and dual array of 64 slice detectors, at the 2005 Radiological Society of North America (RSNA) medical meeting. Dual sources increase the temporal resolution by reducing the rotation angle required to acquire a complete image, thus permitting cardiac studies without the use of heart rate lowering medication, as well as permitting imaging of the heart in systole.

The use of two x-ray units makes possible the use of dual energy imaging, which allows an estimate of the average atomic number in a voxel, as well as the total attenutaion. This permits automatic differentiation of calcium (e.g. in bone, or diseased arteries) from iodine (in contrast medium) or titanium (in stents) - which might otherwise be impossible to differentiate. It may also improve the characterization of tissues allowing better tumor differentiation.

256+ Slice CT

At RSNA 2007, Philips announced a 256 slice scanner, while Toshiba announced a "dynamic volume" scanner based on 320 slices. The majority of published data with regard to both technical and clinical aspects of the systems have been related to the prototype unit made by Toshiba Medical Systems.

The recent 3 month Beta installation at Johns Hopkins Press Release using a Toshiba system tested the clinical capabilities of this technology JHU Gazette.

The technology currently remains in a development phase but has demonstrated the potential to significantly reduce radiation exposure by eliminating the requirement for a helical examination in both cardiac CT angiography and whole brain perfusion studies for the evaluation of stroke.

Inverse Geometry CT

Inverse geometry CT (IGCT) is a novel concept which is being investigated as refinement of the classic third generation CT design. Although the technique has been demonstrated on a laboratory proof-of-concept device, it remains to be seen whether IGCT is feasible for a practical scanner. IGCT reverses the shapes of the detector and X-ray sources.

The conventional third-generation CT geometry uses a point source of X-rays, which diverge in a fan beam to act on a linear array of detectors. In multidetector computed tomography (MDCT), this is extended in 3 dimensions to a conical beam acting on a 2D array of detectors.

The IGCT concept, conversely, uses an array of highly collimated X-ray sources which act on a point detector. By using a principle similar to electron beam tomography (EBCT), the individual sources can be activated in turn by steering an electron beam onto each source target.

The rationale behind IGCT is that it avoids the disadvantages of the cone-beam geometry of third generation MDCT. As the z-axis width of the cone beam increases, the quantity of scattered radiation reaching the detector also increases, and the z-axis resolution is thereby degraded - because of the increasing z-axis distance that each ray must traverse.

This reversal of roles has extremely high intrinsic resistance to scatter; and, by reducing the number of detectors required per slice, it makes the use of better performing detectors (e.g. ultra-fast photon counting detectors) more practical. Because a separate detector can be used for each 'slice' of sources, the conical geometry can be replaced with an array of fans, permitting z-axis resolution to be preserved.

Synchrotron X-ray Tomographic Microscopy

Synchrotron X-ray tomographic microscopy is a 3-D scanning technique that allows non-invasive high definition scans of objects with details as fine as 1,000th of a millimetre, meaning it has two to three thousand times the resolution of a traditional medical CT scan.

Synchrotron X-ray tomographic microscopy has been applied in the field of palaeontology to perform non-destructive internal examination of fossils, including fossil embryos to be made. Scientists feel this technology has the potential to revolutionize the field of paleontology. The first team to use the technique have published their findings in Nature, which they believe "could roll back the evolutionary history of arthropods like insects and spiders."

Archaeologists are increasingly turning to Synchrotron X-ray tomographic microscopy as a non-destructive means to examine ancient specimens.

X-ray Tomography

X-ray Tomography is a branch of X-ray microscopy. A series of projection images are used to calculate a three dimensional reconstruction of an object. The technique has found many applications in materials science and later in biology and biomedical research. In terms of the latter, the National centre for X-ray Tomography (NCXT) is one of the principal developers of this technology, in particular for imaging whole, hydrated cells.

DIAGNOSTIC USE

Since its introduction in the 1970s, CT has become an important tool in medical imaging to supplement X-rays and medical ultrasonography. Although it is still quite expensive, it is the gold standard in the diagnosis of a large number of different disease entities. It has more recently begun to also be used for preventive medicine or screening for disease, for example CT colonography for patients with a high risk of colon cancer.

Although a number of institutions offer full-body scans for the general population, this practice remains controversial due to its lack of proven benefit, cost, radiation exposure, and the risk of finding 'incidental' abnormalities that may trigger additional investigations.

Cranial

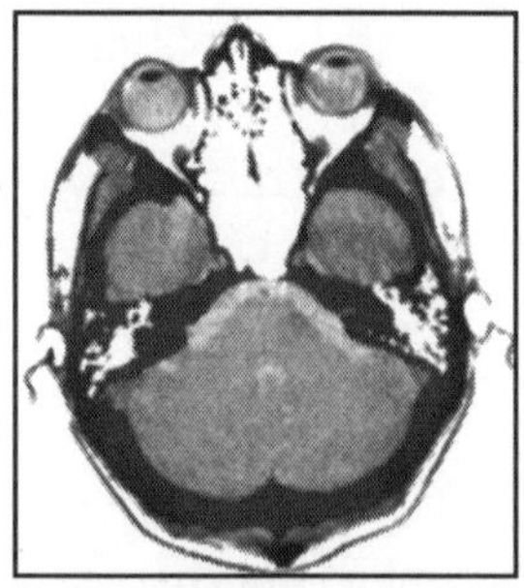

Fig. Normal CT Scan of the Head; this Slice Shows the Cerebellum, a Small Portion of Each Temporal Lobe, the Orbits, and the Ethmoid Sinuses.

Diagnosis of cerebrovascular accidents and intracranial hemorrhage is the most frequent reason for a "head CT" or "CT brain". Scanning is done with or without intravenous contrast agents.

CT generally does not exclude infarct in the acute stage of a stroke. However, CT is useful to exclude an intra-cranial hemorrhage as a cause, or complication of the stroke. For the detection of acute hemorrhage, especially subarachnoid hemorrhage, CT is the test of choice as it is more sensitive than MRI.For detection of tumors, CT scanning with IV contrast is occasionally used but is less sensitive than magnetic resonance imaging (MRI). CT has an important role in evaluation of the functioning of a ventriculoperitoneal shunt by demonstrating the volume of the ventricular system. Although CT cannot assess intracranial pressure, it can demonstrate several important causes of raised intracranial pressure. Despite the limitation that CT may not detect raised intracranial pressure, it may help in the clinical decision to perform lumbar puncture and is often performed in this context. CT is also useful in the setting of trauma for evaluating facial and skull fractures.In the head/neck/mouth area, CT scanning is used for surgical planning for craniofacial and dentofacial deformities, evaluation of cysts and some tumors of the jaws/paranasal sinuses/ nasal cavity/orbits, diagnosis of the causes of chronic sinusitis, and for planning of dental implant reconstruction.

Chest

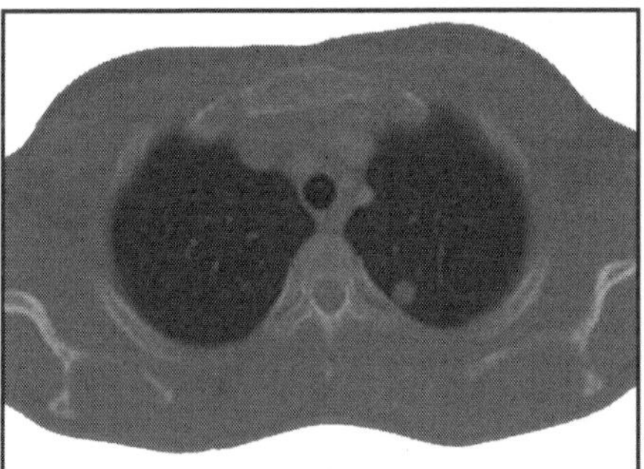

Fig. Chest CT: Axial Slice.

CT is excellent for detecting both acute and chronic changes in the lung parenchyma. A variety of different techniques are used depending on the suspected abnormality. For evaluation of chronic interstitial processes (emphysema, fibrosis, and so forth), thin sections with high spatial frequency reconstructions are used - often scans are performed both in inspiration and expiration. This special technique is called High resolution CT (HRCT).

Note: HRCT is normally done with thin section with skipped areas between the thin sections. Therefore it produces a sampling of the lung and not continuous images. Continuous images are provided in a standard CT of the chest.

For detection of airspace disease (such as pneumonia) or cancer, relatively thick sections and general purpose image reconstruction techniques may be adequate. IV contrast may also be used as it clarifies the anatomy and boundaries of the great vessels and improves assessment of the mediastinum and hilar regions for lymphadenopathy; this is particularly important for accurate assessment of cancer.

CT angiography of the chest is also becoming the primary method for detecting pulmonary embolism (PE) and aortic dissection, and requires accurately timed rapid injections of contrast (Bolus Tracking) and high-speed helical scanners. CT is the standard method of evaluating abnormalities seen on chest X-ray and of following findings of uncertain acute significance.

PULMONARY ANGIOGRAM

CT pulmonary angiogram (CTPA) is a medical diagnostic test used to diagnose pulmonary embolism (PE). It employs computed tomography to obtain an image of the pulmonary arteries.

Diagnostic Use

It is a preferred choice of imaging in the diagnosis of PE due to its minimally invasive nature for the patient, whose only requirement for the scan is a cannula (usually a 20G). Before this test is requested, it is usual for the referring clinician to have carried out a D-dimer blood test and requested a chest X-Ray to rule out any other possible differential diagnosis.

Acquisition

- MDCT (multi detector CT) scanners give the optimum resolution and image quality for this test
- Images are usually taken on a 0.625mm slice thickness, although 2mm is sufficient.
- 50 - 100 mls of contrast is given to the patient at a rate of 4 ml/s.
- The tracker/locator is placed at the level of the Pulmonary Arteries, which sit roughly at the level of the carina.
- Images are acquired with the maximum intensity of radio-opaque contrast in the Pulmonary Arteries. This is done using bolus tracking.

CT machines are now so sophisticated that the test can be done with a patient visit of 5 minutes with an approximate scan time of only 5 seconds or less.

Interpretation

A normal CTPA scan will show the contrast filling the pulmonary vessels, looking bright white. Ideally the aorta should be empty of contrast, to reduce any partial volume artefact which may result in a false positive. Any mass filling defects, such as an embolus, will appear dark in place of the contrast, filling/blocking the space where blood should be flowing into the lungs.

Cardiac

With the advent of subsecond rotation combined with multi-slice CT (up to 64-slice), high resolution and high speed can be obtained at the same time, allowing excellent imaging of the coronary arteries (cardiac CT angiography).

Images with an even higher temporal resolution can be formed using retrospective ECG gating. In this technique, each portion of the heart is imaged more than once while an ECG trace is recorded. The ECG is then used to correlate the CT data with their corresponding phases of cardiac contraction.

Once this correlation is complete, all data that were recorded while the heart was in motion (systole) can be ignored and images can be made from the remaining data that happened to be acquired while the heart was at rest (diastole). In this way, individual frames in a cardiac CT investigation have a better temporal resolution than the shortest tube rotation time.

Because the heart is effectively imaged more than once, cardiac CT angiography results in a relatively high radiation exposure around 12 mSv.

For the sake of comparison, a chest X-ray carries a dose of approximately 0.02 to 0.2 mSv and natural background radiation exposure is around 0.01 mSv/day. Thus, cardiac CTA is equivalent to approximately 100-600 chest X-rays or over 3 years worth of natural background radiation.

Methods are available to decrease this exposure, however, such as prospectively decreasing radiation output based on the concurrently acquired ECG (aka tube current modulation.) This can result in a significant decrease in radiation exposure, at the risk of compromising image quality if there is any arrhythmia during the acquisition.

The significance of radiation doses in the diagnostic imaging range has not been proven, although the possibility of inducing an increased cancer risk across a population is a source of significant concern.

This potential risk must be weighed against the competing risk of not performing a test and potentially not diagnosing a significant health problem such as coronary artery disease. It is uncertain whether this modality will replace invasive coronary catheterization.

Currently, it appears that the greatest utility of cardiac CT lies in ruling out coronary artery disease rather than ruling it in. This is because the test has a high sensitivity (greater than 90 per cent) and thus a negative test result means that a patient is very unlikely to have coronary artery disease and can be worked up for other causes of their chest symptoms.

This is termed a high negative predictive value. A positive result is less conclusive and often will be confirmed (and possibly treated) with subsequent invasive angiography. For the record, the positive predictive value of cardiac CTA is estimated at approximately 82 per cent and the negative predictive value is around 93 per cent.

Dual Source CT scanners, introduced in 2005, allow higher temporal resolution by acquiring a full CT slice in only half a rotation, thus reducing motion blurring at high heart rates and potentially allowing for shorter breath-hold time. This is particularly useful for ill patients who have difficulty holding their breath or who are unable to take heart-rate lowering medication.

The speed advantages of 64-slice MSCT have rapidly established it as the minimum standard for newly installed CT scanners intended for cardiac scanning. Manufacturers are now actively developing 256-slice and true 'volumetric' scanners, primarily for their improved cardiac scanning performance.

The latest MSCT scanners acquire images only at 70-80 per cent of the R-R interval (late diastole). This prospective gating can reduce effective dose from 10-15mSv to as little as 1.2mSv in follow-up patients acquiring at 75 per cent of the R-R interval. Effective doses at a centre with well trained staff doing coronary imaging can average less than the doses for conventional coronary angiography.

Abdominal and Pelvic

CT is a sensitive method for diagnosis of abdominal diseases. It is used frequently to determine stage of cancer and to follow progress. It is also a useful test to investigate acute abdominal pain.

Renal/urinary stones, appendicitis, pancreatitis, diverticulitis, abdominal aortic aneurysm, and bowel obstruction are conditions that are readily diagnosed and assessed with CT. CT is also the first line for detecting solid organ injury after trauma.

Oral and/or rectal contrast may be used depending on the indications for the scan. A dilute (2 per cent w/v) suspension of barium sulfate is most commonly used. The concentrated barium sulfate preparations used for fluoroscopy e.g. barium enema are too dense and cause severe artifacts on CT.

Iodinated contrast agents may be used if barium is contraindicated (e.g. suspicion of bowel injury). Other agents may be required to optimize the imaging of specific organs: e.g. rectally administered gas (air or carbon dioxide) for a colon study, or oral water for a stomach study.

CT has limited application in the evaluation of the *pelvis*. For the female pelvis in particular, ultrasound and MRI are the imaging modalities of choice. Nevertheless, it may be part of abdominal scanning (e.g. for tumors), and has uses in assessing fractures.

CT is also used in osteoporosis studies and research along side DXA scanning. Both CT and DXA can be used to assess bone mineral density (BMD) which is used to indicate bone strength, however CT results do not correlate exactly with DXA (the gold standard of BMD measurement).

CT is far more expensive, and subjects patients to much higher levels of ionizing radiation, so it is used infrequently.

Extremities

CT is often used to image complex fractures, especially ones around joints, because of its ability to reconstruct the area of interest in multiple planes.

Fractures, ligamentous injuries and dislocations can easily be recognised with a 0.2 mm resolution.

Advantages and Hazards

Advantages Over Projection Radiography

First, CT completely eliminates the superimposition of images of structures outside the area of interest. Second, because of the inherent high-contrast resolution of CT, differences between tissues that differ in physical density by less than 1 per cent can be distinguished.

Third, data from a single CT imaging procedure consisting of either multiple contiguous or one helical scan can be viewed as images in the axial, coronal, or sagittal planes, depending on the diagnostic task. This is referred to as multiplanar reformatted imaging.

Radiation Exposure

CT is regarded as a moderate to high radiation diagnostic technique. While technical advances have improved radiation efficiency, there has been simultaneous pressure to obtain higher-resolution imaging and use more complex scan techniques, both of which require higher doses of radiation.

The improved resolution of CT has permitted the development of new investigations, which may have advantages; e.g. Compared to conventional angiography, CT angiography avoids the invasive insertion of an arterial catheter and guidewire; CT colonography may be as useful as a barium enema for detection of tumors, but may use a lower radiation dose.

The greatly increased availability of CT, together with its value for an increasing number of conditions, has been responsible for a large rise in popularity.

So large has been this rise that, in the most recent comprehensive survey in the UK, CT scans constituted 7 per cent of all radiologic examinations, but contributed 47 per cent of the total collective dose from medical X-ray examinations in 2000/2001.

Increased CT usage has led to an overall rise in the total amount of medical radiation used, despite reductions in other areas.The radiation dose for a particular study depends on multiple factors: volume scanned, patient build, number and type of scan sequences, and desired resolution and image quality. Additionally, two helical CT scanning parameters that can be adjusted easily and that have a profound effect on radiation dose are tube current and pitch.

CT scans of children have been estimated to produce non-negligible increases in the probability of lifetime cancer mortality leading to calls for the use of reduced current settings for CT scans of children. A 2007 report in the New England Journal of Medicine suggested that the radiation from current CT-scan use may cause as many as 1 in 50 future cases of cancer.According to the USAToday, and members of the American Heart Association, an average CT scan can expose a patient to between 1,000 to 10,000 millirems of radiation, depending on the exact machine and the examination being performed. However, Japanese people who were 1 mile from ground zero received only 3,000 millirems of radiation, on average.

Adverse Reactions to Contrast Agents

Because CT scans rely on intravenously administered contrast agents in order to provide superior image quality, there is a low but non-negligible level of risk associated with the contrast agents themselves. Certain patients may experience severe and potentially life-threatening allergic reactions to the contrast dye.

The contrast agent may also induce kidney damage. The risk of this is increased with patients who have preexisting renal insufficiency, preexisting diabetes, or reduced intravascular volume.

In general, if a patient has normal kidney function, then the risks of contrast nephropathy are negligible. Patients with mild kidney impairment are usually advised to ensure full hydration for several hours before and after the injection.

For moderate kidney failure, the use of iodinated contrast should be avoided; this may mean using an alternative technique instead of CT e.g. MRI. Perhaps paradoxically, patients with severe renal failure requiring dialysis do not require special precautions, as their kidneys have so little function remaining that any further damage would not be noticeable and the dialysis will remove the contrast agent.

Process

X-ray slice data is generated using an X-ray source that rotates around the object; X-ray sensors are positioned on the opposite side of the circle from the X-ray source. The earliest sensors were scintillation detectors, with photomultiplier tubes excited by (typically) sodium iodide crystals.

Modern detectors use the ionization principle and are filled with low-pressure Xenon gas. Many data scans are progressively taken as the object is gradually passed through the gantry. They are combined together by the mathematical procedures known as tomographic reconstruction. The data are arranged in a matrix in memory, and each data point is convolved with its neighbours according with a seed algorithm using Fast Fourier Transform techniques.

This dramatically increases the resolution of each Voxel (volume element). Then a process known as Back Projection essentially reverses the acquisition geometry and stores the result in another memory array. This data can then be displayed, photographed, or used as input for further processing, such as multi-planar reconstruction. Newer machines with faster computer systems and newer software strategies can process not only individual cross sections but continuously changing cross sections as the gantry, with the object to be imaged, is slowly and smoothly slid through the X-ray circle.

These are called *helical* or *spiral CT* machines. Their computer systems integrate the data of the moving individual slices to generate three dimensional volumetric information (3D-CT scan), in turn viewable from multiple different perspectives on attached CT workstation monitors.

This type of data acquisition requires enormous processing power, as the data are arriving in a continuous stream and must be processed in real-time.In conventional CT machines, an X-ray tube and detector are physically rotated behind a circular shroud; in the electron beam tomography (EBT) the tube is far larger and higher power to support the high temporal resolution. The electron beam is deflected in a hollow funnel shaped vacuum chamber. X-rays are generated when the beam hits the stationary target.

The detector is also stationary. This arrangement can result in very fast scans, but is extremely expensive.The data stream representing the varying radiographic intensity sensed at the detectors on the opposite side of the circle during each sweep is then computer processed to calculate cross-sectional estimations of the radiographic density, expressed in Hounsfield units. Sweeps cover 360 or just over 180 degrees in conventional machines, 220 degrees in EBT.

CT is used in medicine as a diagnostic tool and as a guide for interventional procedures. Sometimes contrast materials such as intravenous iodinated contrast are used. This is useful to highlight structures such as blood vessels that otherwise would be difficult to delineate from their surroundings. Using contrast material can also help to obtain functional information about tissues.Pixels in an image obtained by CT scanning are displayed in terms of relative radiodensity.

The pixel itself is displayed according to the mean attenuation of the tissue(s) that it corresponds to on a scale from -1024 to +3071 on the Hounsfield scale. Pixel is a two dimensional unit based on the matrix size and the field of view. When the CT slice thickness is also factored in, the unit is known as a Voxel, which is a three dimensional unit.

The phenomenon that one part of the detector cannot differ between different tissues is called the *"Partial Volume Effect"*. That means that a big amount of cartilage and a thin layer of compact bone can cause the same attenuation in a voxel as hyperdense cartilage alone.

Water has an attenuation of 0 Hounsfield units (HU) while air is -1000 HU, cancellous bone is typically +400 HU, cranial bone can reach 2000 HU or more (os temporale) and can cause artifacts. The attenuation of metallic implants depends on atomic number of the element used: Titanium usually has an amount of +1000 HU, iron steel can completely extinguish the X-ray and is therefore responsible for well-known line-artifacts in computed tomograms.

Artifacts are caused by abrupt transitions between low- and high-density materials, which results in data values that exceed the dynamic range of the processing electronics.

Windowing

Windowing is the process of using the calculated Hounsfield units to make an image. The display device, as well as the human eye, can only resolve 256 shades of gray. These shades of gray can be distributed over a wide range of HU values to get an overview of structures that attenuate the beam to widely varying degrees.

Alternatively, these shades of gray can be distributed over a narrow range of HU values (called a "narrow window") centered over the average HU value of a particular structure to be evaluated.

In this way, subtle variations in the internal makeup of the structure can be discerned. This is a commonly used image processing technique known as contrast compression. For example, to evaluate the abdomen in order to find subtle masses in the liver, one might use liver windows.

Choosing 70 HU as an average HU value for liver, the shades of gray can be distributed over a narrow window or range. One could use 170 HU as the narrow window, with 85 HU above the 70 HU average value; 85 HU below it. Therefore the liver window would extend from -15 HU to +155 HU.

All the shades of gray for the image would be distributed in this range of Hounsfield values. Any HU value below -15 would be pure black, and any HU value above 155 HU would be pure white in this example.

Using this same logic, bone windows would use a *"wide window"* (to evaluate everything from fat-containing medullary bone that contains the marrow, to the dense cortical bone), and the centre or level would be a value in the hundreds of Hounsfield units.

To an untrained person, these window controls would correspond to the more familiar "Brightness" (Window Level) and "Contrast" (Window Width).

Artifacts

Although CT is a relatively accurate test, it is liable to produce artifacts, such as the following.

- *Aliasing Artifact or Streaks:* These appear as dark lines which radiate away from sharp corners. It occurs because it is impossible for the scanner to 'sample' or take enough projections of the object, which is usually metallic. It can also occur when an insufficient X-ray tube current is selected, and insufficient penetration of the x-ray occurs. These artifacts are also closely tied to motion during a scan. This type of artifact commonly occurs in head images around the pituitary fossa area.

- *Partial Volume Effect:* This appears as 'blurring' over sharp edges. It is due to the scanner being unable to differentiate between a small amount of high-density material (e.g. bone) and a larger amount of lower density (e.g. cartilage). The processor tries to average out the two densities or structures, and information is lost. This can be partially overcome by scanning using thinner slices.
- *Ring Artifact:* Probably the most common mechanical artifact, the image of one or many 'rings' appears within an image. This is usually due to a detector fault.
- *Noise Artifact:* This appears as graining on the image and is caused by a low signal to noise ratio. This occurs more commonly when a thin slice thickness is used. It can also occur when the kV or mA of the X-ray tube is insufficient to penetrate the anatomy.
- *Motion Artifact:* This is seen as blurring and/or streaking which is caused by movement of the object being imaged.
- *Windmill:* Streaking appearances can occur when the detectors intersect the reconstruction plane. This can be reduced with filters or a reduction in pitch.
- *Beam Hardening:* This can give a 'cupped appearance'. It occurs when there is more attenuation in the centre of the object than around the edge. This is easily corrected by filtration and software.

Three Dimensional (3D) Image Reconstruction

The Principle

Because contemporary CT scanners offer isotropic, or near isotropic, resolution, display of images does not need to be restricted to the conventional axial images.

Instead, it is possible for a software programme to build a volume by 'stacking' the individual slices one on top of the other. The programme may then display the volume in an alternative manner.

Multiplanar Reconstruction

Multiplanar reconstruction (MPR) is the simplest method of reconstruction. A volume is built by stacking the axial slices.

The software then cuts slices through the volume in a different plane (usually orthogonal). Optionally, a special projection method, such as maximum-intensity projection (MIP) or minimum-intensity projection (mIP), can be used to build the reconstructed slices.

MPR is frequently used for examining the spine. Axial images through the spine will only show one vertebral body at a time and cannot reliably show the intervertebral discs. By reformatting the volume, it becomes much easier to visualise the position of one vertebral body in relation to the others.

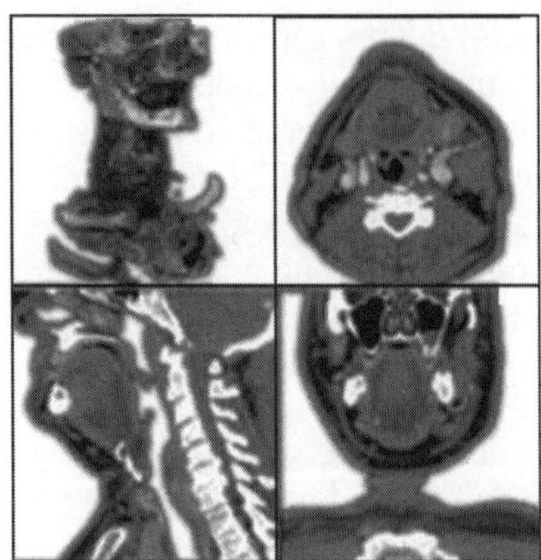

Fig. Typical Screen Layout for Diagnostic Software, Showing One 3D and Three MPR Views

Modern software allows reconstruction in non-orthogonal (oblique) planes so that the optimal plane can be chosen to display an anatomical structure. This may be particularly useful for visualising the structure of the bronchi as these do not lie orthogonal to the direction of the scan. For vascular imaging, curved-plane reconstruction can be performed.

This allows bends in a vessel to be 'straightened' so that the entire length can be visualised on one image, or a short series of images. Once a vessel has been 'straightened' in this way, quantitative measurements of length and cross sectional area can be made, so that surgery or interventional treatment can be planned. MIP reconstructions enhance areas of high radiodensity, and so are useful for angiographic studies. mIP reconstructions tend to enhance air spaces so are useful for assessing lung structure.

3D Rendering Techniques

Surface Rendering

A threshold value of radiodensity is chosen by the operator (e.g. a level that corresponds to bone). A threshold level is set, using edge detection image processing algorithms. From this, a 3-dimensional model can be constructed and displayed on screen. Multiple models can be constructed from various different thresholds, allowing different colors to represent each anatomical component such as bone, muscle, and cartilage. However, the interior structure of each element is not visible in this mode of operation.

Volume Rendering

Surface rendering is limited in that it will only display surfaces which meet a threshold density, and will only display the surface that is closest to the imaginary viewer. In volume rendering, transparency and colors are used to allow a better representation of the volume to be shown in a single image - e.g.

the bones of the pelvis could be displayed as semi-transparent, so that even at an oblique angle, one part of the image does not conceal another.

3D Rendering Software

Image Segmentation

Where different structures have similar radiodensity, it can become impossible to separate them simply by adjusting volume rendering parameters. The solution is called segmentation, a manual or automatic procedure that can remove the unwanted structures from the image.

Example

Some slices of a cranial CT scan are shown below. The bones are whiter than the surrounding area. (Whiter means higher radiodensity.) Note the blood vessels (arrowed) showing brightly due to the injection of an iodine-based contrast agent.

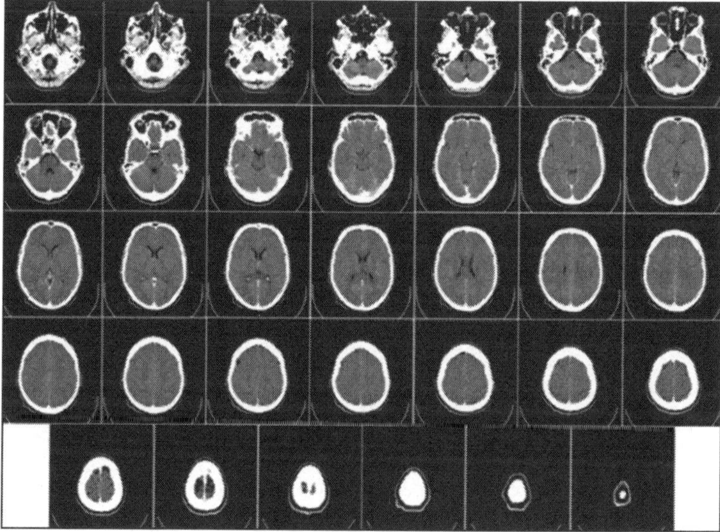

Fig. Computed Tomography of Human Brain, From Base of the Skull to Top. Taken with Intravenous Contrast Medium.

6

Role of Medicinal Lab in Clinical Pathology

SURGERY

Modern surgery works only because cells have a remarkable ability to regroup, bury their dead and heal over the injury. Nanotechnology, "the manufacturing technology of the 21st century," should let us economically build a broad range of complex molecular machines (including, not incidentally, molecular computers). It will let us build fleets of computer controlled molecular tools much smaller than a human cell and built with the accuracy and precision of drug molecules. Such tools will let medicine, for the first time, intervene in a sophisticated and controlled way at the cellular and molecular level.

They could remove obstructions in the circulatory system, kill cancer cells, or take over the function of subcellular organelles. Just as today we have the artifical heart, so in the future we could have the artificial mitochondrion. Equally dramatic, nanotechnology will give us new instruments to examine tissue in unprecedented detail. Sensors smaller than a cell would give us an inside and exquisitely precise look at ongoing function.

Tissue that was either chemically fixed or flash frozen could be analysed literally down to the molecular level, giving a completely detailed "snapshot" of cellular, subcellular and molecular activities. There is broad agreement (though not consensus) that we will at some point in the future be able to inexpensively fabricate essentially any structure that is consistent with chemical and physical law and specified in molecular. The most direct route to achieving this capability involves positioning and assembling individual atoms and molecules in a fashion conceptually similar to snapping together LEGO blocks. By designing and building programmable self replicating manufacturing systems that incorporate these principles we should be able to achieve very low manufacturing costs.

While the design and development of such programmable self replicating molecular manufacturing systems will be a major task and will likely require many years or a few decades, it appears that this kind of capability, to quote Feynman.

Design concepts for general purpose self replicating manufacturing systems have been discussed for many years, and their utility in manufacturing has been emphasized recently. These proposals draw on a body of work started by von Neumann. A wide range of methods have been considered. The von Neumann architecture for a self replicating system is the ancestral and archetypal proposal.

GENERAL MANUFACTURING SYSTEM

Von Neumann's proposal consisted of two central elements: a universal computer and a universal constructor. The universal computer contains a programme that directs the behaviour of the universal constructor.

The universal constructor, in turn, is used to manufacture both another universal computer and another universal constructor. Once construction is finished the programme contained in the original universal computer is copied to the new universal computer and programme execution is started.

Von Neumann worked out the details for a constructor that worked in a theoretical two-dimensional cellular automata world (parts of his proposal have since been modeled computationally[REF24]). The constructor had an arm which it could move about and which could be used to change the state of the cell at the tip of the arm.

By progressively sweeping the arm back and forth and changing the state of the cell at the tip, it was possible to create "objects" consisting of regions of the two-dimensional cellular automata world which were fully specified by the programme that controlled the constructor.

While this solution demonstrates the theoretical validity of the idea, von Neumann's kinematic constructor (which was not worked out in such detail) has had perhaps a greater influence, for it is a model of general manufacturing which can more easily be adapted to the three-dimensional world in which we live. The kinematic constructor was a robotic arm which moved in three-space and which grasped parts from a sea of parts around it. These parts were then assembled into another kinematic constructor and its associated control computer.

An important point to notice is that self replication, while important, is not by itself an objective. A device able to make copies of itself but unable to make anything else would not be very valuable. Von Neumann's proposals centered around the combination of a universal constructor, which could make anything it was directed to make, and a universal computer, which could compute anything it was directed to compute.

It is this ability to make any one of a broad range of structures under flexible programmatic control that is of value. The ability of the device to make copies of itself is simply a means to achieve low cost, rather than an end in itself.

DREXLER'S ARCHITECTURE FOR AN ASSEMBLER

Drexler's assembler follows the von Neumann kinematic architecture, but is specialized for dealing with systems made of atoms.

The emphasis here (in contrast to von Neumann's proposal) is on small size. The computer and constructor both shrink to the molecular scale, while the constructor takes on additional detail consistent with the desire to manipulate molecular structures with atomic precision.

The molecular constructor has two major subsystems:

1. A positional capability and
2. The tip chemistry.

The positional capability might be provided by one or more small robotic arms, or alternatively might be provided by any one of a wide range of devices that provide positional control[REF09, REF15, REF25]. The emphasis, though, is on a positional device that is very small in scale: perhaps 0.1 microns (100 nanometers) or so in size.

The tip chemistry is logically similar to the ability of the von Neumann universal constructor to alter the state of a cell at the tip of the arm, but now the change in "state" corresponds to a change in molecular structure. That is, we must specify a set of well defined chemical reactions that take place at the tip of the arm, and this set must be sufficient to allow the synthesis of the structures of interest. It is worth noting that current methods in computational chemistry are sufficient to model the kinds of structures that will appear in a broad class of molecular machines, including all of the structures and reactions needed for some assemblers.

SIZE OF DEVICES

Drexler's proposal for molecular mechanical logic [REF06] is the most compact and, from the system point of view, the best worked out. The logic elements ("locks," roughly the equivalent of a single transistor) need occupy a volume of only a few cubic nanometers.

Even including system overhead (power, connections, etc). the volume per element should still be less than 100 cubic nanometers. A 10,000 element logic system (enough to hold a small processor) would occupy a cube no more than 100 nanometers on a side.

That is, a volume only slightly larger than 0.001 cubic microns would be sufficient to hold a small computer. This compares favourably with the volume of a typical cell (thousands of cubic microns) and is even substantially smaller than subcellular organelles.

Operating continuously at a gigahertz such a computer would use less than 10 ^ *-9* watts. By comparison, the human body uses about 100 watts at rest and more during exercise. Slower operation and the use of reversible logic would reduce power consumption, quite possibly dramatically[REF19, REF31]. A variety of molecular sensors and actuators would also fit in such a volume.

A molecular "robotic arm" less than 100 nanometers long should be quite feasible, as well as molecular binding sites 10 nanometers in size or less. By contrast, a single red blood cell is about 8 microns in diameter (over 80 times larger in linear dimensions than our 100 nanometer processor). Devices of the size range suggested above (~0.1 microns) would easily fit in the circulatory system and would even be able to enter individual cells.

CANCER CELLS

Given such molecular tools, we could design a small device able to identify and kill cancer cells. The device would have a small computer, several binding sites to determine the concentration of specific molecules, and a supply of some poison which could be selectively released and was able to kill a cell identified as cancerous. The device would circulate freely throughout the body, and would periodically sample its environment by determining whether the binding sites were or were not occupied.

Occupancy statistics would allow determination of concentration. Today's monoclonal antibodies are able to bind to only a single type of protein or other antigen, and have not proven effective against most cancers. The cancer killing device suggested here could incorporate a dozen different binding sites and so could monitor the concentrations of a dozen different types of molecules. The computer could determine if the profile of concentrations fit a pre-programmed "cancerous" profile and would, when a cancerous profile was encountered, release the poison.

Beyond being able to determine the concentrations of different compounds, the cancer killer could also determine local pressure. A pressure sensor little more than 10 nanometers on a side would be sufficient to detect pressure changes of less than 0.1 atmospheres (a little over a pound per square inch.

See, for example, the discussion on page 472 et sequitur of *Nanosystems*[REF06] for the kind of analysis involved. One atmosphere is ~10^*5* Pascals, so PV in this case would be (0.1 × 10^*5)* × (10^*–8*)^*3* or 10^*4* × 10^ *–24* or 10^*–20* joules. Multiple samples would be required to achieve reliable operation, as kT is ~4 × 10^*–21* joules at body temperature.

Linear increases in sensor volume would produce exponential increases in immunity to thermal noise and linear improvements in pressure sensitivity if that were to prove useful. Doubling the linear dimensions of the sensor would produce an eight-fold increase in both volume and pressure sensitivity).

As acoustic signals in the megahertz range are commonly employed in diagnostics (ultrasound imaging of pregnant women, for example), the ability to detect such signals would permit the cancer killer to safely receive broadcast instructions. By using several macroscopic acoustic signal sources, the cancer killer could determine its location within the body much as a radio receiver on earth can use the transmissions from several satellites to determine its position (as in the widely used GPS system).

Megahertz transmission frequencies would also permit multiple samples of the pressure to be taken from the pressure sensor, as the CPU would be operating at gigahertz frequencies.

The cancer killer could thus determine that it was located in (say) the big toe. If the objective was to kill a colon cancer, the cancer killer in the big toe would not release its poison. Very precise control over location of the cancer killer's activities could thus be achieved.

The cancer killer could readily be reprogrammed to attack different targets (and could, in fact, be reprogrammed via acoustic signals transmitted while it was in the body). This general architecture could provide a flexible method of destroying unwanted structures (bacterial infestations, etc).

OXYGEN

A second application would be to provide metabolic support in the event of impaired circulation. Poor blood flow, caused by a variety of conditions, can result in serious tissue damage. A major cause of tissue damage is inadequate oxygen. A simple method of improving the levels of available oxygen despite reduced blood flow would be to provide an "artificial red blood cell." We will consider a simple design here: a sphere with an internal diameter of 0.1 microns (100 nanometers) filled with high pressure oxygen at ~1,000 atmospheres (about 10^8 pascals).

The oxygen would be allowed to trickle out from the sphere at a constant rate (without feedback). Diamond has a Youngs modulus of about 10 ^ *12* pascals. An atomically precise diamondoid structure should be able to tolerate a stress of greater than 5×10^{10} pascals (5% of the modulus).

Thus, a 0.1 micron sphere of oxygen at a pressure of 10 ^ *8* pascals could be contained by a hollow diamondoid sphere with an internal diameter of 0.1 microns and a thickness of less than one nanometer. This thickness, thin as it is, results in an applied stress on the diamond of well under 1% of its modulus—from a purely structural point of view we should be able to use a very large "bucky ball," i.e., a sphere whose surface is a single layer of graphite.

Perhaps the most complex issue involved in the selection of the material is the reaction of the body's immune system. While some suitable surface structure should exist which does not trigger a response by the immune system—after all, there are many surfaces in the body that are not attacked—the selection of a specific surface structure will require further research.

To give a feeling for the range of possible surface structures, the hydrogenated diamond (111) surface could have a variety of "camouflauge" molecules covalently bound to its surface. A broad range of biological molecules could be anchored to the surface, either directly or via polymer tethers.

The Van der Waals' equation of state is (p+a/v^2) (v–b) = RT, where p is the pressure, v is the volume per mole, R is the universal gas constant, T is the temperature in Kelvins, and a and b are constants specific to the particular gas involved. For oxygen, a = 1.36 atm liter^*2*/mole^*2* and b = 0.03186 liter/mole and R = 0.0820568 liter-atmospheres/mole-kelvin. A mole of oxygen at 1,000 atmospheres and at body temperature (310 Kelvins) occupies 0.048 liters, or about 21 moles/liter. A mole of oxygen at 1 atmosphere and 310 Kelvins occupies 25.4 liters, or about 0.04 moles/liter. This implies a compression of ~530 to 1. A resting human uses ~240 cc/minute of oxygen, so a liter of oxygen compressed to 1,000 atmospheres should be sufficient to maintain metabolism for about 36 hours (a day and a half).

It might be desirable to replace less than a liter of blood with our microspheres of compressed oxygen, but it should still be quite feasible to provide oxygen to tissue even when circulation is severely compromised for periods of at least many hours from a single infusion.

Transport in the "wrong" direction (for this application), but simply reversing the direction of rotor motion would result in transport from inside the reservoir to the external fluid. By driving a rotor at the right speed, oxygen could be released from the internal reservoir into the external environment at the desired rate.

More sophisticated systems would release oxygen only when the measured external partial pressure of oxygen fell below a threshold level, and so could be used as an emergency reserve that would come into play only when normal circulation was (for some reason) interupted.

Full replacement of red blood cells would involve the design of devices able to absorb and compress oxygen when the partial pressure was above a high threshold (as in the lungs) while releasing it when the partial pressure was below a lower threshold (as in tissues using oxygen).

In this case, selective transport of oxygen into an internal reservoir would be required. If a single stage did not provide a sufficiently selective transport system, a multi-staged or cascaded system could be used. Compression of oxygen would presumably require a power system, perhaps taking energy from the combustion of glucose and oxygen (thus permitting free operation in tissue).

Release of the compressed oxygen should allow recovery of a significant fraction of the energy used to compress it, so the total power consumed by such a device need not be great. If the device were to simultaneously absorb carbon dioxide when it was present at high concentrations (in the tissue) and release it when it was at low concentrations (in the lungs), then it would also provide a method of removing one of the major products of metabolic activity.

Calculations similar to those given above imply a human's oxygen intake and carbon dioxide output could both be handled for a period of about a day by about a liter of small spheres. As oxygen is being absorbed by our artificial red blood cells in the lungs at the same time that carbon dioxide is being released, and oxygen is being released in the tissues when carbon dioxide is being absorbed, the energy needed to compress one gas can be provided by decompressing the other. The power system need only make up for losses caused by inefficiencies in this process. These losses could presumably be made small, thus allowing our artificial red blood cells to operate with little energy consumption. By comparison, a liter of blood normally contains ~0.2 liters of oxygen while one liter of our spheres contained ~530 liters of oxygen (where "liter of oxygen" means, as is common in the literature on human oxygen consumption, one liter of the gas under standard conditions of temperature and pressure).

Thus, our spheres are over 2,000 times more efficient per unit volume than blood; taking into account that blood is only about half occupied by red blood cells, our spheres are over 1,000 times more efficient than red blood cells.

Failure of a 0.1 micron sphere would result in creation of a bubble of oxygen less than 1 micron in diameter. Occasional failures could be tolerated. Given the extremely low defect rates projected for nanotechnology, such failures should be very infrequent.

ARTIFICIAL MITOCHONDRIA

While providing oxygen to healthy tissue should maintain metabolism, tissues already suffering from ischemic injury (tissue injury caused by loss of blood flow) might no longer be able to properly metabolize oxygen. In particular, the mitochondria will, at some point, fail. Increased oxygen levels in the presence of nonfunctional or partially functional mitochondria will be ineffective in restoring the tissue. However, more direct metabolic support could be provided.

The direct release of ATP, coupled with selective release or absorption of critical metabolites (using the kind of selective transport system mentioned earlier), should be effective in restoring cellular function even when mitochondrial function had been compromised.

The devices restoring metabolite levels, injected into the body, should be able to operate autonomously for many hours (depending on power requirements, the storage capacity of the device and the release and uptake rates required to maintain metabolite levels).

FURTHER POSSIBILITIES

While levels of critical metabolites could be restored, other damage caused during the ischemic event would also have to be dealt with. In particular, there might have been significant free radical damage to various molecular structures within the cell, including its DNA.

If damage was significant restoring metabolite levels would be insufficient, by itself, to restore the cell to a healthy state. Various options could be pursued at this point. If the cellular condition was deteriorating (unchecked by the normal homeostatic mechanisms, which presumably would cease to function when cellular energy levels fell below a critical value), some general method of slowing further deterioration would be desirable.

Cooling of the tissue, or the injection of compounds that would slow or block deteriorative reactions would be desirable. As autonomous molecular machines with externally provided power could be used to restore function, maintaining function in the tissue itself would no longer be critical. Deliberately turning off the metabolism of the cell to prevent further damage would become a feasible option. Following some interval of reduced (or even absent) metabolic activity during which damage was repaired, tissue metabolism could be restarted again in a controlled fashion. It is clear that this approach should be able to reverse substantially greater damage than can be dealt with today.

A primary reason for this is that autonomous molecular machines using externally provided power would be able to continue operating even when the tissue itself was no longer functional. We would finally have an ability to heal injured cells, instead of simply helping injured cells to heal themselves.

NANOTECHNOLOGY AND MEDICAL RESEARCH

Advances in medical technology necessarily depend on our understanding of living systems. With the kind of devices discussed earlier, we should be able to explore and analyse living systems in greater detail than ever before considered possible. Autonomous molecular machines, operating in the human body, could monitor levels of different compounds and store that information in internal memory.

They could determine both their location and the time. Thus, information could be gathered about changing conditions inside the body, and that information could be tied to both the location and the time of collection. Physical samples of small volumes (nano tissue samples) could likewise be taken. These molecular machines could then be filtered out of the blood supply and the stored information (and samples) could be analysed. This would provide a picture of activities within healthy or injured tissue. This new knowledge would give us new insights and new approaches to curing the sick and healing the injured.

TAKING SNAPSHOTS OF THE ENTIRE SYSTEM

More dramatically, it should be feasible to take "snapshots" of tissue samples and analyse the structure down to the molecular level. First, a small tissue sample could be either fixed or frozen. Chemical fixation can be used to rapidly block most tissue changes. Ultra fast freezing of small tissue samples is an effective method of halting essentially all chemical processes and diffusion of all molecules. Once fixed or frozen, the tissue sample could be analysed in a leisurely fashion. With nanotechnology (and indeed, to some extent with current STM and AFM technologies, though rather more expensively) it should be feasible to scan the tissue surface in molecular detail, and store that information in a computer. Once the surface had been scanned, it could be removed in a very selective and precise fashion, and scanned again.

As an example, the use of a positionally controlled carbene has been proposed for use in the synthesis of complex diamondoid structures [REF06, REF21]. Such a positionally controlled carbene is highly reactive and, if positioned at an appropriate site on the surface of the tissue being analysed, would readily react with a surface molecule.

This surface molecule could then be removed. A wide variety of other "sticky" molecular tools could be brought up to the surface and allowed to react with surface molecules, which could then be removed, exposing the layers beneath. The use of a positionally controlled carbene implies that the environment in which it is used must be inert.

This requirement could be satisfied by analyzing the tissue sample at very low temperature (a few Kelvins) and in a very good vacuum. Under these conditions the tissue specimen would remain stable during even a protracted analysis process.

While this process can readily be envisioned for very small structures, nanotechnology should make massive parallelism feasible. That is, a single positional device could be used at a certain speed to provide information about a certain (rather small) volume of tissue in a reasonable time.

Nanotechnology should permit the manufacture of a large number of small devices, each able to analyse a small volume. Given enough such devices operating in parallel, larger volumes could be analysed and the information from many individual devices integrated to provide a coherent picture of the larger whole. Effective use of this option will require massive computational power—which will also be made feasible with nanotechnology.

Estimates of the computational power that should be provided by nanotechnology exceed 10 ^ *24* logic operations per second for a single desktop computer[REF06]. This amount of raw computational power should make control of a large number of parallel devices feasible, and should permit integration and analysis of the information so obtained. In short, tissue samples could be "frozen" (either literally by ultrafast cooling or figuratively by chemical fixation) and the entire resulting tissue sample could be analysed down to the level of individual molecules.

The information so obtained could be processed by computers able to handle the flood of data produced. The resulting "snapshots" will provide us with an instantaneous look at metabolic and cellular activities across even relatively large volumes of tissue. Such an ability should revolutionize our understanding of the complex processes that take place in living systems.

The possibility of truly revolutionary advances in our medical abilities has also created renewed interest in cryonics. The abilities discussed here might well take years or decades to develop. It is quite natural to ask: "When might we see these systems actually used?" The scientifically correct answer is, of course, "We don't know."

That said, it is worth noting that if progress in computer hardware continues as the trend lines of the last 50 years suggest, we should have some form of molecular manufacturing in the 2010 to 2020 time frame. After this, the medical applications will require some additional time to develop. The remarkably steady trend lines in computer hardware, however, give a false sense that there is a "schedule" and that developments will spontaneously happen at their appointed time.

This is incorrect. How long it will take to develop these systems depends very much on what we do. If focused efforts to develop molecular manufacturing and its medical applications are pursued, we will have such systems well within our lifetimes. If we make no special efforts the schedule will slip, possibly by a great deal.

POSITIONAL CONTROL

Manufactured products are made from atoms. The properties of those products depend on how those atoms are arranged. Viewed from the molecular level today's macroscopic manufacturing methods are crude and imprecise. Casting, milling, welding and all the other traditional manufacturing methods spray atoms about in great statistical herds. Even lithography (which already lets us put millions of transistors on a chip no bigger than your fingernail) is fundamentally statistical and random.

Exactly how many dopant atoms are in a single transistor and exactly where each individual dopant atom is located is neither specified nor known: if we have roughly the right number in roughly the right place, we can make a working transistor. For today, that is good enough.

The exception is chemistry. Large high purity crystals can have almost every atom in the right place. So, too, can many long polymers. The structures of proteins with hundreds and even thousands of amino acids can be specified down to the last atom. Most dramatically (and fortunately for us!) DNA strands with many tens of millions of bases can be copied with almost perfect accuracy.

And it seems that almost any small molecule (with perhaps several dozens of atoms) can be synthesized, if only we have the skill and patience. Yet the laws of physics and chemistry in principle permit arranging and rearranging the elements in so many combinations and permutations that all of our manufacturing skills and all of our chemical skills barely suffice to scratch the surface of what is possible.

THE UTILITY OF DIAMOND

Almost any manufactured product could be improved, often by several orders of magnitude, if we could precisely control its structure at the molecular level. We often want our products to be light and strong. Diamond is light and strong: the strength-to-weight ratio of diamond is over 50 times that of steel. Yet we do not today have diamond spars in airplanes nor diamond hulls for rockets. Today we can't economically make diamond. Even if we could, simple diamond crystals can shatter. We'd have to modify the structure to make it tough and shatter proof: perhaps diamond fibres. While easily done in principle, we can't do this in practice today. Great strength and light weight are not the exclusive province of diamond: graphite can be stronger. And if we consider the many ways in which carbon atoms can be arranged and rearranged, then it's obvious that there are a host of other possibilities.

Yet all share a common problem: we can't yet economically make them in the exact shapes that we want. Great strength is only one property that we prize highly: when we make computers we are more concerned by electrical properties. Here, too, diamond excels.

Today's computers are made of semiconductors, and the semiconductor of choice is silicon. This is not because silicon is the ideal semiconductor from which to make computers, but because we know how to make devices from it. The computer industry has strong opinions about what makes a good logic device and what makes a good computer, and diamond will let us make better computers than silicon.

Diamond has a wider bandgap, hence electrical devices will work at higher temperatures. It has greater thermal conductivity, so devices can be more easily cooled. It has a greater breakdown field, hence devices can be smaller. It has higher electron and hole mobility which, when combined with higher electric fields, will result in higher speed.

But again, we see no diamond computers, just as we see no diamond airplanes: we can't economically manufacture them yet. Large pure crystals of silicon can be made relatively easily, but large pure crystals of diamond are scarce.

We can etch the silicon surface and add dopants with a precision measured in tenths of microns, while the corresponding steps for diamond are more difficult. Not more difficult in principle: just more difficult today.

LONG RANGE COMPLEX ORDER

Making computers highlights another problem. It's not enough to make a pure crystal, it must also have an extremely precise and complex pattern of impurities. The exact location of the dopant atoms in the semiconductor lattice controls how devices function and where signals can propagate. Local order is crucial to make each device work, but long range complex order is crucial to make the computer as a whole work. While we can make some things today that are highly precise and have simple long range order (*e.g.*, crystals), it is the requirement for complex long range order that prevents us from making computers of the kind we'd like to make. While it's plausible we could make high density memory from crystals and perhaps some types of cellular automatons, we couldn't make anything that resembled the computers on the market today.

Today's high speed semiconductor-based digital computers (like the 80486 or the Pentium) have millions of logic elements wired together in complex and highly idiosyncratic patterns. This is well beyond the capabilities of crystal growth or bio-polymer synthesis. It will require a fundamentally new manufacturing technology: molecular manufacturing.

A Gap

Today, there is a gap in our synthetic abilities: we can make complex mechanical machinery and electronic devices (including computers, which have millions of transistors), but we can't make such devices with the precision with which the chemist can synthesize a crystal, a bio-polymer, or a relatively small molecule.

With chemistry we can make precise molecular structures and compounds, but we haven't been able to scale up that success to molecular computers (and other macroscopic products as precise as molecules).

Molecular manufacturing will, by definition, let us economically manufacture almost any specified structure that is consistent with the laws of chemistry and physics. To simplify the problem somewhat we can narrow our focus to structures that resemble diamond in a broad sense: the diamondoid structures as defined by Drexler.

This class includes (among other things) diamond crystals of arbitrary shape but with stably terminated surfaces (*e.g.*, hydrogenated (111) or the like) and with impurities at precise locations in the diamond lattice (*e.g.*, substitutional boron). Our objective is to manufacture particular diamondoid structures once the location and type of every atom has been specified by design.

THE INTEREST OF THE COMPUTER INDUSTRY

The attraction of molecular manufacturing for the computer industry should be clear. It should let us make computers at a manufacturing cost of less than a dollar per pound, operating at frequencies of tens of gigahertz or more, with linear dimensions for a single device of roughly 10 nanometers, high reliability, and energy dissipation (using conventional methods) of roughly 10 ^ –18 joules per logic operation.

If we make thermodynamically reversible computers (which the author and others have recently shown can be made from conventional electronic devices, *e.g.*, CMOS) then the energy dissipation per logic operation can be reduced to well below kT at T = 300 Kelvins (well below 10^–21 joules).

The computer industry is spending billions of dollars to make better computers. It is widely acknowledged within the industry that lithography is approaching its limits. Articles like *The Future of the Transistor, Miniaturization of Electronics and its Limits* and *Outlook for VLSI: Will the Balloon Burst?* quite clearly show that conventional lithography will run out of steam (in perhaps a decade, though there is less agreement about the exact time frame).

There is already interest in molecular logic devices and that interest will increase sharply as improvements in conventional manufacturing methods become increasingly difficult. However, any new proposal for manufacturing molecular computers will be weighed against (at least) the criteria mentioned above. If it cannot easily beat conventional methods after they have been pushed to their uttermost limits, then it will be rejected. The computer industry will soon be pouring vast sums into research aimed at molecular computing, but the great bulk of funding will go towards well thought out proposals that offer a realistic possibility of substantially exceeding the performance of the ultimately evolved silicon VLSI technology that we expect to develop over the next decade. If you can't beat tomorrow's mainstream computers, you might as well not try.

The Problem

For this and many other reasons the class of diamondoid structures is a reasonable one to consider. The problem of building a diamondoid electronic computer captures many of the fundamental issues in molecular manufacturing, and poses clearly the issue of building large structures that cannot be made by regular repetition of some substructure (*e.g.*, the unit cell of a crystal or the monomeric unit in a bio-polymer). This brings us to a core issue in molecular manufacturing: how do we synthesize such things? Today, we can synthesize diamond at low pressure and low temperature by using CVD (Chemical Vapour Deposition) methods. Diamond CVD growth involves highly reactive species (radicals, carbenes, etc.) in a gas over the growing diamond surface that bombard and react with that surface at random. Because reaction sites are random, growth of many defect structures occurs (dislocations, etc.) as well as the desired perfect diamond structure.

Two fundamental mechanisms in the growth process include:

1. Abstraction of hydrogens from the diamond surface leaving behind reactive sites (dangling bonds, radicals) and
2. Interaction of carbon species (both reactive (CH_2, CH_3, etc.) as well as relatively unreactive species (C_2H_2)) with the surface, thus depositing carbon.

If we are to synthesize diamondoid structures it is plausible that we begin our search for the basic reaction steps involved in this synthesis by looking at existing reactions that occur in the CVD growth of diamond. The use of a reactive gas in the synthesis process, however, would seem to defeat any hope of making precisely patterned diamondoid structures, for the gas will interact with the growing surface at random.

POSITIONAL CONTROL IS FUNDAMENTAL

Here, we introduce the fundamental concept of molecular manufacturing: positional control over the site of reactions. To take a specific example we consider site specific hydrogen abstraction from the diamond (111) surface.

The ability to remove specific hydrogen atoms from the surface of the diamondoid work piece under construction is likely to be a fundamental unit operation in any attempt to make atomically precise diamondoid structures.

Hydrogen abstraction during CVD diamond growth typically involves a radical reaction between atomic H from the gas with H bonded to carbon on the surface producing H2.

It is unclear how to make this process site specific. However, there are other structures with a high affinity for hydrogen which offer greater possibilities for positional control. In particular, the propynyl radical C3H3 has a great affinity for hydrogen.

Further, this radical has the very useful property that it has two ends: one end is a highly reactive radical while the other end is a stable sp3 carbon. Thus, we could synthesize a larger molecule with the propynyl radical at its end. The larger molecule would be held at the tip of a positional device.

The positional device would provide control over the orientation and position of this hydrogen abstraction tool (*e.g.*, a six degrees of freedom manipulator) and thus control the site of abstraction by controlling the position of the tool.

Ab initio quantum chemical analysis of the abstraction of hydrogen from isobutane using an ethynyl abstraction tool supports the idea that the barrier to this reaction is zero. The reaction will proceed rapidly and, because of the large exothermicity, irreversibly. Calculated barriers for abstraction from several other molecules were also small, suggesting that this hydrogen abstraction tool could be used to abstract hydrogen from a wide range of different molecules. Molecular dynamics simulations provide evidence that the abstraction reaction will select the correct hydrogen atom in the face of thermal noise at room temperature, as well as providing further support for the basic mechanism.

The site specific abstraction of hydrogen illustrates the core concept in molecular manufacturing: selecting the reaction site by controlling the position and orientation of the reactants. The (relatively stiff) diamondoid workpiece is held in place, while a tool (in our example, a hydrogen abstraction tool) is positioned using a rather conventional (if also rather small) robotic arm.

The ideas of using tools, controlling the position of those tools with a general purpose manipulator, and building complex structures by putting together components using those positionally controlled tools are rather common and even mundane at the macroscopic level. At the molecular level, they are new and almost shocking: yet it is simply mapping onto the molecular world the concepts and ideas that have proven so useful and powerful in macroscopic manufacturing. By adding positional control we should be able to develop a method of molecular manufacturing which combines the best features of both conventional macroscopic manufacturing and chemical synthesis.

OTHER MOLECULAR TOOLS

If we are to grow diamond, we must also have carbon deposition tools. Drexler has suggested the use of positionally controlled carbenes and alkynes and proposed reaction pathways and surface structures where these tools would apply.In both cases, the tools are positioned at a precise point on the growing diamondoid structure and are used to deposit one or more carbon atoms at a desired location.

These deposition reactions parallel proposals in the CVD literature except for the addition of positional control (*e.g.*, at least one portion of the moiety must be part of an extended "handle" which can be held by a positional device). These are only two examples from the wide range of tools that are capable of depositing carbon on a surface. The broad range of possible tools coupled with the great power of ab initio computational chemistry should let us define and verify a complete set of molecular tools capable of synthesizing essentially any diamondoid structure. The work by Musgrave et. al. and Sinnott et. al. are first steps towards this objective. Modern ab initio methods can produce results that are sufficiently accurate for this type of analysis. Further research in this area is feasible and should be pursued.

THE CONTEXT OF TOOL USE

For such tools to be usable in a system context we must satisfy certain constraints. First and foremost, we must have a device capable of positioning the tool to within something like an atomic diameter. On the diamond (111) surface, the distance between adjacent hydrogens is about 2.5 Angstroms.

Thus, positional accuracy of 1 to 2 angstroms for the hydrogen abstraction tool is required to prevent abstraction of the wrong hydrogen. Second, because the tools can be highly reactive, we require an inert environment. A simple inert environment is vacuum. Compressed helium or some other inert gas would also work. Third, because it is the relative tool-workpiece position that must be controlled, the workpiece under construction must be relatively rigid (*e.g.*, not subject to vibrational motions that would exceed about an angstrom). Fourth and last, we must have some way of generating the sometimes highly reactive tools (*e.g.*, we need to define a precursor to the hydrogen abstraction tool, as well as precursors to the other tools).

In some sense, the analysis that we will now pursue is similar in type to retrosynthetic analysis. We start with the final product that we wish to build (a macroscopic diamondoid computer, for example), and then consider the possible predecessor structures which would yield the final product in one step. Then we consider the predecessor structures to those structures, and so on. We extend retrosynthetic analysis beyond its traditional bounds, but the general concept remains the same: given the finished product we deduce the possible ways in which it could have been constructed. This approach has been called "backwards chaining" by Drexler.

Positional Devices and Molecular "Arms"

Work with SPMs (Scanning Probe Microscopes) clearly show that it is possible to achieve positional accuracies of a small fraction of an angstrom. Small (~0.1 microns) diamondoid "arms" or positional devices with similar positional accuracy are in principle quite feasible.

The field of robotics provides a broad range of designs for positional devices which are largely scale independent. Shrinking these designs to submicron size is conceptually straightforwards.

A factor of crucial importance in the design of molecular-scale positional devices is the accuracy with which the tip can be positioned, particularly in the face of thermal noise. While atomically precise bearings and joints will not suffer from chatter, backlash, wear, tooth-to-tooth errors and other sources of inaccuracy caused by imprecise manufacturing, they will still suffer from positional errors caused by thermal noise. To control this source of error, it is essential that the robotic arm be very stiff, and so the use of stiff materials is desirable.

The Young's modulus for diamond is about 10 ^ 12 Pascals (very stiff), and back-of-the-envelope calculations show that a hollow cylinder of such material that is perhaps 100 nanometers long and 30 nanometers in diameter should have a positional accuracy at the tip, in the face of thermal noise at room temperature, of a small fraction of an atomic diameter.

A more detailed design and analysis of a jointed tubular robotic arm taking into account the bending and rocking motions of joints in the arm further supports this conclusion. Alternatives to the simple robotic arm are available which might be more attractive.

Other Requirements for Tool Use

Creating an inert environment also presents no fundamental problems: high quality vacuums are common in laboratories today. If our objective is to have a very small very high quality vacuum, then a relatively thin wall of diamondoid material could be used as a barrier to keep a volume which was a modest fraction of a cubic micron free of any contaminants.

If the volume were initially constructed free of contaminants then such a barrier would keep the inside free of any contaminants with high probability. Because we are building diamondoid structures, they will be very stiff. As a consequence, it is relatively easy to meet the requirement that the objects that are being manufactured must themselves be stiff. Finally, generation of "activated" tools from relatively stable precursors can be done by a variety of methods. Because we are assuming an environment in which we have positional control we can use particularly simple precursors.

If we pull on the two handles with sufficient force, something will break. Because the X–C bond was deliberately selected to be weaker than the other bonds in the structure, it will break. This gives us the activated hydrogen abstraction tool. A related question is: how can we get the hydrogen off the tip of the abstraction tool? A simple answer is: don't. Throw the tool away after one use. In a system design using this approach, it would be necessary to provide a continuous stream of precursors. These would be activated, used once, and then discarded.

A more elegant approach would be to remove the hydrogen from the tip and recycle the tool, as discussed by Drexler and Musgrave et. al. More generally the activation of relatively stable precursors can be done by using any of several forms of energy: mechanical, optical, chemical or other. While the use of mechanical means to provide the activation energy for chemical reactions is relatively novel, in an environment where positional control is already available it is quite natural.

SELECTIVE TRANSPORT ACROSS A BARRIER

Having introduced a diamondoid barrier to keep unwanted contaminants out (much as the bacterial wall allows bacteria to maintain an appropriate internal environment in the face of a fluctuating external environment) we must now solve the problem of getting desired raw materials through the barrier.

We might, for example, wish to transport the hydrogen abstraction tool precursor across the diamondoid barrier. After use we will also need to eject the spent tool.

Several ways to solve this problem are feasible. A proposal by Drexler is to use a rotor embedded in the diamondoid wall which moves binding sites from the outside of the wall to the inside of the wall. By modulating the affinity of the binding site so that it will have high affinity for the desired molecule outside the barrier and low affinity inside the barrier, efficient transport across the barrier can be achieved.

The desired molecule will bind to the binding site when it is outside the barrier, the binding site will be rotated to the inside of the barrier and the binding affinity reduced (in the illustrated proposal by mechanically pushing a rod into the binding site, thus physically precluding occupancy), and the molecule will be released on the inside of the barrier.

The result is to increase the concentration of the desired molecule. A few stages of such a filtration system can achieve extremely high purities. The final stage, rather than ejecting the molecule into a liquid, would deliver the molecule into the inert internal environment in a well defined orientation where it could be further processed.

One simple method of further processing would be for the oriented molecule to be directly transferred to the tip of the positional device.

CONTROL SIGNALS

Finally, we will need a source of control signals for our molecular arm. One general approach would be to use a molecular computer. We will not consider a particular design for a molecular computer here, it is sufficient to note that many proposals for molecular computation have been considered in the literature and it is generally expected that some type of very small computational device will be feasible in a few decades.

This completes our (all too brief) outline of a small device able to manufacture a broad class of diamondoid materials. Basically, the design is driven by the desire to provide the environment needed to synthesize diamond and diamondoid materials using the kinds of reactions that occur naturally during CVD growth of diamond. The device is itself made from diamondoid materials, which means that one such device can manufacture a second such device.

This ability to self replicate is crucial in achieving low manufacturing costs. As the reader might appreciate, the design and construction of one such general purpose device might well prove to be a time consuming and expensive undertaking. This cost cannot be justified unless the resulting device has great value.

If the device can self replicate then the successful design and development of one such device can be used to build an entirely new manufacturing technology. The manufacturing costs for the second, third, fourth.... 10 ^ 10.... etc. devices will consist largely of the raw materials and energy costs. Thus, a very large R&D cost can (if necessary) be justified.

A number of technical issues involved in self replicating systems are discussed in *Self Replicating Systems and Molecular Manufacturing* while some of the obvious safety issues are discussed in *The Risks of Nanotechnology*.

REVERSIBLE LOGIC

In a conventional computer the logical state of the system at time t (denoted S_t) will uniquely determine the state of the system at time t+1. If the function F maps the system state onto the successor state, then $S_{t+1} = F(S_t)$.

The requirement that the successor of a state be unique can be expressed as: if $F(S_t)$!= $F(S'_t)$, then S_t != S'_t. In a logically reversible system, the state of the system at time t will uniquely determine the state of the system at both time t–1 and t+1. This can be expressed as: if $F(S_t)$!= $F(S'_t)$, then S_t != S'_t *and* if $F^{-1}(S_t)$!= $F^{-1}(S'_t)$, then S_t != S'_t. By contrast, in an irreversible system it will sometimes be the case that $F^{-1}(S_t)$!= $F^{-1}(S'_t)$ and $S_t = S'_t$. That is, a given state might have two (or more) distinct and different predecessor states.

This neglects any special handling that might be required for the initial and final states of the computation. The initial logical state might not have a predecessor, and the final logical state might not have a successor. Alternatively, the predecessor of the initial state might be the final state, and the successor of the final state might be the initial state (i.e., the computation could be a giant loop). These states are rare in most computations.

The laws of physics are fully reversible at the microscopic scale, and so a physical system implementing a logically irreversible system is faced with a problem: when the logically irreversible system maps two logical states onto a single result state, the physical system must somehow map two physical states onto a single result state, as well. This, of course, is impossible (for the underlying laws of physics are reversible, and hence the physical system is reversible), and so something has to give.

In today's computational systems, a single logical state will be represented not by a single physical state, but by any one of several possible physical states (which differ from each other in only trivial ways). We can rephrase this by saying that each logical state of the system is represented by a certain volume of phase space, *e.g.*, by a certain range of possible physical states.

When we perform a logically irreversible operation and merge logical states, we must either compress the representation in phase space or increase the volume of phase space that represents a logical state.

If we ban indefinite growth in phase space then we are forced (at some point) to compress the phase space representation of the logical state. Phase space, however, is incompressible (which corresponds to the statement that merging two physical states is impossible, for the laws of physics are reversible). As a consequence, irreversible operations force an increase in the volume of phase space occupied by the system. However, if the allowed computational degrees of freedom in the system are not allowed to expand, then this increase in phase space must take place in the non-computational degrees of freedom, *e.g.*, waste heat.

Because mapping two logical states onto a single output state effectively erases a bit of information, the fact that irreversible logic must dissipate heat can also be stated as: erasing information must dissipate heat. Erasing a single bit of information generates at least ln(2) x kT joules of heat. By contrast a logically reversible system can be mapped onto the reversible physical world without the mismatch that occurs with logically irreversible systems. There is no need to compress phase space, and the mapping between logical and physical representations need not perform a basically non-physical act, *e.g.*, the erasure of information. As a consequence, there is no fundamental need to dissipate heat during the course of a computation.

This discussion of reversible logic has been given in terms of a computing system, rather than in terms of individual logic elements. This avoids a problem which can cause confusion: one and the same logic element can be viewed as either reversible or as irreversible, depending on the system context in which it is used. For example, AND gates are often cited as "irreversible" logic devices.

As commonly implemented and used, AND gates are indeed irreversible. However, it is possible to use some types of AND gates in a reversible fashion. All we need to do is insure that the operation of the AND gate takes place in a system context which does not erase information.

If the two inputs to an AND gate are erased following computation of the result then we must dissipate heat. If, however, the two inputs are *not* erased, then we have *not* erased any information and the computation need not be irreversible nor fundamentally dissipative.

This is a general principle: any irreversible combinational function F can be embedded in a larger reversible function F'. We might define F' as: $F'(x) = <x,F(x)>$. The new function F' simply computes F and then concatenate the input x onto the output, insuring that we have not erased information.

We could, if convenient, retain even more information. If, during the course of computing F, we happen to compute various intermediate results $i_0, i_1 \ldots i_n$, then we could retain these intermediate results as well. We could define

$$F'' = <x, i_0, i_1 \ldots i_n, F(x)>.$$

F" is also reversible, and by keeping the additional information its implementation might be simplified. As a consequence it is possible (in the proper context) to use AND and OR operations in a reversible computation. The physical instantiation of such a logical computation can be done in a way which preserves local reversibility and is asymptotically nondissipative. Later in this paper we will sometimes compute irreversible functions F in a manner which is logically and thermodynamically reversible.

The actual implementation is done by retaining the intermediate values of the computation, as well as the input. This insures logical reversibility. In actual fact, the computation of F has been embedded in the computation of F", where F" is logically reversible. In summary, reversible computations are consistent with the basic laws of physics at a microscopic scale, while irreversible computations are in some sense fundamentally incompatible.

The price we must pay for this incompatibility is heat. If we don't want to pay the price then we must learn to compute in harmony with the natural laws of physics, *e.g.*, we must learn how to design reversible computers.

MECHANICAL COMPUTATION

The earliest example of a mechanical computer is Babbage's Analytical Engine. This device, had it been built, would have carried out the functions of a rather conventional computer but would have done so mechanically.

Remarkably, it was designed in the early 1800's. A working model of the simpler Difference Engine No. 2 was recently built by the British Museum of Science from Babbage's original blueprints using parts that would have been available in the 1800's, both in terms of the materials used and the precision of the milling.

A more recent reason for interest in mechanical logic has been that several proposals for reversible computation were basically mechanical in nature. Two mechanical designs that are well known in the reversible logic community are Fredkins "billiard ball" model of computation and Bennett's "Brownian Clockwork Turing Machine".

Drexler's "rod logic" also implements combinational logic in a reversible manner. In the billiard ball model, billiard balls are fired into the computer and their ballistic trajectory—they bounce off each other and off fixed "mirrors"-defines an arbitrary reversible computation. This is an example of a computation which dissipates as little energy as desired while rapidly computing an answer. In the clockwork Turing machine, the state of the computation can "drift" either forwards or backwards, subject to a small "driving force."

The energy dissipation can be made arbitrarily small by making the driving force smaller and smaller, though at the cost of reducing the computational speed.

More recently there has been interest in mechanical logic devices because:

- It should be possible to scale them to the molecular size range,
- At such sizes the speed of operation becomes reasonable (sub nanosecond switching times) and
- Analyzing molecular mechanical logic devices is relatively simple (an important point when the devices can't yet be built).

Further, it should be possible to make molecular mechanical devices that are much smaller than molecular electronic devices (though the ultimate speed of operation of molecular mechanical devices will almost certainly be slower than that of molecular electronic devices).

TRENDS IN ENERGY DISSIPATION

Whether mechanical, electronic, electromechanical, or whatever; the trends in energy dissipation will drive computer hardware ever more strongly towards the use of reversible computation. For the last 50 years the energy dissipation per gate operation has been declining with remarkable regularity.

Extrapolation of this trend shows the energy dissipation per device operation reaching kT (where k is Boltzmann's constant and T is the temperature in Kelvin) by the year 2015. (This assumes that T is 300 Kelvin-more on this later). To gain some perspective on this consider that an "AND" gate which has a power supply of one volt and which allows a single electron to go from that one volt supply to ground during the course of a switching operation, will dissipate one electron volt.

Although one electron volt is about forty times kT (and well above the theoretical limit), it will be difficult for simple improvements of current devices to reach even this level of energy dissipation. Extrapolating present trends, we should reach forty kT between the year 2000 and 2010, *e.g.*, within ten to twenty years.

As a consequence, we can state quite confidently that one of three things will occur:

- The historic rate of decreasing energy dissipation per device operation will slow or halt in the next one or two decades or
- We will operate computers at lower temperatures or
- We will develop new, novel, reversible computer systems that can beat the kT barrier.

The first option is quite unattractive. The heroic cooling methods used in the Cray 3 supercomputer to remove the heat generated by the computer's operation suggest that failure to reduce energy dissipation per gate operation would be a major limiting factor in future computer performance.

Further, although the raw cost of electrical power is not yet a major limitation, it would become so in the future if reductions in energy dissipation did not keep pace with advances in other areas.

The Wall Street Journal said "Computer systems currently account for 5% of commercial electricity use in the U.S., with the potential to grow to 10% by the year 2000." The second option will not reduce overall energy dissipation. If we operated future devices at 3 Kelvin we could reduce energy dissipation by a factor of 100-but for fundamental thermodynamic reasons the coefficient of performance of the refrigerator for the system can be at best 3K/(300K–3K ~ 0.01. Thus, the lower energy required per gate operation will be balanced by the increased energy needed by the refrigerator.

Further, in many applications low temperature operation is not an option. The use of liquid nitrogen in laptop computers or many embedded applications is not attractive. However, factors other than net energy savings can make low temperature operation worthwhile. Some potentially attractive devices don't operate at higher temperatures: they have to be refrigerated or they don't work. A large mainframe computer made from such devices and operated at a low temperature might be the most economical method of delivering computational power in some cases. Refrigeration *per se*, however, does not seem too attractive. Finally, and most attractively, we could develop reversible logic devices. Such devices would, in theory, allow energy dissipations indefinitely below kT per logic operation. While *some* barrier will likely eventually be encountered, the use of reversible logic should allow us to continue current trends in energy dissipation per logic operation for the longest possible time. Further research in this area is the most appropriate response to the rather limited range of possibilities that face us.

REVERSIBLE COMPUTER ARCHITECTURES

One problem is the need to develop novel "reversible" computer architectures. Such architectures have been discussed elsewhere. A wide variety of computations can be done in a reversible manner. Bennett concluded: "...for any $e > 0$, ordinary multitape Turing machines using time T and space S can be simulated by reversible ones using time $O(T^{1+e})$ and space $O(S \log T)$ or in linear time and space $O(ST^e)$."

Even if we do not adopt new and novel computer architectures, simple applications of reversible computation could be made within the framework of existing architectures. A typical computer executes a sequence of instructions, and each instruction will typically change the contents of a single register or memory operation. Although loading the result of the instruction into a register will normally be irreversible (it destroys the previous contents of the register) it is still the case that all *other* operations performed by the computer during instruction execution could in principle be made reversible.

Thus, although we would have to dissipate roughly kT energy for each bit in the output register for each instruction execution, we need not use energy-dissipative logic devices throughout the computer. We can go one step further without making any changes in computer architecture: the simple register-register add instruction R1 = R1 + R2 is logically reversible. With proper hardware, this particular instruction could in principle be made to dissipate as little energy as we desired.

While irreversible instructions (*e.g.*, R1 = 0) would still dissipate greater energy, the overall energy dissipation of the computer could be reduced significantly if a reversible system were developed and used to implement the reversible instructions. Of course, once the energy-wasting irreversible instructions were identified, compilers would learn to avoid using them. This would provide an entirely evolutionary path from the current irreversible designs to computer architectures that were as reversible as was practically feasible. While there is debate about how far this trend can go it is clear that a significant percentage of computer operations can be made reversible-perhaps a remarkably high percentage.

SOME OTHER PROPOSALS

To be successful, we must develop appropriate fully reversible switching devices that are physically realizable. We shall use the term "physically realizable" to mean "implementable by an appropriate configuration of atoms."

Many of the earlier proposals do not appear to be physically realizable, although recent reversible proposals, particularly those based on conventional technologies such as CMOS or CCD's, are very clearly physically realizable.

An early electronic proposal by Likharev based on Josephson junctions"...is particularly significant, because it is a genuine example... of a system that has frictional forces proportional to velocity" according to Landauer. Likharev's "parametric quantron" is directly analogous to the second proposal made later in this paper. The parametric quantron is based on Josephson junctions and operates at low temperatures. Modern "high temperature" superconductors should allow operation at liquid nitrogen temperatures (although Josephson junctions have not yet been demonstrated to work at that temperature), but the low temperature of operation is still a significant disadvantage.

The parametric quantron uses magnetic fields to transmit logic information from device to device. It cannot be scaled to the size range considered here for molecular mechanical devices, and the speed-power trade-off in the parametric quantron might not be significantly better than the speed-power trade-off in molecular mechanical devices.

The first proposal discussed here is derived from the work of Drexler, who has argued persuasively that mechanical logic devices can be scaled to the molecular level. The scaling properties of current electronic devices are unlikely to be as good. Drexler's proposed "rod logic" is also reversible. Drexler concluded that rod logic, when scaled to molecular size, should eventually be able to achieve an energy dissipation of somewhat less than kT at 300 Kelvins with gate delay times of 50 picoseconds.

Reducing the speed of operation would further reduce energy dissipation. Drexler, however, also argues that electronic devices will very likely prove superior in speed of operation, a conclusion supported by recent work by Merkle and Drexler. The primary reason for pessimism about the speed of mechanical logic is that the nuclei of atoms have greater mass than electrons, and so any device which depends on movement of the nuclei seems doomed to be slower than a device that uses the motions of electrons.

The carbon nucleus is over 20,000 times as massive as an electron, and will normally accelerate roughly 20,000 times more slowly. An alternative view is that the speed of sound in solids is roughly 10^4 meters per second, whereas the speed of electronic signals is roughly 10^8 meters per second.

Speed is not the only important criterion for evaluating logic devices. If small size is the deciding criterion then molecular mechanical reversible logic is more attractive. Small size might make it competitive for some applications (high density memory, for example) where speed is not paramount. While the greater mass of nuclei as compared with electrons results in slower speed, it also greatly reduces the distance through which the nuclei can tunnel.

One of the major limitations in scaling electronic devices to the smallest possible size is the ability of electrons to tunnel distances of a few nanometers. By contrast, devices whose function depends on the position of nuclei can be scaled to linear dimensions of two nanometers or less. It might be that an electronic device only two nanometers across will be forever infeasible because a single electron can tunnel this distance (though such a claim must be viewed with caution).

Thus, molecular mechanical devices might enjoy a fundamental advantage in terms of small size. Another limitation of mechanical devices is the sliding motion of one surface upon another.

This is not a significant problem if atomically perfect surfaces can be used as Drexler assumes, but current manufacturing techniques are not able to achieve this level of perfection. Drexler and others have argued that we will eventually be able to build most physically realizable structures, including complex molecular logic elements which are atomically precise. While electromechanical logic devices employing sliding silicon parts have been built and are radiation resistant, the friction and wear caused when imperfect silicon surfaces slide over each other is a major drawback.

As we will demonstrate, a mechanical logic device need not involve a sliding motion of one surface past another. Elimination of the sliding motion results in several advantages. First, it simplifies the analysis of molecular-scale mechanical logic devices.

Because such devices cannot be built with current technology, any claims about their performance must rest on theoretical analysis.

By eliminating the sliding motion the analysis becomes simpler and more fool proof. A second more practical advantage is the elimination of the sliding motion when larger devices are built with current technology. The use of non-sliding logic in silicon eliminates the wear and friction that the sliding action creates. The energy dissipation of the device can therefore be substantially reduced, and the operational lifetime extended.

BASIC IDEA

Drexler's rod logic is based on the observation that two objects cannot occupy the same place at the same time. If two objects both have parts that can occupy the same place when the objects move, then the motion of one object can be used to limit the motion of the other. In rod logic the interacting objects are rods and the parts that interact are called "knobs.". Normally, a rod has one degree of mechanical freedom: it can move back and forth along its own axis. Two rods that are set at right angles to each other can interact if they can be moved so that their "knobs" can occupy the same position.

This common region of space that both knobs can attempt to occupy is called the "lock." One rod can be moved so that its knob occupies the lock, but when this is attempted with the second rod, the knobs will collide and the motion of the second rod will be blocked. The first knob to reach the lock is the "gate knob," and the second knob is the "probe knob." Using this terminology, if the gate knob occupies the lock, the probe knob is blocked and thus the motion of the second rod is also blocked.

The rods must be constrained in their motions so that they cannot move except along the specified axis, nor rotate and change the location of the knob. Either of these illegal motions would let one rod slip past the other and cause a logic failure. Drexler constrained the rods by embedding them in a "matrix," a solid block of material with "channels" in which the rods are obliged to slide.

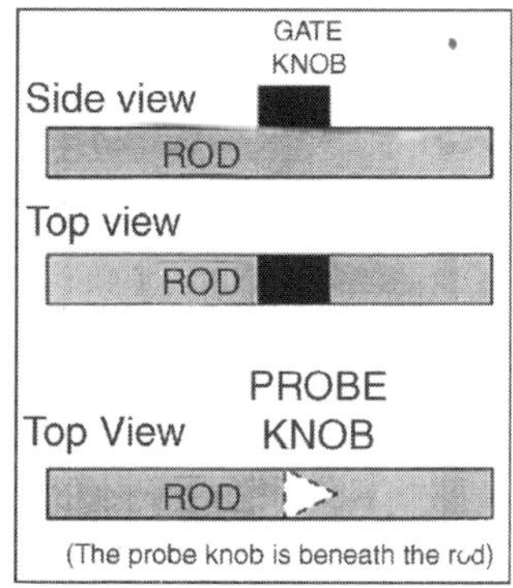

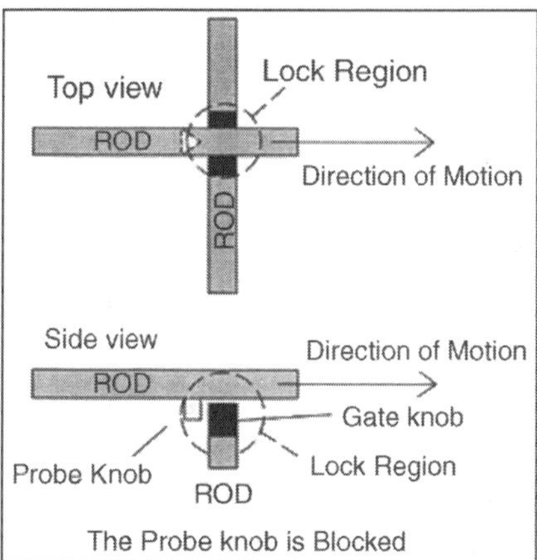

We eliminate the matrix by the simple expedient of mounting the rods on flexible supports, which hold the rods in position. When a rod is pulled, the supports are elastically deformed (which allows rod motion).

If the supports prevent lateral motion of the second rod then the collision of the probe knob with the gate knob will block the further motion of the probe knob. If the supports do not sufficiently prevent lateral motion of the second rod during the collision, then a fixed "lock support" can be placed behind the lock to prevent the gate knob from being pushed out of position by the force of the probe knob.

The probe knob would then force the gate knob against the lock support, and the further motion of the probe knob would be prevented. The elastic supports are illustrated only in figure. For the sake of clarity, further illustrations of non-sliding logic will not show the elastic supports.

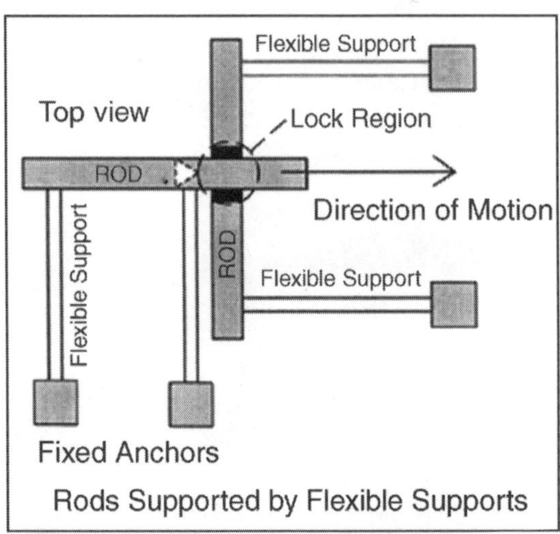

Rods Supported by Flexible Supports

However, the reader should presume that each rod is held in position by an appropriate set of supports, even though they are not shown. The length of the rods must also be controlled. Stretching of the rods would change the positions of the gate knobs.

Should the gate knobs move a sufficient distance from their correct location from this cause, even though they continued to move only in the channel, the probe knobs would slip past them.

While stretching is usually insignificant at the macroscopic scale, it is significant and must be taken into account on the molecular scale. Drexler reduced this source of error by applying tension to the ends of the rods. When this is done the material from which the "rods" are made can be both flexible and compressible, and might be better described as string. The term "rod" should thus be viewed with some caution, as many rather un-rod-like structures can be used quite effectively.

Rod logic is somewhat different from many popular logic systems. In most current systems, the output signal from a typical gate is available shortly after the input signals are applied. This does not occur in rod logic, which is fundamentally a clocked system.

Rods do not move unless pulled, and only when a rod is pulled can we tell if it is blocked or unblocked. The output signal is not available until after the input signals are applied and the output rod is pulled. For this reason, the temporal pattern used to pull the rods (the clocking sequence) is of critical importance in the operation of a rod-logic circuit.

At each point in time a given rod can be:

- Pulled or
- Released or
- Left unchanged.

If it is pulled, it either moves or does not move, depending on whether or not the locks associated with the rod are blocked or unblocked. Because the rod might or might not move when it is pulled, it is convenient to put a spring between the rod and the source of the motion used to pull the rod. This spring is called the "drive spring." The source of motion is called the "driver." If the rod does not move when the driver moves, then the drive spring extends. Although we refer to "releasing" the rod, a better description might be "unpulling" the rod. The force applied to the rod should be gradually relaxed and the rod gradually allowed to resume its original position to minimize energy dissipation.

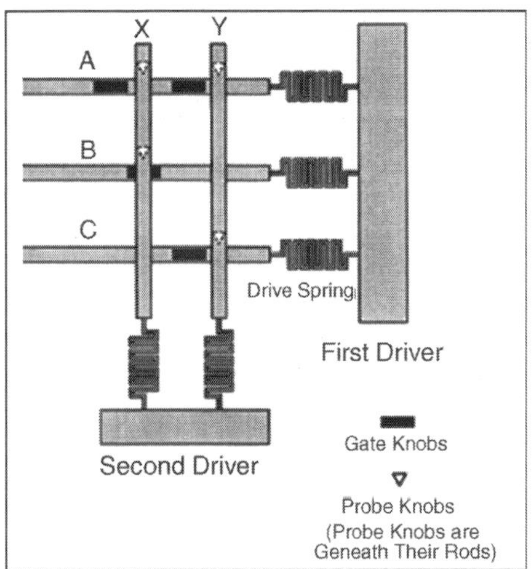

We now give an example of a complete cycle of operation for a simple logic function. Three inputs, A, B, and C, enter from the left along the three horizontal rods. The first driver is on the right, and three drive springs connect rods A, B, and C to the driver.

Two outputs, X and Y, exit downwards along the two vertical rods. Two drive springs connect the bottoms of the rod to the top of the second driver. At the intersection of each horizontal rod with each vertical rod, there can be a lock. Note that each lock can initially be either blocked (occupied by the gate knob) or unblocked (not occupied by the gate knob).

The cycle of operations proceeds as follows. First, the first driver moves to the right. This applies force to the three rods A, B, and C through the three drive springs. Rods B and C are free to move, while rod A is blocked (by a lock not shown on the diagram). The drive spring for rod A extends, while the drive springs for rods B and C do not. The motion of rods B and C unblocks the gate at the intersection of B and X, but blocks the gate at the intersection of C and Y.

The two locks controlled by rod A continue to be unblocked. This is illustrated in Figure. Second, the second driver moves downwards. This applies force to the two output rods X and Y. X is free to move, and does so, while Y is blocked. The drive spring for Y extends.

This is illustrated in Figure. Third, the second driver is released and rods X and Y resume their original positions. Fourth, the first driver is released and rods A, B and C resume their original positions.

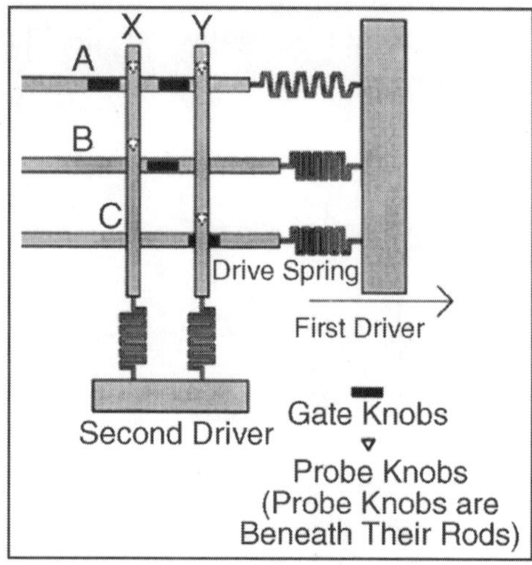

Note that cycles 1 and 2 compute an output, while cycles 3 and 4 reverse the motions involved in cycles 1 and 2, thereby "uncomputing" the output. Therefore this clocked sequence of actions is entirely reversible.

The energy dissipation per operation could, in principle, be made less than kT. If we attempted to change this sequence, *e.g.*, we interchanged cycles 3 and 4 and released driver 1 before releasing driver 2, then the probe knob and gate knob would slide past each other at the lock at the intersection of C and Y. That is, the wrong sequence of clock signals would introduce sliding motion.

The clock sequence in rod logic must be carefully specified to prevent this kind of problem. In general, if we have an N level logic circuit, then we will need to divide the rods into N groups numbered from 1 to N. Each rod in a group will be connected to the corresponding driver.

The drivers will be moved in sequence, starting with driver 1 and terminating with driver N.

The rods in group i will control the motion of the rods in group i+1. After the Nth level rods have been pulled, the drivers will be released in reverse sequence, starting with driver N and terminating with driver 1. What has been described so far will allow the construction of an N level reversible combinational logic circuit.

To be useful, we must also specify a latch which can store the output of the combinational circuit. This can be done relatively easily by modifying the basic rod logic design described so far. We define a set of "latch rods" which, in essence, are the N+1st logic level rods.

For pedagogical purposes we will refer to the Nth level rods as either "Nth level rods" or "output rods," whichever seems clearer. In essence, the latch rods are used to "latch up" or remember the state of the output rods. The proper latch rods will be moved when the output rods move. The latch rods will then be locked into position. This arrangement is described in more detail in the next few paragraphs.

Each output rod will be lengthened and a new "drive knob" will be added near the end away from the drive spring.

A "drive knob" is a knob whose purpose is to pull a "driven knob," and in consequence to move the rod to which the driven knob is attached, also called the "driven rod."

The driven rod, like all rods, will move along its axis. As a consequence, the driver rod and the driven rod must be parallel, for the motion of the drive rod will be transferred directly to the driven rod.

The action of the driver knob is unlike the action of either a "probe knob," which is used to determine whether or not a lock is blocked, or a "gate knob," which is used to block and unblock a lock.

The drive knob on the output rod will be used to pull on the driven knob which is attached to the latch rod. In this case, the output rod is the driver rod and the latch rod is the driven rod. The latch rod is parallel to the output rod, not at right angles.

If the output rod is pulled and moves, then the driver knob on the output rod will pull on the driven knob on the latch rod, and the latch rod will also be pulled. Because the latch rod will not be blocked, it will also move.

Once the latch rods have been moved into their proper positions, they are held in place by the "holding rod." The holding rod is at right angles to the latch rods, and is always free to move. The holding rod has gate knobs at all positions. All the locks between the latch rods and the holding rod are initially unblocked.

After the latch rods are in their correct position, the holding rod moves and all the gate knobs on the holding rod block all the gates. In those latch rods which have not moved, the probe knob on the latch rod is clear of the lock and has not moved through it.

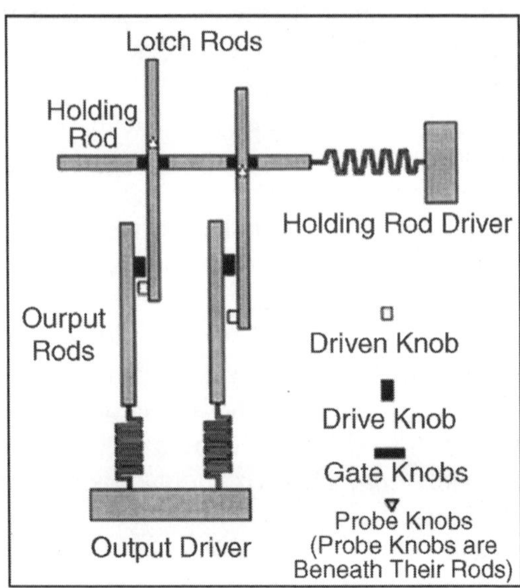

On those latch rods which have moved, the probe knob has been moved through the lock and is also clear of it.

Thus, in either case, the holding rod is free to move and the gate knobs on the holding rod can occupy all the corresponding locks. Once the locks are blocked, the output driver is released. The output rods move back to their original positions.

Those latch rods that were moved are now held in place by the gate knobs on the holding rod and cannot return to their original positions. The output rods are free to move at this point in the cycle, whether or not the latch rods have been blocked, because the motion of the driver knobs on the output rods is now away from the driven knobs.

Although this method will correctly latch up the output, it now presents the problem of releasing the holding rod driver and restoring the holding rod to its original position.

If we simply release the holding rod driver, then the probe knobs on the latch rods which bear upon the gate knobs on the holding rod will cause friction when the holding rod moves. This will work, but will result in greater energy dissipation both because of the friction between the probe knobs and gate knobs and because the energy stored in the latch rod supports will be dissipated when the latch rods spring free.

The latch rod supports are, in effect, springs that attempt to restore the latch rod to its "normal" position.

When the latch rod probe knobs are unblocked as the holding rod gate knobs move out of the locks, the latch rod will snap back to this position and oscillate, thus dissipating energy.

This is in keeping with the irreversible nature of the operation: the information held in the latch rods will be destroyed, which requires dissipation of about kT per latch rod. A more clever method would be to "unwrite" the information held in the latch rods.

This differs fundamentally from erasing the information. In this technique, the information held in the latch rods is recomputed (by any method we might find convenient) and the output rods are driven with this freshly recomputed information. This recomputed information is identical to the actual contents of the latch. In this way, the pressure on the holding rod gate knobs will be released, and the holding rod will again be free to move. The holding rod driver can then be released, and the output driver (and all preceding drivers) can be released as usual. The information in the latch rods is "unwritten" in a reversible manner (no step in the unwriting process destroys information) and the energy dissipated per latch rod operation can in principle be less than kT during this process.

This allows us to remember the value computed by a combinational logic circuit in a set of latches. With some additional mechanism, we can compute an iterated reversible computation. This will allow us to perform the more or less normal sequence of operations in a computer. That is, the state of a computation in a normal CPU is held in a series of latches (flip-flops) and that state is used as the input to a combinational logic circuit which computes the next state. The next state is then clocked into the flip-flops while the previous state is destroyed.

This sequence allows a conventional computer to execute a series of instructions by repeatedly computing the next state from the current state, and repeatedly replacing the current state with the next state. Of course, in a reversible computation, we not only need to compute the next state from the current state, we must also be able to uniquely determine the current state from the next state, *e.g.*, the computation must be reversible. There are many ways of designing such a reversible computer. In the following paragraphs we describe a simple architecture for carrying out a reversible computation. We assume that we have a reversible combinational function whose iteration we feel is computationally useful (*e.g.*, the function implements a single instruction or step of a reversible computation). We shall call this function F. We start with the initial state of the computation stored in a set of initial latch rods which are held in position by a driven holding rod. We then compute F(initial latch rods), and store the result in a set of output latch rods, which are assumed to be initially empty.

Having once computed the next state and stored it in the output latch rods, we must unwrite the initial latch rods. To do this, we compute F^{-1}(output latch rods), which should be identical to the state already stored in the initial latch rods. Thus, not only do we have combinational logic for computing F, we have combinational logic for computing F^{-1}. This additional logic is absolutely necessary.

If we did not have a method of computing F^{-1}, we would not be able to re-compute the contents of the input latches. If we could not re-compute the contents of the input latches, we could not unwrite them (which can be done in an asymptotically non-dissipative fashion) but would instead be forced to erase the input latches (which is an inherently dissipative operation).

7

Core Diseases

BREAST DISEASE

Breast diseases can be classified either with disorders of the integument, or disorders of the reproductive system. A majority of breast diseases are noncancerous.

Breast awareness is a goal of the breast health movement. Rather than promoting the largely ineffective, formally structured breast self-examinations, breast awareness promotes informal familiarity with the normal state of a woman's breasts.

NEOPLASMS

A *breast neoplasm* is an abnormal mass of tissue in the breast as a result of neoplasia. A breast neoplasm may be benign, as in fibroadenoma, or it may be malignant, in which case it is termed breast cancer. Either case commonly presents as a breast lump. Approximately 7% of breast lumps are fibroadenomas and 10% are breast cancer, the rest being other benign conditions or no disease. Phyllodes tumor is a fibroepithelial tumor which can either benign, borderline or malignant.

Malignant neoplasms (breast cancer)

Among women worldwide, breast cancer is the most common cause of cancer death. Breast self-examination (BSE) is an easy but unreliable method for finding possible breast cancer. Factors that appear to be implicated in decreasing the risk of, early diagnosis of. or recurrence of breast cancer are regular breast examinations by health care professionals, regular mammograms, self-examination of breasts, healthy diet, and exercise to decrease excess body fat.

FIBROCYSTIC BREAST CHANGES

Also called: fibrocystic breast disease, chronic cystic mastitis, diffuse cystic mastopathy, mammary dysplasia

INFECTIONS AND INFLAMMATIONS

These may be caused among others by trauma, secretory stasis/milk engorgement, hormonal stimulation, infections or autoimmune reactions. Repeated occurrence unrelated to lactation requires endocrinological examination. Main article: Mastitis

- bacterial mastitis
- mastitis from milk engorgement or secretory stasis
- mastitis or mumps
- chronic subareolar abscess
- tuberculosis of the breast
- syphilis of the breast
- retromammary abscess
- actinomycosis of the breast
- duct ectasia syndrome
- breast engorgement

ABNORMAL NIPPLE CONDITIONS

Abnormal nipple conditions include:

- nipple discharge
- inverted nipples
- supernumerary nipples

OTHER BREAST CONDITIONS

- supernumerary breasts
- gynecomastia (males)
- Mondor's disease
- Paget's disease of the breast
- nipple discharge, galactorrhea
- breast cyst
- mastalgia
- galactocoele

GYNECOLOGICAL DISORDERS

The NICHD (National Institute of Child Health and Human Development) funds and conducts research on many disorders that affect the organs in a woman's abdominal and pelvic areas. In general, most of these disorders don't directly affect a woman's changes of getting pregnant naturally. Some of these conditions include:

- Vulvodynia
- Vaginitis
- Pelvic Floor Disorders
- Pelvic Pain

VULVODYNIA

Vulvodynia (vul-voh-DINN-nee-uh) is the term used to describe chronic discomfort or pain of the vulva, especially burning, stinging, irritation, or rawness of the area. Health care providers don't agree on the exact definition of vulvodynia. Currently, the term is used to describe a variety of conditions.

The NICHD is also supporting other research on vulvodynia.

VAGINITIS

- smaller
- medium
- larger
- 1
- 2
- 3
- Next

Gynecological Disorders

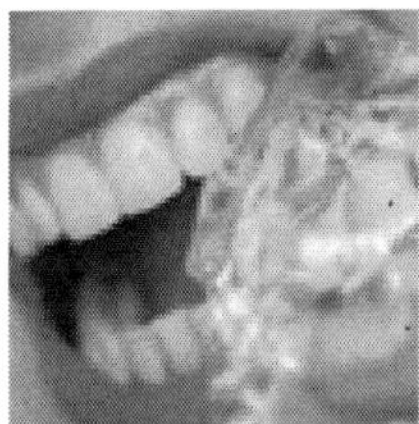

1. Slideshow: 19 Habits That Wreck Your Teeth
2. Dental (Oral) Health Quiz
3. Slideshow: Top Problems in Your Mouth

Facebook Twitter Email Print Article

The NICHD (National Institute of Child Health and Human Development) funds and conducts research on many disorders that affect the organs in a woman's abdominal and pelvic areas. In general, most of these disorders don't directly affect a woman's changes of getting pregnant naturally. Some of these conditions include:

- Vulvodynia
- Vaginitis
- Pelvic Floor Disorders
- Pelvic Pain

Vulvodynia

Vulvodynia is the term used to describe chronic discomfort or pain of the vulva, especially burning, stinging, irritation, or rawness of the area. Health care providers don't agree on the exact definition of vulvodynia. Currently, the term is used to describe a variety of conditions.

The NICHD is also supporting other research on vulvodynia.

Vaginitis

Vaginitis (va-jinn-EYE-tiss) is a term used to describe any disorder that causes swelling or infection of both the vulva and the vagina. Vaginitis is different from vulvodynia because it affects the vagina, which is inside the woman's body; vulvodyina only affects the vulva, which is outside the woman's body.

The most common types of vaginitis include:

- "Yeast" infections—Infections caused by the fungus Candida. The most apparent symptom of a yeast infection is a thick, white vaginal discharge; some women also experience a red, itchy vulva. There are many over-the-counter and prescription treatments for yeast infections. If you think you have a yeast infection, talk to your health care provider about how to treat it.
- Bacterial vaginosis—Caused by an overgrowth of bacteria that are normally present in the vagina. This type of vaginosis is the most common vaginal infection for women of reproductive age. The most common symptom is a vaginal discharge, which is usually thin and milky; it may also have a "fishy" odor. Your health care provider can recommend medications to treat bacterial vaginosis.
- Sexually transmitted forms of vaginitis—These types of vaginitis are most often spread through sexual contact (vaginal, oral, or anal intercourse or intimate contact), and are also called sexually transmitted diseases or sexually transmitted infections (STIs). Some types of sexually transmitted vaginitis include:
- Trichomoniasis—Is a curable infection. Many women with this condition don't have any symptoms; but some women do. Common symptoms include: vaginal discharge that is bubbly, greenish-yellow, and has an odor; itching and soreness of the vulva and the vagina; and burning when you urinate. Most health care providers will prescribe an antibiotic to treat and cure trichomoniasis; however, for treatment to work properly, sexual partners should be treated at the same time.
- Chlamydia—Is a curable infection. Because chlamydia does not make most people sick, you can have the infection and not even know it. Symptoms of chlamydia include a mucus-like or pus-like vaginal discharge or pain when you urinate. But these symptoms can be mild. The bacteria can also infect your throat, if you've had oral physical contact with an infected partner. A pregnant woman infected with chlamydia can transmit the infection to her infant during delivery. In the infant, the infection can cause the lining of the eye to become swollen and red (often called pink eye). If left untreated, chlamydia can move inside the body and cause pelvic inflammatory disease (PID),

which can be serious. Health care providers will prescribe an antibiotic to treat and cure chlamydia; however, penicillin, an antibiotic used to treat other infections, won't cure chlamydia.

- Herpes simplex virus —Also called "genital herpes," is caused by a virus. Genital herpes can be controlled, but not cured. Most women with genital herpes will have sores or lesions on the vulva, or on the outside of the vagina; sometimes these sores are found within the vagina, and can only be seen during a gynecological exam. The sores are often the source of pain for women infected with genital herpes. Your health care provider can recommend ways to control the symptoms of genital herpes.
- Human papilloma virus (HPV)—Is caused by a virus. It can be controlled, but not cured. Some women with HPV don't have any symptoms; they don't find out they have the virus until they get the results of their annual pap smear. Other women with HPV have genital warts, usually gray, white, or purple, that grow in their vagina or rectum, or on their vulva or groin.
- Genital warts can be painful. Some types of HPV are known to lead to certain types of cervical cancer and other cervical problems. Efforts are now underway to develop a vaccine to protect women from HPV, which could also prevent certain types of cervical cancer.
- Noninfectious vaginitis—Is typically the result of an allergic reaction or an irritation to vaginal sprays, creams, and spermacides, or to soaps, detergents, and fabric softeners. Once you stop using the product that caused the reaction, your symptoms should go away. But, your health care provider may suggest a medicated cream to reduce the symptoms until the reaction goes away.

PELVIC FLOOR DISORDERS

The term "pelvic floor" refers to the group of muscles that form a sling or hammock across the opening of the pelvis. These muscles, together with their surrounding tissues, keep all of the pelvic organs (bladder, uterus, and rectum) in place so that the organs function correctly.

A "pelvic floor disorder," then, is a problem with these muscles or the surrounding tissues that leads to dysfunction of one or more of the pelvic organs.

This understudied area of women's health includes a variety of problems, the most common of which are:

- Pelvic Organ Prolapse—Includes: Uterine prolapse—A woman's uterus drops down into her vagina. Vaginal prolapse—Often occurs after a hysterectomy (when the uterus is removed); the top of the vagina loses its support and drops.

- Urinary Incontinence—Can occur when the bladder drops down into the vagina. Because the bladder is not in its proper location, urine can leak out easily and without a woman's control.
- Anal Incontinence—Can occur when the rectum bulges into or out of the vagina. The rectum's location makes it difficult for a woman to control leakage. Anal incontinence can also occur when there is damage to the anal sphincter, the ring of muscle that keeps the anus closed. An estimated one-third of all women are affected by one type of pelvic floor disorder. Nearly 10 percent of that group will undergo surgery to correct a pelvic floor disorder.

While some pelvic floor disorders may result from pelvic surgery or radiation treatments, in some of cases, the initial trigger for the problem is vaginal delivery of a child. However, researchers don't clearly understand how vaginal delivery is related to pelvic floor disorders; they can't determine which women will develop pelvic floor disorders based on length or intensity of labor.

Many women with pelvic floor disorders also reported chronic pain as a symptom of their condition. These women noted that the pain's frequency and intensity had a major affect on their quality of life. Because of its chronic pain feature, vulvodynia is sometimes included as a pelvic floor disorder.

Although researchers know little about the causes or features of pelvic floor disorders, research in underway on a variety of topics related to pelvic floor disorders. In July 2001, the NICHD established the Pelvic Floor Disorders Network (PFDN) to support research projects that examine problems related to pelvic floor disorders. The PFDN includes seven clinical sites around the country, and a central data collection center. Through this research, the NICHD hopes to learn more about: normal pelvic floor function, the characteristics of known pelvic floor disorders, the effects of hormones on these conditions, injury during vaginal delivery and how it is related to these conditions, and the development of tools to help health care providers understand the level of function, dysfunction, or pain.

PELVIC PAIN

Pelvic pain is a general term that health care providers use to describe steady pain, or pain that comes and goes, that occurs mostly or only in the lower abdomen area. In some cases, the pain might be severe and might get in the way of daily activities; in other cases, the pain might be dull and occur only during the menstrual cycle. Pelvic pain also describes pain that occurs during sexual intercourse.

In general, pelvic pain signals that there may be a problem with one of the organs in your pelvic area: uterus, ovaries, fallopian tubes, cervix, vagina, lower intestines, or rectum. Or, it might be a symptom of an infection. Your health care provider will likely conduct a number of tests to find the cause of your pain. Treatment varies by what the cause is, how intense the pain is, and how often the pain occurs. Sometimes pain medication is the best option. Other times, an antibiotic may be necessary. If the pain results from a problem with one of your pelvic organs, for example, if you find out that you have endometriosis, then your treatment may be more involved.

The International Pelvic Pain Society offers patient information about pelvic pain and chronic pelvic pain, as well as some suggestions for how to talk with your health care provider about pelvic pain.

UROLOGIC DISEASE

Urologic disease can involve congenital or acquired dysfunction of the urinary system. Kidney diseases are normally investigated and treated by nephrologists, while the specialty of urology deals with problems in the other organs. Gynecologists may deal with problems of incontinence in women. Diseases of other bodily systems also have a direct effect on urogenital function. For instance, it has been shown that protein released by the kidneys in diabetes mellitus sensitises the kidney to the damaging effects of hypertension. Diabetes also can have a direct effect on urination due to peripheral neuropathies which occur in some individuals with poorly controlled diabetics.

Renal failure is defined by functional impairment of the kidney. Renal failure can be acute or chronic, and can be further broken down into categories of pre-renal, intrinsic renal and post-renal. Pre-renal failure refers to impairment of supply of blood to the functional nephrons including renal artery stenosis. Intrinsic renal diseases are the classic diseases of the kidney including drug toxicity and nephritis. Post-renal failure is outlet obstruction after the kidney, such as a kidney stone or prostatic bladder outlet obstruction. Renal failure may require medication, dietary and lifestyle modification and dialysis. Primary renal cell carcinomas as well as metastatic cancers can affect the kidney.

NON-RENAL URINARY TRACT DISEASE

The causes of diseases of the body are common to the urinary tract. Structural and or traumatic change can lead to hemorrhage, functional blockage or inflammation. Colonisation by bacteria, protozoa or fungi can cause infection. Uncontrolled cell growth can cause neoplasia. For example:

- Urinary tract infections (UTIs), interstitial cystitis
- incontinence (involuntary loss of urine), benign prostatic hyperplasia (where the prostate overgrows), prostatitis (inflammation of the prostate).
- Urinary retention, which is a common complication of benign prostatic hyperplasia (BPH), though it can also be caused by other types of urinary tract obstruction, nerve dysfunction, tethered spinal cord syndrome, constipation, infection and certain medications.

- Transitional cell carcinoma (bladder cancer), renal cell carcinoma (kidney cancer), and prostate cancer are examples of neoplasms affecting the urinary system.
- Urinary tract obstruction

The term "uropathy" refers to a disease of the urinary tract, while "nephropathy" refers to a disease of the kidney.

TESTING

Biochemical blood tests determine the amount of typical markers of renal function in the blood serum, for instance serum urea and serum creatinine. Biochemistry can also be used to determine serum electrolytes. Special biochemical tests (arterial blood gas) can determine the amount of dissolved gases in the blood, indicating if pH imbalances are acute or chronic.

Urinalysis is a test that studies urine for abnormal substances such as protein or signs of infection.

- A Full Ward Test, also known as dipstick urinalysis, involves the dipping of a biochemically active test strip into the urine specimen to determine levels of tell-tale chemicals in the urine.
- Urinalysis can also involve MC&S microscopy, culture and sensitivity

Urodynamic tests evaluate the storage of urine in the bladder and the flow of urine from the bladder through the urethra. It may be performed in cases of incontinence or neurological problems affecting the urinary tract. Ultrasound is commonly performed to investigate problems of the kidney and/or urinary tract. Radiology:

- KUB is plain radiography of the urinary system, e.g. to identify kidney stones.
- An intravenous pyelogram studies the shape of the urinary system.
- CAT scans and MRI can also be useful in localising urinary tract pathology.
- A voiding cystogram is a functional study where contrast "dye" is injected through a catheter into the bladder. Under x-ray the radiologist asks the patient to void (usually young children) and will watch the contrast exiting the body on the x-ray monitor. This examines the child's bladder and lower urinary tract. Typically looking for vesicoureteral reflux, involving urine backflow up into the kidneys.

PANCREATIC DISEASE

Pancreatitis is inflammation of the pancreas. There are two forms of pancreatitis, which are different in causes and symptoms, and require different treatment:

- Acute pancreatitis is a rapid-onset inflammation of the pancreas, most frequently caused by alcoholism or gallstones.

- Chronic pancreatitis is a long-standing inflammation of the pancreas.

The pancreas is central in the pathophysiology of both major types of diabetes mellitus. In type 1 diabetes mellitus, there is direct damage to the endocrine pancreas that results in insufficient insulin synthesis and secretion. Type 2 diabetes mellitus, which begins with insulin resistance, is characterized by the ultimate failure of pancreatic â cells to match insulin production with insulin demand.Exocrine pancreatic insufficiency (EPI) is the inability to properly digest food due to a lack of digestive enzymes made by the pancreas. EPI is found in humans afflicted with cystic fibrosis and Shwachman-Diamond syndrome.

It is caused by a progressive loss of the pancreatic cells that make digestive enzymes. Chronic pancreatitis is the most common cause of EPI in humans. Loss of digestive enzymes leads to maldigestion and malabsorption of nutrients.Cystic fibrosis, also known as mucoviscidosis, is a hereditary disease that affects the entire body, causing progressive disability and early death. It is caused by a mutation in the cystic fibrosis transmembrane conductance regulator (CFTR) gene.

The product of this gene helps create sweat, digestive juices, and mucus. The name *cystic fibrosis* refers to the characteristic 'fibrosis' (tissue scarring) and cyst formation within the pancreas, causing irreversible damage, and often resulting in painful inflammation (pancreatitis).

A pancreatic pseudocyst is a circumscribed collection of fluid rich in amylase and other pancreatic enzymes, blood and necrotic tissue, typically located in the lesser sac.

X-ray computed tomography (CT scan) findings of cysts in the pancreas are common, and often are benign. In a study of 2,832 patients without pancreatic disease, 73 patients (2.6%) had cysts in the pancreas. About 85% of these patients had a single cyst. Cysts ranged in size from 2 to 38 mm (mean, 8.9 mm). There was a strong correlation between the presence of cysts and age. No cysts were identified among patients less than 40 years of age, while 8.7 percent of the patients aged 80 to 89 years had a pancreatic cyst.

Cysts also may be present due to intraductal papillary mucinous neoplasm.

CONGENITAL MALFORMATIONS

- Pancreas divisum: Pancreas divisum is a malformation in which the pancreas fails to fuse. It is a rare condition that affects only 6% of the world's population, and of these few, only 1% ever have symptoms that require surgery.
- Annular pancreas: Annular pancreas is characterized by a pancreas that encircles the duodenum. It results from an embryological malformation in which the early pancreatic buds undergo inappropriate rotation and fusion, which can lead to small bowel obstruction.

NEOPLASMS

Benign:

- Serous cystadenoma of the pancreas
- Solid pseudopapillary neoplasm

Zollinger-Ellison syndrome:

- Zollinger-Ellison syndrome is a collection of findings in individuals with gastrinoma, a tumor of the gastrin-producing cells of the pancreas. Unbridled gastrin secretion results in elevated levels of the hormone, and increased hydrochloric acid secretion from parietal cells of the stomach. It can lead to ulceration and scarring of the stomach and intestinal mucosa.

HEMOSUCCUS PANCREATICUS

Hemosuccus pancreaticus, also known as pseudohematobilia or Wirsungorrhage, is a rare cause of hemorrhage in the gastrointestinal tract. It is caused by a bleeding source in the pancreas, pancreatic duct, or structures adjacent to the pancreas, such as the splenic artery, that bleed into the pancreatic duct. Patients with hemosuccus may develop symptoms of gastrointestinal hemorrhage, such as blood in the stools, maroon stools, or melena. They may also develop abdominal pain.

Hemosuccus pancreaticus is associated with pancreatitis, pancreatic cancer and aneurysms of the splenic artery. Angiography may be used to diagnose hemosuccus pancreaticus, where the celiac axis is injected to determine the blood vessel that is bleeding.

Concomitant embolization of the end vessel may terminate the hemorrhage. Alternatively, a distal pancreatectomy may be required to stop the hemorrhage.

HEPATOBILIARY DISEASES

LIVER DISEASES

Viral hepatitis

- Acute hepatitis A
- Acute hepatitis B
- Acute hepatitis C
- Acute Hepatitis D – this is a superinfection with the delta-agent in a patient already infected with hepatitis B
- Acute hepatitis E
- Chronic viral hepatitis
- Other viral hepatitis viruses may exist but their relation to the disease is not firmly established like the previous ones (Hepatitis F, GB virus C, Hepatitis X)

Other infectious diseases

- Hepatitis:
  - cytomegalovirus infection
  - herpesviral: herpes simplex infection
- Toxoplasmosis
- Hepatosplenic schistosomiasis
- Portal hypertension in schistosomiasis
- Liver disease in syphilis
- Epstein-Barr virus infection
- yellow fever virus infection
- rubella virus infection
- leptospirosis
- Echinococcosis
- Amoebiasis

Other inflammatory diseases

- liver abscess
- autoimmune hepatitis
- primary biliary cholangitis (primary biliary cirrhosis)
- phlebitis of the portal vein
- granulomatous hepatitis
  - berylliosis
  - sarcoidosis
- nonalcoholic steatohepatitis (NASH)

Alcohol

This may cause fatty liver, hepatitis, fibrosis and sclerosis leading to cirrhosis and finally liver failure.

Toxins:

This includes mostly drug-induced hepatotoxicity, (DILI) which may generate many different patterns over liver disease, including

- cholestasis
- necrosis
- acute hepatitis and chronic hepatitis of different forms,
- cirrhosis
- Effects of Acetaminophen (Tylenol)
- other rare disorders like focal nodular hyperplasia, Hepatic_fibrosis, peliosis hepatis and veno-occlusive disease.

Liver damage is part of Reye's syndrome.

Tumours:

Malignant neoplasm of liver and intrahepatic bile ducts. The most frequent forms are metastatic malignant neoplasm of liver)

- liver cell carcinoma
  - hepatocellular carcinoma

    - hepatoma
- cholangiocarcinoma
- hepatoblastoma
- angiosarcoma of liver
- Kupffer cell sarcoma
- other sarcomas of liver

Benign neoplasm of liver include hepatic hemangiomas, hepatic adenomas, and focal nodular hyperplasia (FNH).

End-stage liver disease:

Chronic liver diseases like chronic hepatitis, chronic alcohol abuse or chronic toxic liver disease may cause

- liver failure and hepatorenal syndrome
- fibrosis and cirrhosis of liver

Cirrhosis may also occur in primary biliary cirrhosis. Rarely, cirrhosis is congenital.

Metabolic diseases:

- metabolic diseases (chapter E in ICD-10)
    - haemochromatosis
    - Wilson's disease
    - Gilbert's syndrome
    - Crigler-Najjar syndrome
    - Dubin-Johnson syndrome
    - Rotor's syndrome

Vascular disorders:

- chronic passive congestion of liver
- central haemorrhagic necrosis of liver
- infarction of liver
- peliosis hepatis
- veno-occlusive disease
- portal hypertension
- Budd-Chiari syndrome

Cysts:

- Congenital cystic disease of the liver
- Cysts caused by Echinococcus
- Polycystic liver disease

Others:

Amyloid degeneration of liver

GALLBLADDER AND BILIARY TRACT DISEASES

- malignant neoplasm of the gallbladder
- malignant neoplasm of other parts of biliary tract
    - extrahepatic bile duct

  — ampulla of Vater
- cholelithiasis
- cholecystitis
- others (excluding postcholecystectomy syndrome), but including
  — other obstructions of the gallbladder
  — hydrops, perforation, fistula
  — cholesterolosis
  — biliary dyskinesia
- K83: other diseases of the biliary tract:
  — cholangitis (including ascending cholangitis and primary sclerosing cholangitis)
  — obstruction, perforation, fistula of biliary tract
  — spasm of sphincter of Oddi
  — biliary cyst
  — biliary atresia

GASTROINTESTINAL DISEASE

Gastrointestinal diseases refer to diseases involving the gastrointestinal tract, namely the esophagus, stomach, small intestine, large intestine and rectum, and the accessory organs of digestion, the liver, gallbladder, and pancreas.

ORAL DISEASE

Even though anatomically part of the GI tract, diseases of the mouth are often not considered alongside other gastrointestinal diseases. By far the most common oral conditions are plaque-induced diseases (e.g. gingivitis, periodontitis, dental caries). Some diseases which involve other parts of the GI tract can manifest in the mouth, alone or in combination, including:

- Gastroesophageal reflux disease can cause acid erosion of the teeth and halitosis.
- Gardner's syndrome can be associated with failure of tooth eruption, supernumerary teeth, and dentigerous cysts.
- Peutz–Jeghers syndrome can cause dark spots on the oral mucosa or on the lips or the skin around the mouth.
- Several GI diseases, especially those associated with malabsorption can cause recurrent mouth ulcers, atrophic glossitis, angular cheilitis. E.g. Crohn's disease is sometimes termed orofacial granulomatosis when it involves the mouth alone.
- Sideropenic dysphagia can cause glossitis, angular cheilitis.

OESOPHAGEAL DISEASE

Oesophageal diseases include a spectrum of disorders affecting the oesophagus. The most common condition of the oesophagus in Western countries is gastroesophageal reflux disease, which in chronic forms is thought to result in changes to the epithelium of the oesophagus, known as Barrett's oesophagus.

Acute disease might include infections such as oesophagitis, trauma caused ingestion of corrosive substances, or rupture of veins such as oesophageal varices, Boerhaave syndrome or Mallory-Weiss tears. Chronic diseases might include congenital diseases such as Zenker's diverticulum and esophageal webbing, and oesophageal motility disorders including the Nutcracker oesophagus, achalasia, diffuse oesophageal spasm, and oesophageal stricture.

Oesophageal disease may result in a sore throat, throwing up blood, difficulty swallowing or vomiting. Chronic or congenital diseases might be investigated using Barium swallows, endoscopy and biopsy, whereas acute diseases such as reflux may be investigated and diagnosed based on symptoms and a medical history alone.

GASTRIC DISEASE

Stomach diseases refer to diseases affecting the stomach. Inflammation of the stomach by infection from any cause is called gastritis, and when including other parts of the gastrointestinal tract called gastroenteritis. When gastritis is persists in a chronic state, it is associated with several diseases, including atrophic gastritis, pyloric stenosis, and gastric cancer. Another common condition is gastric ulceration, peptic ulcers. Ulceration erodes the gastric mucosa, which protects the tissue of the stomach from the stomach acids. Peptic ulcers are most commonly caused by a bacterial *Helicobacter pylori* infection.

As well as peptic ulcers, vomiting blood may result from abnormal arteries or veins that have ruptured, including Dieulafoy's lesion and Gastric antral vascular ectasia. Congenital disorders of the stomach include pernicious anaemia, in which a targeted immune response against parietal cells results in an inability to absorb vitamin B12. Other common symptoms that stomach disease might cause include indigestion or dyspepsia, vomiting, and in chronic disease, digestive problems leading to forms of malnutrition. In addition to routine tests, an endoscopy might be used to examine or take a biopsy from the stomach.

INTESTINAL DISEASE

The small and large intestines may be affected by infectious, autoimmune, and physiological states. Inflammation of the intestines is called enterocolitis, which may lead to diarrhoea.

Acute conditions affecting the bowels include infectious diarrhoea and mesenteric ischaemia. Causes of constipation may include faecal impaction and bowel obstruction, which may in turn be caused by ileus, intussusception, volvulus. Inflammatory bowel disease is a condition of unknown aetiology, classified as either Crohn's disease or ulcerative colitis, that can affect the intestines and other parts of the gastrointestinal tract. Other causes of illness include intestinal pseudoobstruction, and necrotizing enterocolitis.

Diseases of the intestine may cause vomiting, diarrhoea or constipation, and altered stool, such as with blood in stool. Colonoscopy may be used to examine the large intestine, and a person's stool may be sent for culture and microscopy. Infectious disease may be treated with targeted antibiotics, and inflammatory bowel disease with immunosuppression. Surgery may also be used to treat some causes of bowel obstruction.

Small intestine

The small intestine consists of the duodenum, jejunum and ileum. Inflammation of the small intestine is called enteritis, which if localised to just part is called duodenitis, jejunitis and ileitis, respectively. Peptic ulcers are also common in the duodenum.

Chronic diseases of malabsorption may affect the small intestine, including the autoimmune coeliac disease, infective Tropical sprue, and congenital or surgical short bowel syndrome. Other rarer diseases affecting the small intestine include Curling's ulcer, Blind loop syndrome, Milroy disease and Whipple's disease. Tumours of the small intestine include gastrointestinal stromal tumours, lipomas, hamartomas and carcinoid syndromes

Diseases of the small intestine may present with symptoms such as diarrhoea, malnutrition, fatigue and weight loss. Investigations pursued may include blood tests to monitor nutrition, such as iron levels, folate and calcium, endoscopy and biopsy of the duodenum, and barium swallow. Treatments may include renutrition, and antibiotics for infections.

Large intestine

Diseases that affect the large intestine may affect it in whole or in part. Appendicitis is one such disease, caused by inflammation of the appendix. Generalised inflammation of the large intestine is referred to as colitis, which when caused be the bacteria *Clostridium difficile* is referred to as Pseudomembranous colitis. Diverticulitis is a common cause of abdominal pain resulting from outpouchings that particularly affects the colon. Functional colonic diseases refer to disorders without a known cause, and include irritable bowel syndrome and Intestinal pseudoobstruction. Constipation may result from lifestyle factors, impaction of a rigid stool in the rectum, or in neonates, Hirschprung's disease.

Diseases affecting the large intestine may cause to be passed with stool, may cause constipation, or may result in abdominal pain or a fever. Tests that specifically examine the function of the large intestine include barium swallows, abdominal x-rays, and colonoscopy.

Rectum and anus

Diseases affecting the rectum and anus are extremely common, especially in older adults. Hemorrhoids, vascular outpouchings of skin, are very common, as is pruritis ani, referring to anal itchiness. Other conditions, such as anal cancer may be associated with ulcerative colitis or with sexually transmitted infections such as HIV. Inflammation of the rectum is known as proctitis, one cause of which is radiation damage associated with radiotherapy to other sites such as the prostate. Faecal incontinence can result from mechanical and neurological problems, and when associated with a lack of voluntary voiding ability is described as encopresis. Pain on passing stool may result from anal abscesses, small inflamed nodules, anal fissures, and anal fistulas.

Rectal and anal disease may be asymptomatic, or may present with pain when passing stools, fresh blood in stool, a feeling of incomplete emptying, or pencil-thin stools. In addition to regular tests, medical tests used to investigate the anus and rectum include the digital rectal exam and proctoscopy.

ACCESSORY DIGESTIVE GLAND DISEASE

Hepatic

Hepatic diseases refers to those affecting the liver. Hepatitis refers to inflammation of liver tissue, and may be acute or chronic. Infectious viral hepatitis, such as Hepatitis A, B and C, affect in excess of (X) million people worldwide. Liver disease may also be a result of lifestyle factors, such as Fatty liver and NASH. Alcoholic liver disease may also develop as a result of chronic alcohol use, which may also cause Alcoholic hepatitis. Cirrhosis may develop as a result of chronic hepatic fibrosis in a chronically inflamed liver, such as one affected by alcohol or viral hepatitis.

Liver abscesses are often acute conditions, with common causes being pyogenic and amoebic. Chronic liver disease, such as cirrhosis, may be a cause of liver failure, a state where the liver is unable to compensate for chronic damage, and unable to meet the metabolic demands of the body. In the acute setting, this may be a cause of hepatic encephalopathy and hepatorenal syndrome. Other causes of chronic liver disease are genetic or autoimmune disease, such as Hemochromatosis, Wilson's Disease, autoimmune hepatitis, and primary biliary cirrhosis.

Acute liver disease rarely results in pain, but may result in jaundice. Infectious liver disease may cause a fever. Chronic liver disease may result in a buildup of fluid in the abdomen, yellowing of the skin or eyes, easy bruising, immunosuppression, and feminsation

In order to investigate liver disease, a medical history, including regarding a person's family history, travel to risk-prone areas, alcohol use and food consumption, may be taken. A medical examination may be conducted to investigate for symptoms of liver disease. Blood tests may be used, particularly liver function tests, and other blood tests may be used to investigate the presence of the Hepatitis viruses in the blood, and ultrasound used. If ascites is present, abdominal fluid may be tested for protein levels.

Pancreatic

Pancreatic diseases that affect digestion refers to disorders affecting the exocrine pancreas, which is a part of the pancreas involved in digestion.

One of the most common conditions of the exocrine pancreas is acute pancreatitis, which in the majority of cases relates to gallstones that have impacted in the pancreatic part of the biliary tree, or due to acute or chronic alcohol abuse or as a side-effect of ERCP. Other forms of pancreatitis include chronic and hereditary forms. Chronic pancreatitis may predispose to pancreatic cancer and is strongly linked to alcohol use. Other rarer diseases affecting the pancreas may include pancreatic pseudocysts, exocrine pancreatic insufficiency, and pancreatic fistulas. Pancreatic disease may present with or without symptoms. When symptoms occur, such as in acute pancreatitis, a person may suffer from acute-onset, severe mid-abdominal pain, nausea and vomiting. In severe cases, pancreatitis may lead to rapid blood loss and systemic inflammatory response syndrome. When the pancreas is unable to secrete digestive enzymes, such as with a pancreatic cancer occluding the pancreatic duct, result in jaundice. Pancreatic disease might be investigated using abdominal x-rays, MRCP or ERCP, CT scans, and through blood tests such as measurement of the amylase and lipase enzymes.

Gallbladder and biliary tract

Diseases of the hepatobiliary system affect the biliary tract , which secretes bile in order to aid digestion of fats. Diseases of the gallbladder and bile ducts are commonly diet-related, and may include the formation of gallstones that impact in the gallbladder (Cholecystolithiasis) or in the common bile duct (Choledocholithiasis). Gallstones are a common cause of inflammation of the gallbladder, called Cholecystitis. Inflammation of the biliary duct is called Cholangitis, which may be associated with autoimmune disease, such as primary sclerosing cholangitis, or a result of bacterial infection, such as ascending cholangitis. Disease of the biliary tree may cause pain in the upper right abdomen, particularly when pressed. Disease might be investigated using ultrasound or ERCP, and might be treated with drugs such as antibiotics or UDCA, or by the surgical removal of the gallbladder.

RESPIRATORY DISEASE

Respiratory disease is a medical term that encompasses pathological conditions affecting the organs and tissues that make gas exchange possible in higher organisms, and includes conditions of the upper respiratory tract, trachea, bronchi, bronchioles, alveoli, pleura and pleural cavity, and the nerves and muscles of breathing. Respiratory diseases range from mild and self-limiting, such as the common cold, to life-threatening entities like bacterial pneumonia, pulmonary embolism, and lung cancer.

The study of respiratory disease is known as pulmonology. A doctor who specializes in respiratory disease is known as a pulmonologist, a chest medicine specialist, a respiratory medicine specialist, a respirologist or a thoracic medicine specialist.

UBET Respiratory diseases can be classified in many different ways, including by the organ or tissue involved, by the type and pattern of associated signs and symptoms, or by the cause (aetiology) of the disease.

INFLAMMATORY LUNG DISEASE

Characterized by a high neutrophil count, e.g. asthma, cystic fibrosis, emphysema, chronic obstructive pulmonary disorder or acute respiratory distress syndrome.

RESTRICTIVE LUNG DISEASES

Restrictive lung diseases are a category of respiratory disease characterized by a loss of lung compliance, causing incomplete lung expansion and increased lung stiffness, such as in infants with respiratory distress syndrome.

RESPIRATORY TRACT INFECTIONS

Infections can affect any part of the respiratory system. They are traditionally divided into upper respiratory tract infections and lower respiratory tract infections.

Upper respiratory tract infection

The most common upper respiratory tract infection is the common cold. However, infections of specific organs of the upper respiratory tract such as sinusitis, tonsillitis, otitis media, pharyngitis and laryngitis are also considered upper respiratory tract infections.

Lower respiratory tract infection

The most common lower respiratory tract infection is pneumonia, an infection of the lungs which is usually caused by bacteria, particularly *Streptococcus pneumoniae* in Western countries. Worldwide, tuberculosis is an important cause of pneumonia.

Other pathogens such as viruses and fungi can cause pneumonia for example severe acute respiratory syndrome and pneumocystis pneumonia. A pneumonia may develop complications such as a lung abscess, a round cavity in the lung caused by the infection, or may spread to the pleural cavity. Poor oral care may be a contributing factor to lower respiratory disease. New research suggests bacteria from gum disease travel through airways and into the lungs.

Malignant tumors

Malignant tumors of the respiratory system, particularly primary carcinomas of the lung, are a major health problem responsible for 15% of all cancer diagnoses and 30% of all cancer deaths. The majority of respiratory system cancers are attributable to smoking tobacco.

The major histological types of respiratory system cancer are:

- Small cell lung cancer
- Non-small cell lung cancer
  - — Adenocarcinoma of the lung
  - — Squamous cell carcinoma of the lung
  - — Large cell lung carcinoma
- Other lung cancers (carcinoid, Kaposi's sarcoma, melanoma)
- Lymphoma
- Head and neck cancer
- Pleural mesothelioma, almost always caused by exposure to asbestos dust.

In addition, since many cancers spread via the bloodstream and the entire cardiac output passes through the lungs, it is common for cancer metastases to occur within the lung. Breast cancer may invade directly through local spread, and through lymph node metastases. After metastasis to the liver, colon cancer frequently metastasizes to the lung. Prostate cancer, germ cell cancer and renal cell carcinoma may also metastasize to the lung.

Treatment of respiratory system cancer depends on the type of cancer. Surgical removal of part of a lung (lobectomy, segmentectomy, or wedge resection) or of an entire lung pneumonectomy), along with chemotherapy and radiotherapy, are all used. The chance of surviving lung cancer depends on the cancer stage at the time the cancer is diagnosed, and to some extent on the histology, and is only about 14-17% overall. In the case of metastases to the lung, treatment can occasionally be curative but only in certain, rare circumstances.

Benign tumors

Benign tumors are relatively rare causes of respiratory disease. Examples of benign tumors are:

- Pulmonary hamartoma
- Congenital malformations such as pulmonary sequestration and congenital cystic adenomatoid malformation (CCAM).

Pleural cavity diseases

Pleural cavity diseases include pleural mesothelioma which are mentioned above.

A collection of fluid in the pleural cavity is known as a pleural effusion. This may be due to fluid shifting from the bloodstream into the pleural cavity due to conditions such as congestive heart failure and cirrhosis. It may also be due to inflammation of the pleura itself as can occur with infection, pulmonary embolus, tuberculosis, mesothelioma and other conditions.

A pneumothorax is a hole in the pleura covering the lung allowing air in the lung to escape into the pleural cavity. The affected lung "collapses" like a deflated balloon. A tension pneumothorax is a particularly severe form of this condition where the air in the pleural cavity cannot escape, so the pneumothorax keeps getting bigger until it compresses the heart and blood vessels, leading to a life-threatening situation.

Pulmonary vascular disease

Pulmonary vascular diseases are conditions that affect the pulmonary circulation. Examples are:

- Pulmonary embolism, a blood clot that forms in a vein, breaks free, travels through the heart and lodges in the lungs (thromboembolism). Large pulmonary emboli are fatal, causing sudden death. A number of other substances can also embolise (travel through the blood stream) to the lungs but they are much more rare: fat embolism (particularly after bony injury), amniotic fluid embolism (with complications of labour and delivery), air embolism (iatrogenic - caused by invasive medical procedures).
- Pulmonary arterial hypertension, elevated pressure in the pulmonary arteries. Most commonly it is idiopathic (i.e. of unknown cause) but it can be due to the effects of another disease, particularly COPD. This can lead to strain on the right side of the heart, a condition known as cor pulmonale.
- Pulmonary edema, leakage of fluid from capillaries of the lung into the alveoli (or air spaces). It is usually due to congestive heart failure.
- Pulmonary hemorrhage, inflammation and damage to capillaries in the lung resulting in blood leaking into the alveoli. This may cause blood to be coughed up. Pulmonary hemorrhage can be due to auto-immune disorders such as granulomatosis with polyangiitis and Goodpasture's syndrome.

Neonatal diseases

Pulmonary diseases may also impact newborns, such as pulmonary hyperplasia and Infant respiratory distress syndrome.

DIAGNOSIS

Respiratory diseases may be investigated by performing one or more of the following tests

- Biopsy of the lung or pleura
- Blood test
- Bronchoscopy
- Chest x-ray
- Computed tomography scan
- Culture of microorganisms from secretions such as sputum
- Ultrasound scanning can be useful to detect fluid such as pleural effusion
- Pulmonary function test
- Ventilation—perfusion scan

EPIDEMIOLOGY

Respiratory disease is a common and significant cause of illness and death around the world. In the US, approximately 1 billion "common colds" occur each year.

A study found that in 2010, there were approximately 6.8 million emergency department visits for respiratory disorders in the U.S. for patients under the age of 18. In 2012, respiratory conditions were the most frequent reasons for hospital stays among children.

In the UK, approximately 1 in 7 individuals are affected by some form of chronic lung disease, most commonly chronic obstructive pulmonary disease, which includes asthma, chronic bronchitis and emphysema. Respiratory diseases (including lung cancer) are responsible for over 10% of hospitalizations and over 16% of deaths in Canada. In 2011, respiratory disease with ventilator support accounted for 93.3% of ICU utilization in the United States.

CARDIOVASCULAR DISEASE

Cardiovascular disease (CVD) is a class of diseases that involve the heart or blood vessels. Cardiovascular disease includes coronary artery diseases (CAD) such as angina and myocardial infarction (commonly known as a heart attack). Other CVDs are stroke, hypertensive heart disease, rheumatic heart disease, cardiomyopathy, atrial fibrillation, congenital heart disease, endocarditis, aortic aneurysms, peripheral artery disease and venous thrombosis.

The underlying mechanisms vary depending on the disease in question. Coronary artery disease, stroke, and peripheral artery disease involve atherosclerosis. This may be caused by high blood pressure, smoking, diabetes, lack of exercise, obesity, high blood cholesterol, poor diet, and excessive alcohol consumption, among others. High blood pressure results in 13% of CVD deaths, while tobacco results in 9%, diabetes 6%, lack of exercise 6% and obesity 5%. Rheumatic heart disease may follow untreated strep throat.

It is estimated that 90% of CVD is preventable. Prevention of atherosclerosis is by decreasing risk factors through: healthy eating, exercise, avoidance of tobacco smoke and limiting alcohol intake. Treating high blood pressure and diabetes is also beneficial. Treating people who have strep throat with antibiotics can decrease the risk of rheumatic heart disease. The effect of the use of aspirin in people who are otherwise healthy is of unclear benefit. The United States Preventive Services Task Force recommends against its use for prevention in women less than 55 and men less than 45 years old; however, in those who are older it is recommends in some individuals. Treatment of those who have CVD improves outcomes.

Cardiovascular diseases are the leading cause of death globally. This is true in all areas of the world except Africa. Together they resulted in 17.3 million deaths (31.5%) in 2013 up from 12.3 million (25.8%) in 1990. Deaths, at a given age, from CVD are more common and have been increasing in much of the developing world, while rates have declined in most of the developed world since the 1970s. Coronary artery disease and stroke account for 80% of CVD deaths in males and 75% of CVD deaths in females. Most cardiovascular disease affects older adults. In the United States 11% of people between 20 and 40 have CVD, while 37% between 40 and 60, 71% of people between 60 and 80, and 85% of people over 80 have CVD. The average age of death from coronary artery disease in the developed world is around 80 while it is around 68 in the developing world. Disease onset is typically seven to ten years earlier in men as compared to women.

TYPES

There are many cardiovascular diseases involving the blood vessels. They are known as vascular diseases:

- Coronary artery disease (also known as coronary heart disease and ischemic heart disease)
- Peripheral arterial disease – disease of blood vessels that supply blood to the arms and legs
- Cerebrovascular disease – disease of blood vessels that supply blood to the brain (includes stroke)
- Renal artery stenosis
- Aortic aneurysm

There are also many cadiovascular diseases that involve the heart.

- Cardiomyopathy – diseases of cardiac muscle
- Hypertensive heart disease – diseases of the heart secondary to high blood pressure or hypertension
- Heart failure

- Pulmonary heart disease – a failure at the right side of the heart with respiratory system involvement
- Cardiac dysrhythmias – abnormalities of heart rhythm
- Inflammatory heart disease
  - Endocarditis – inflammation of the inner layer of the heart, the endocardium. The structures most commonly involved are the heart valves.
  - Inflammatory cardiomegaly
  - Myocarditis – inflammation of the myocardium, the muscular part of the heart.
- Valvular heart disease
- Congenital heart disease – heart structure malformations existing at birth
- Rheumatic heart disease – heart muscles and valves damage due to rheumatic fever caused by *Streptococcus pyogenes* a group A streptococcal infection.

RISK FACTORS

There are several risk factors for heart diseases: age, gender, tobacco use, physical inactivity, excessive alcohol consumption, unhealthy diet, obesity, family history of cardiovascular disease, raised blood pressure (hypertension), raised blood sugar (diabetes mellitus), raised blood cholesterol (hyperlipidemia), psychosocial factors, poverty and low educational status, and air pollution. While the individual contribution of each risk factor varies between different communities or ethnic groups the overall contribution of these risk factors is very consistent.

Some of these risk factors, such as age, gender or family history, are immutable; however, many important cardiovascular risk factors are modifiable by lifestyle change, social change, drug treatment and prevention of hypertension, hyperlipidemia, and diabetes.

Age

Age is by far the most important risk factor in developing cardiovascular or heart diseases, with approximately a tripling of risk with each decade of life. It is estimated that 82 percent of people who die of coronary heart disease are 65 and older. At the same time, the risk of stroke doubles every decade after age 55.

Multiple explanations have been proposed to explain why age increases the risk of cardiovascular/heart diseases. One of them is related to serum cholesterol level. In most populations, the serum total cholesterol level increases as age increases. In men, this increase levels off around age 45 to 50 years. In women, the increase continues sharply until age 60 to 65 years.

Aging is also associated with changes in the mechanical and structural properties of the vascular wall, which leads to the loss of arterial elasticity and reduced arterial compliance and may subsequently lead to coronary artery disease.

Sex

Men are at greater risk of heart disease than pre-menopausal women. Once past menopause, it has been argued that a woman's risk is similar to a man's although more recent data from the WHO and UN disputes this. If a female has diabetes, she is more likely to develop heart disease than a male with diabetes.

Coronary heart diseases are 2 to 5 times more common among middle-aged men than women. In a study done by the World Health Organization, sex contributes to approximately 40% of the variation in sex ratios of coronary heart disease mortality. Another study reports similar results finding that gender differences explains nearly half the risk associated with cardiovascular diseases One of the proposed explanations for gender differences in cardiovascular diseases is hormonal difference. Among women, estrogen is the predominant sex hormone. Estrogen may have protective effects through glucose metabolism and hemostatic system, and may have direct effect in improving endothelial cell function. The production of estrogen decreases after menopause, and this may change the female lipid metabolism toward a more atherogenic form by decreasing the HDL cholesterol level while increasing LDL and total cholesterol levels.

Among men and women, there are notable differences in body weight, height, body fat distribution, heart rate, stroke volume, and arterial compliance. In the very elderly, age-related large artery pulsatility and stiffness is more pronounced among women than men. This may be caused by the women's smaller body size and arterial dimensions which are independent of menopause.

Tobacco

Cigarettes are the major form of smoked tobacco. Risks to health from tobacco use result not only from direct consumption of tobacco, but also from exposure to second-hand smoke. Approximately 10% of cardiovascular disease is attributed to smoking; however, people who quit smoking by age 30 have almost as low a risk of death as never smokers.

Physical inactivity

Insufficient physical activity (defined as less than 5 x 30 minutes of moderate activity per week, or less than 3 x 20 minutes of vigorous activity per week) is currently the fourth leading risk factor for mortality worldwide. In 2008, 31.3% of adults aged 15 or older (28.2% men and 34.4% women) were insufficiently physically active. The risk of ischemic heart disease and diabetes mellitus is reduced by almost a third in adults who participate in 150 minutes of moderate physical activity each week (or equivalent). In addition, physical activity assists weight loss and improves blood glucose control, blood pressure, lipid profile and insulin sensitivity. These effects may, at least in part, explain its cardiovascular benefits.

Diet

High dietary intakes of saturated fat, trans-fats and salt, and low intake of fruits, vegetables and fish are linked to cardiovascular risk, although whether all these associations are a cause is disputed. The World Health Organization attributes approximately 1.7 million deaths worldwide to low fruit and vegetable consumption. The amount of dietary salt consumed is also an important determinant of blood pressure levels and overall cardiovascular risk. Frequent consumption of high-energy foods, such as processed foods that are high in fats and sugars, promotes obesity and may increase cardiovascular risk. High trans-fat intake has adverse effects on blood lipids and circulating inflammatory markers, and elimination of trans-fat from diets has been widely advocated. There is evidence that higher consumption of sugar is associated with higher blood pressure and unfavorable blood lipids, and sugar intake also increases the risk of diabetes mellitus. High consumption of processed meats is associated with an increased risk of cardiovascular disease, possibly in part due to increased dietary salt intake.

The relationship between alcohol consumption and cardiovascular disease is complex, and may depend on the amount of alcohol consumed. There is a direct relationship between high levels of alcohol consumption and risk of cardiovascular disease. Drinking at low levels without episodes of heavy drinking may be associated with a reduced risk of cardiovascular disease. Overall alcohol consumption at the population level is associated with multiple health risks that exceed any potential benefits.

Socioeconomic disadvantage

Cardiovascular disease affects low- and middle-income countries even more than high-income countries. There is relatively little information regarding social patterns of cardiovascular disease within low- and middle-income countries, but within high-income countries low income and low educational status are consistently associated with greater risk of cardiovascular disease. Policies that have resulted in increased socio-economic inequalities have been associated with greater subsequent socio-economic differences in cardiovascular disease implying a cause and effect relationship. Psychosocial factors, environmental exposures, health behaviours, and health-care access and quality contribute to socio-economic differentials in cardiovascular disease. The Commission on Social Determinants of Health recommended that more equal distributions of power, wealth, education, housing, environmental factors, nutrition, and health care were needed to address inequalities in cardiovascular disease and non-communicable diseases.

Air pollution

Particulate matter has been studied for its short- and long-term exposure effects on cardiovascular disease. Currently, $PM_{2.5}$ is the major focus, in which gradients are used to determine CVD risk. For every 10 ìg/m of $PM_{2.5}$ long-term exposure, there was an estimated 8–18% CVD mortality risk. Women had a higher relative risk (RR) (1.42) for $PM_{2.5}$ induced coronary artery disease than men (0.90) did. Overall, long-term PM exposure increased rate of atherosclerosis and inflammation.

In regards to short-term exposure (2 hours), every 25 ìg/m of $PM_{2.5}$ resulted in a 48% increase of CVD mortality risk. In addition, after only 5 days of exposure, a rise in systolic and diastolic (2.7 mmHg) blood pressure occurred for every 10.5 ìg/m of $PM_{2.5}$. Other research has implicated $PM_{2.5}$ in irregular heart rhythm, reduced heart rate variability (decreased vagal tone), and most notably heart failure. $PM_{2.5}$ is also linked to carotid artery thickening and increased risk of acute myocardial infarction.

Tests

- Coronary artery calcification
- Carotid total plaque area
- Elevated Low-density lipoprotein-p
- Elevated blood levels of brain natriuretic peptide (also known as B-type) (BNP)

PATHOPHYSIOLOGY

Population-based studies show that atherosclerosis, the major precursor of cardiovascular disease, begins in childhood. The Pathobiological Determinants of Atherosclerosis in Youth Study demonstrated that intimal lesions appear in all the aortas and more than half of the right coronary arteries of youths aged 7–9 years.

This is extremely important considering that 1 in 3 people die from complications attributable to atherosclerosis. In order to stem the tide, education and awareness that cardiovascular disease poses the greatest threat, and measures to prevent or reverse this disease must be taken.

Obesity and diabetes mellitus are often linked to cardiovascular disease, as are a history of chronic kidney disease and hypercholesterolaemia. In fact, cardiovascular disease is the most life-threatening of the diabetic complications and diabetics are two- to four-fold more likely to die of cardiovascular-related causes than nondiabetics.

SCREENING

Screening ECGs (either at rest or with exercise) are not recommended in those without symptoms who are at low risk. This includes those who are young without risk factors. In those at higher risk the evidence for screening with ECGs is inconclusive.

Additionally echocardiography, myocardial perfusion imaging, and cardiac stress testing is not recommended in those at low risk who do not have symptoms.

Some biomarkers may add to conventional cardiovascular risk factors in predicting the risk of future cardiovascular disease; however, the clinical value of some biomarkers is questionable.

PREVENTION

Currently practiced measures to prevent cardiovascular disease include:

- A low-fat, high-fiber diet including whole grains and fruit and vegetables. Five portions a day reduces risk by about 25%.
- Tobacco cessation and avoidance of second-hand smoke
- Limit alcohol consumption to the recommended daily limits; consumption of 1–2 standard alcoholic drinks per day may reduce risk by 30%. However, excessive alcohol intake increases the risk of cardiovascular disease.
- Lower blood pressures, if elevated
- Decrease body fat if overweight or obese
- Increase daily activity to 30 minutes of vigorous exercise per day at least five times per week ;
- Reduce sugar consumptions
- Decrease psychosocial stress. This measure may be complicated by imprecise definitions of what constitute psychosocial interventions. Mental stress–induced myocardial ischemia is associated with an increased risk of heart problems in those with previous heart disease. Severe emotional and physical stress leads to a form of heart dysfunction known as Takotsubo syndrome in some people. Stress, however, plays a relatively minor role in hypertension. Specific relaxation therapies are of unclear benefit.

For adults without a known diagnosis of hypertension, diabetes, hyperlipidemia, or cardiovascular disease, routine counseling to advise them to improve their diet and increase their physical activity has not been found to significantly alter behavior, and thus is not recommended. It is unclear whether or not dental care in those with periodontitis affects the risk of cardiovascular disease. Exercise in those who are at high risk of heart disease has not been well studied as of 2014.

Diet

A diet high in fruits and vegetables decreases the risk of cardiovascular disease and death. Evidence suggests that the Mediterranean diet may improve cardiovascular outcomes. There is also evidence that a Mediterranean diet may be more effective than a low-fat diet in bringing about long-term changes to cardiovascular risk factors (e.g., lower cholesterol level and blood pressure). The DASH diet (high in nuts, fish, fruits and vegetables, and low in sweets, red meat and fat) has been shown to reduce blood pressure, lower total and low density lipoprotein cholesterol and improve metabolic syndrome; but the long-term benefits outside the context of a clinical trial have been questioned. A high fiber diet appears to lower the risk.

Total fat intake does not appear to be an important risk factor. A diet high in trans fatty acids, however, does appear to increase rates of cardiovascular disease. Worldwide, dietary guidelines recommend a reduction in saturated fat. However, there are some questions around the effect of saturated fat on cardiovascular disease in the medical literature. Reviews from 2014 and 2015 did not find evidence of harm from saturated fats. A 2012 Cochrane review found suggestive evidence of a small benefit from replacing dietary saturated fat by unsaturated fat.

A 2013 meta analysis concludes that substitution with omega 6 linoleic acid (a type of unsaturated fat) may increase cardiovascular risk. Replacement of saturated fats with carbohydrates does not change or may increase risk. Benefits from replacement with polyunsaturated fat appears greatest; however, supplementation with omega-3 fatty acids (a type of polysaturated fat) does not appear to have an effect.

The effect of a low-salt diet is unclear. A Cochrane review concluded that any benefit in either hypertensive or normal-tensive people is small if present. In addition, the review suggested that a low-salt diet may be harmful in those with congestive heart failure. However, the review was criticized in particular for not excluding a trial in heart failure where people had low-salt and -water levels due to diuretics. When this study is left out, the rest of the trials show a trend to benefit. Another review of dietary salt concluded that there is strong evidence that high dietary salt intake increases blood pressure and worsens hypertension, and that it increases the number of cardiovascular disease events; the latter happen both through the increased blood pressure *and*, quite likely, through other mechanisms. Moderate evidence was found that high salt intake increases cardiovascular mortality; and some evidence was found for an increase in overall mortality, strokes, and left ventricular hypertrophy.

Supplements

While a healthy diet is beneficial, in general the effect of antioxidant supplementation (vitamin E, vitamin C, etc.) or vitamins has not been shown to protection against cardiovascular disease and in some cases may possibly result in harm. Mineral supplements have also not been found to be useful. Niacin, a type of vitamin B3, may be an exception with a modest decrease in the risk of cardiovascular events in those at high risk. Magnesium supplementation lowers high blood pressure in a dose dependent manner. Magnesium therapy is recommended for patients with ventricular arrhythmia associated with torsades de pointes who present with long QT syndrome as well as for the treatment of patients with digoxin intoxication-induced arrhythmias. Evidence to support omega-3 fatty acid supplementation is lacking.

Medication

Aspirin has been found to be of only modest benefit in those at low risk of heart disease as the risk of serious bleeding is almost equal to the benefit with respect to cardiovascular problems. In those at really low risk it is not recommended.

Statins are effective in preventing further cardiovascular disease in people with a history of cardiovascular disease. As the event rate is higher in men than in women, the decrease in events is more easily seen in men than women. In those without cardiovascular disease but risk factors statins appear to also be beneficial with a decrease in mortality and further heart disease. The time course over which statins provide prevention against death appears to be long, of the order of one year, which is much longer than the duration of their effect on lipids. The medications niacin, fibrates and CETP Inhibitors, while they may increase HDL cholesterol do not affect the risk of cardiovascular disease in those who are already on statins. The use of vasoactive agents for people with pulmonary hypertension with left heart disease or hypoxemic lung diseases may cause harm and unnecessary expense.

MANAGEMENT

Cardiovascular disease is treatable with initial treatment primarily focused on diet and lifestyle interventions.

EPIDEMIOLOGY

Cardiovascular diseases are the leading cause of death. In 2008, 30% of all global death is attributed to cardiovascular diseases. Death caused by cardiovascular diseases are also higher in low- and middle-income countries as over 80% of all global death caused by cardiovascular diseases occurred in those countries. It is also estimated that by 2030, over 23 million people will die from cardiovascular diseases each year.

It is estimated that 60% of the world's cardiovascular disease burden will occur in the South Asian subcontinent despite only accounting for 20% of the world's population. This may be secondary to a combination of genetic predisposition and environmental factors. Organizations such as the Indian Heart Association are working with the World Heart Federation to raise awareness about this issue.

RESEARCH

The first studies on cardiovascular health were performed in year 1949 by Jerry Morris using occupational health data and were published in year 1958. The causes, prevention, and/or treatment of all forms of cardiovascular disease remain active fields of biomedical research, with hundreds of scientific studies being published on a weekly basis.

A fairly recent emphasis is on the link between low-grade inflammation that hallmarks atherosclerosis and its possible interventions. C-reactive protein is a common inflammatory marker that has been found to be present in increased levels in patients who are at risk for cardiovascular disease. Also osteoprotegerin, which is involved with regulation of a key inflammatory transcription factor called NF-êB, has been found to be a risk factor of cardiovascular disease and mortality. Some areas currently being researched include the possible links between infection with *Chlamydophila pneumoniae* (a major cause of pneumonia) and coronary artery disease. The *Chlamydia* link has become less plausible with the absence of improvement after antibiotic use.

Several research also investigated the benefits of melatonin on cardiovascular diseases prevention and cure. Melatonin is a pineal gland secretion and it is shown to be able to lower total cholesterol, very-low-density and low-density lipoprotein cholesterol levels in the blood plasma of rats. Reduction of blood pressure is also observed when pharmacological doses are applied. Thus, it is deemed to be a plausible treatment for hypertension. However, further research needs to be conducted to investigate the side-effects, optimal dosage, etc. before it can be licensed for use.

ENDOCRINE DISORDERS

The endocrine system is a network of glands that produce and release hormones that help control many important body functions, including the body's ability to change calories into energy that powers cells and organs. The endocrine system influences how your heart beats, how your bones and tissues grow, even your ability to make a baby. It plays a vital role in whether or not you develop diabetes, thyroid disease, growth disorders, sexual dysfunction, and a host of other hormone-related disorders.

GLANDS OF THE ENDOCRINE SYSTEM

Each gland of the endocrine system releases specific hormones into your bloodstream. These hormones travel through your blood to other cells and help control or coordinate many body processes.

Endocrine glands include:

- Adrenal glands: Two glands that sit on top of the kidneys that release the hormone cortisol.
- Hypothalamus: A part of the lower middle brain that tells the pituitary gland when to release hormones.
- Ovaries: The female reproductive organs that release eggs and produce sex hormones.
- Islet cells in the pancreas: Cells in the pancreas control the release of the hormones insulin and glucagon.
- Parathyroid: Four tiny glands in the neck that play a role in bone development.
- Pineal gland: A gland found near the center of the brain that may be linked to sleep patterns.
- Pituitary gland: A gland found at the base of brain behind the sinuses. It is often called the "master gland" because it influences many other glands, especially the thyroid. Problems with the pituitary gland can affect bone growth, a woman's menstrual cycles, and the release of breast milk.
- Testes: The male reproductive glands that produce sperm and sex hormones.
- Thymus: A gland in the upper chest that helps develop the body's immune system early in life.
- Thyroid: A butterfly-shaped gland in the front of the neck that controls metabolism.

Even the slightest hiccup with the function of one or more of these glands can throw off the delicate balance of hormones in your body and lead to an endocrine disorder, or endocrine disease.

CAUSES OF ENDOCRINE DISORDERS

Endocrine disorders are typically grouped into two categories:

- Endocrine disease that results when a gland produces too much or too little of an endocrine hormone, called a hormone imbalance.
- Endocrine disease due to the development of lesions (such as nodules or tumors) in the endocrine system, which may or may not affect hormone levels.

The endocrine's feedback system helps control the balance of hormones in the bloodstream. If your body has too much or too little of a certain hormone, the feedback system signals the proper gland or glands to correct the problem. A hormone imbalance may occur if this feedback system has trouble keeping the right level of hormones in the bloodstream, or if your body doesn't clear them out of the bloodstream properly. Increased or decreased levels of endocrine hormone may be caused by:

- A problem with the endocrine feedback system
- Failure of a gland to stimulate another gland to release hormones (for example, a problem with the hypothalamus can disrupt hormone production in the pituitary gland)
- A genetic disorder, such as multiple endocrine neoplasia (MEN) or congenital hypothyroidism
- Infection
- Injury to an endocrine gland
- Tumor of an endocrine gland

Most endocrine tumors and nodules (lumps) are noncancerous. They usually do not spread to other parts of the body. However, a tumor or nodule on the gland may interfere with the gland's hormone production.

TYPES OF ENDOCRINE DISORDERS

There are many different types of endocrine disorders. Diabetes is the most common endocrine disorder diagnosed in the U.S.

Other endocrine disorders include:

- Adrenal insufficiency. The adrenal gland releases too little of the hormone cortisol and sometimes, aldosterone. Symptoms include fatigue, stomach upset, dehydration, and skin changes. Addison's disease is a type of adrenal insufficiency.
- Cushing's disease. Overproduction of a pituitary gland hormone leads to an overactive adrenal gland. A similar condition called Cushing's syndrome may occur in people, particularly children, who take high doses of corticosteroid medications.
- Gigantism (acromegaly) and other growth hormone problems. If the pituitary gland produces too much growth hormone, a child's bones and body parts may grow abnormally fast. If growth hormone levels are too low, a child can stop growing in height.
- Hyperthyroidism. The thyroid gland produces too much thyroid hormone, leading to weight loss, fast heart rate, sweating, and nervousness. The most common cause for an overactive thyroid is an autoimmune disorder called Grave's disease.
- Hypothyroidism. The thyroid gland does not produce enough thyroid hormone, leading to fatigue, constipation, dry skin, and depression. The underactive gland can cause slowed development in children. Some types of hypothyroidism are present at birth.
- Hypopituitarism. The pituitary gland releases little or no hormones. It may be caused by a number of different diseases. Women with this condition may stop getting their periods.
- Multiple endocrine neoplasia I and II (MEN I and MEN II). These rare, genetic conditions are passed down through families. They cause

tumors of the parathyroid, adrenal, and thyroid glands, leading to overproduction of hormones.
- Polycystic ovary syndrome (PCOS). Overproduction of androgens interfere with the development of eggs and their release from the female ovaries. PCOS is a leading cause of infertility.
- Precocious puberty. Abnormally early puberty that occurs when glands tell the body to release sex hormones too soon in life.

TESTING FOR ENDOCRINE DISORDERS

If you have an endocrine disorder, your doctor may refer you to a specialist called an endocrinologist. An endocrinologist is specially trained in problems with the endocrine system.

The symptoms of an endocrine disorder vary widely and depend on the specific gland involved. However, most people with endocrine disease complain of fatigue and weakness. Blood and urine tests to check your hormone levels can help your doctors determine if you have an endocrine disorder. Imaging tests may be done to help locate or pinpoint a nodule or tumor. Treatment of endocrine disorders can be complicated, as a change in one hormone level can throw off another. Your doctor or specialist may order routine blood work to check for problems or to determine if your medication or treatment plan needs to be adjusted.

NERVOUS SYSTEM DISEASES

- Multiple Sclerosis – Literally, "many hardenings," MS is a disease of unknown cause that manifests as multiple hard plaques of degeneration of the insulating layer of nerve fibers in the central nervous system. The loss of insulation allows "short circuiting" of nerve impulses. Depending upon where the degeneration occurs, patients may suffer paralysis, sensory disturbances or blindness.
- Cerebrovascular accident (CVA) – the fancy name for a "stroke". A blood vessel in the brain may burst causing internal bleeding. Or, a clot may arise in a brain blood vessel (a thrombus), or arise elsewhere (embolus) and travel to get stuck in a brain vessel which then deprives brain tissue of oxygen. Depending upon the area of the brain involved, the patient may suffer paralysis, loss of speech or loss of vision.
- Transient Ischemic Attack (TIA) – "Ischemia" was introduced previously in the circulatory diseases module referring to the heart. It literally means "not quite enough blood". A short period of insufficient blood supply to the brain can have the same signs and symptoms as a stroke such as weakness in an arm, a partial loss of vision, but the problem lasts less than 24 hours. People who get TIA's are at increased risk of having a stroke in the future.

- Epilepsy – a Greek word for "seizure." Convulsions is another term used. Seizures may have many causes and not all seizures are epilepsy. High fevers in young children may trigger seizures which are short in duration, easily controlled and, typically, have no permanent aftereffects. Epilepsy is a specific condition which may occur at any age, seizures are more intense, longer lasting in duration, and recur with some frequency. The condition may be controlled with medication, or if unresponsive to drugs, may require surgery.
- Aphasia – loss of speech. The speech centers are located on the left side of the brain in a majority of people. If someone suffers a "stroke" (cerebrovascular accident-CVA), or traumatic brain injury, and it involves the left side of the brain, they may suffer speech impediments that vary over a spectrum of problems from difficulty in finding the right word, speaking slowly and with difficulty, or complete loss of speech. Actually, there are two speech centers. Injury described above involves the motor speech area, the area of the brain that produces language by integrating thoughts of speech with the movements of the larynx, lips and tongue. There is a second speech area, the receptive or sensory area, that enables us to understand speech. Injury to the latter results in still fluent speech, but the individual does not understand what they are hearing.

CENTRAL NERVOUS SYSTEM DISEASE

A central nervous system disease can affect either the spinal cord (myelopathy) or brain (encephalopathy), both of which are part of the central nervous system.Functions

- Spinal cord: The spinal cord transmits sensory reception from the peripheral nervous system. It also conducts motor information to the body's skeletal muscles, cardiac muscles, smooth muscles, and glands. There are 31 pairs of spinal nerves along the spinal cord. These nerves each contain both sensory and motor axons. The spinal cord is protected by vertebrae and connects the peripheral nervous system to the brain, and it acts as a "minor" coordinating center.
- Brain: It allows the body to function. The brain is protected by the skull; however, if the brain is damaged, the results to the human body can be very consequential.

Types of disease

- Bipolar disorder: Bipolar disorder is a serious illness of the nervous system. Symptoms can include both signs of major depression & mania. Mood swings from the highs of mania to the lows of deep depression usually occurs over several weeks to months. New research suggests that bipolar disorder is actually a neurological disease genetically related to Parkinson's disease

- Catalepsy: Catalepsy is a nervous disorder characterized by immobility and muscular rigidity, along with a decreased sensitivity to pain. Catalepsy is considered a symptom of serious diseases of the nervous system (e.g., Parkinson's disease, Epilepsy, etc.) rather than a disease by itself. Cataleptic fits can range in duration from several minutes to weeks. Catalepsy often responds to Benzodiazepines (e.g., Lorazepam) in pill & I.V. form.
- Epilepsy/Seizures: Epilepsy is an unpredictable, serious, and potentially fatal disorder of the nervous system, thought to be the result of faulty electrical activity in the brain. Epileptic seizures result from abnormal, excessive, or hypersynchronous neuronal activity in the brain. About 50 million people worldwide have epilepsy, and nearly 80% of epilepsy occurs in developing countries. Epilepsy becomes more common as people age. Onset of new cases occurs most frequently in infants and the elderly. Epileptic seizures may occur in recovering patients as a consequence of brain surgery.
- Encephalitis: Encephalitis is an inflammation of the brain. It is usually caused by a foreign substance or a viral infection. Symptoms of this disease include headache, neck pain, drowsiness, nausea, and fever. If caused by the West Nile virus, it may be lethal to humans, as well as birds and horses.
- Meningitis: Meningitis is an inflammation of the meninges (membranes) of the brain and spinal cord. It is most often caused by a bacterial or viral infection. Fever, vomiting, and a stiff neck are all symptoms of meningitis.
- Migraine: A chronic, often debilitating neurological disorder characterized by recurrent moderate to severe headaches, often in association with a number of autonomic nervous system symptoms.
- Tropical spastic paraparesis: Troby, a virus that can also cause leukemia, is a disease of the bone marrow.
- Arachnoid cysts: Arachnoid cysts are cerebrospinal fluid covered by arachnoidal cells that may develop on the brain or spinal cord. They are a congenital disorder, and in some cases may not show symptoms. However, if there is a large cyst, symptoms may include headache, seizures, ataxia (lack of muscle control), hemiparesis, and several others. Macrocephaly and ADHD are common among children, while presenile dementia, hydrocephalus (an abnormality of the dynamics of the cerebrospinal fluid), and urinary incontinence are symptoms for elderly patients (65 and older).

- Huntington's: Huntington's disease is a degenerative neurological disorder that is inherited. Degeneration of neuronal cells occurs throughout the brain, especially in the striatum. There is a progressive decline that results in abnormal movements. Statistics show that Huntington's disease may affect 10 per 100,000 people of Western European descent.
- Alzheimer's: Alzheimer's is a neurodegenerative disease typically found in people over the age of 65 years. Worldwide, approximately 24 million people have dementia; 60% of these cases are due to Alzheimer's. The ultimate cause is unknown. The clinical sign of Alzheimer's is progressive cognition deterioration.
- Attention deficit/hyperactivity disorder (ADHD): ADHD (often highly debated & controversial) is now largely considered to be a genuine organic disorder of the nervous system, according to the United States government. ADHD, which in severe cases can be debilitating, has symptoms thought to be caused by structural as well as biochemical imbalances in the brain; in particular, low levels of the neurotransmitters dopamine and norepinephrine, which are responsible for controlling and maintaining attention and movement. Many people with ADHD continue to have symptoms well into adulthood. Also of note is an increased risk of the development of Dementia with Lewy bodies, or (DLB), & a direct genetic association of Attention deficit disorder to Parkinson's disease two progressive, and serious, neurological diseases whose symptoms,often occur in people over age 65.
- Locked-in syndrome: A medical condition, usually resulting from a stroke that damages part of the brainstem, in which the body and most of the facial muscles are paralysed but consciousness remains and the ability to perform certain eye movements is preserved.
- Parkinson's: Parkinson's disease, or PD, is a progressive illness of the nervous system. Caused by the death of dopamine-producing brain cells that affect motor skills and speech. Symptoms may include bradykinesia (slow physical movement), muscle rigidity, and tremors. Behavior, thinking, sensation disorders, and the sometimes co-morbid skin condition Seborrheic dermatitis are just some of PD's numerous nonmotor symptoms. Interestingly, Parkinson's disease, Attention deficit/hyperactivity disorder (ADHD) & Bi-polar disorder, all appear to have some connection to one another, as all three nervous system disorders involve lower than normal levels of the brain chemical dopamine(In ADHD, Parkinson's, & the depressive phase of Bi-polar disorder.) or too much dopamine(In,Mania or Manic states of Bi-polar disorder.) in different areas of the brain:

- Tourette's: Tourette's syndrome is an inherited neurological disorder. Early onset may be during childhood, and it is characterized by physical and verbal tics. The exact cause of Tourette's, other than genetic factors, is unknown.
- Multiple sclerosis: Multiple sclerosis (MS) is a chronic, inflammatory demyelinating disease, meaning that the myelin sheath of neurons is damaged. Symptoms of MS include visual and sensation problems, muscle weakness, and depression.

Causes

- Trauma: Any type of traumatic brain injury (TBI) or injury done to the spinal cord can result in a wide spectrum of disabilities in a person. Depending on the section of the brain or spinal cord that suffers the trauma, the outcome may be anticipated.
- Infections: Infectious diseases are transmitted in several ways. Some of these infections may affect the brain or spinal cord directly. Generally, an infection is a disease that is caused by the invasion of a microorganism or virus.
- Degeneration: Degenerative spinal disorders involve a loss of function in the spine. Pressure on the spinal cord and nerves may be associated with herniation or disc displacement. Brain degeneration also causes central nervous system diseases. Studies have shown that obese people may have severe degeneration in the brain due to loss of tissue affecting cognition.
- Structural defects: Common structural defects include birth defects, anencephaly, hypospadias, and spina bifida. Children born with structural defects may have malformed limbs, heart problems, and facial abnormalities.
- Tumors: A tumor is an abnormal growth of body tissue. In the beginning, tumors can be noncancerous, but if they become malignant, they are cancerous. In general, they appear when there is a problem with cellular division. Problems with the body's immune system can lead to tumors.
- Autoimmune disorders: An autoimmune disorder is a condition where in the immune system attacks and destroys healthy body tissue. This is caused by a loss of tolerance to proteins in the body, resulting in immune cells recognising these as 'foreign' and directing an immune response against them.
- Stroke: A stroke is an interruption of the blood supply to the brain. Approximately every 40 seconds, someone in the US has a stroke. This is can happen when a blood vessel is blocked by a blood clot or when a blood vessel ruptures, causing blood to leak to the brain. If

the brain cannot get enough oxygen and blood, brain cells can die, leading to permanent damage.

Signs and symptoms

Every disease has different signs and symptoms. Some of them are persistent headache; pain in the face, back, arms, or legs; an inability to concentrate; loss of feeling; memory loss; loss of muscle strength; tremors; seizures; increased reflexes, spasticity, tics; paralysis; and slurred speech. One should seek medical attention if affected by these.

Treatments

There is a wide range of treatments for central nervous system diseases. These can range from surgery to rehabilitation or prescribed medications.

Bibliography

A V S S Sambamurty: *Textbook of Plant Pathology*, I K Publications, Delhi, 2006.

A.B.A.M. Baudoin: *Laboratory Exercises in Plant Pathology: An Instructional Kit-Teachers Manual and Students Manual (2 Vols)*, Scientific Publications, Delhi, 2011.

A.K. Agarwal: *Plant Sciences and Genetics in Agriculture*, Monalisa Enterprises, Delhi, 2011.

A.K. Zingare: *Microbiology and Plant Pathology*, Satyam Publications, Delhi, 2013.

Amar Tyagi: *Plant Pathology*, Anmol Publications, Delhi, 2006

Ashok K. Mishra, A. Bohra and Akhilesh Mishra: *Plant Pathology: Diseases and Management*, Agrobios Publications, Jaipur, 2005.

Awani Kr. Singh: *Encyclopaedia of Bacterial Plant Pathology*, Anmol Publications, Delhi, 2010.

B P Chakravarti: *Methods of Bacterial Plant Pathology*, Agrotech Publications, Jodhpur, 2008.

C. Manoharachary, D.K. Purohit, S. Ram Reddy, M.A. Singara Charya and S. Girisham: *Frontiers in Microbial Biotechnology and Plant Pathology*, Scientific Publications, Delhi, 2002.

Chandra Shekhar Sharma: *Plant Pathology*, Agrotech Press, Rajasthan, 2013.

D P Tripathi: *Plant Pathology at a Glance (Encyclopedia of Plant Pathology)*, Scientific Publications, Delhi, 2008.

D.K. Jha: *Laboratory Manual on Plant Pathology*, Pointer Publications, Jaipur, 2004.

A.C. Shuttleworth and R.H. Smythe : *Clinical Veterinary Surgery*, Greenworld Publication, Delhi, 2000.

Ajay Kumar Upadhyaya : *Text Book of Preventive Veterinary Medicine*, International Book, Delhi, 2005.

Ajit Kumar Santra : *A Treatise for Students of Veterinary, Zoology*, International Book Distributing Company, Delhi, 2008.

Anuj Sharma : *Encyclopaedia of Veterinary Science*, Anmol Publication, Delhi, 2006.

Ashis Kumar Ghosh : *Ethnomedicine for Human and Veterinary Development*, Daya Publication, Delhi, 2009.

Debasis Jana and Nilotpal Ghosh : *Essentials of Veterinary Practice*, Daya Publication, Delhi, 2011.

Dinesh Arora : *Biotech's Dictionary of Veterinary*, Biotech, Delhi, 2004.

F W Nicholas : *Introduction to Veterinary Genetics*, Blackwell Science, 2004.

G.D. Bagchi and Sushil Kumar : *Indian Traditional Veterinary Medicinal Plants*, Central Institute of Medicinal and Aromatic Plants, 2000.

Gary R. Mullen and Lance A. Durden : *Medical and Veterinary Entomology*, Academic Press an imprint of Elsevier, Delhi, 2013.

Geo F. Boddie : *Diagnostic Methods in Veterinary Medicine*, Greenworld Publication, Delhi, 2005.

J L Vegad : *A Textbook of Veterinary General Pathology*, International, Delhi, 2012.

J.F. Craig : *Flemings's Veterinary Obstetrics*, Greenworld, Delhi, 2000.

J.L. Vegad and A.K. Katiyar : *A Textbook of Veterinary Special Pathology*, IBDCO Publication, Delhi, 2005.

J.L. Vegad and Madhu Swamy : *A Textbook of Veterinary Systemic Pathology*, IBDC Publishers, 2010.

John T. Abrams : *Linton's Animal Nutrition and Veterinary Dietetics*, Greenworld, Delhi, 2000.

Jules J. Haberman : *The Farmer's Veterinary Handbook* , Greenworld, Delhi, 2001.

M.K. Shukla : *Applied Veterinary Andrology and Frozen Semen Technology*, New India Publication, Delhi, 2011.

M.V. Thrusfield and E.A.M. Graat : *Application of Quantitative Methods in Veterinary Epidemiology*, International Publication, Delhi, 2003.

Mahesh Kumar and R.D. Sharma : *Textbook of Clinical Veterinary Medicine*, Indian Council of Agri Res, 2009.

Manual of Veterinary Helminthology : S S Chaudhri; S K Gupta; D P Banerjee; P K Bhatnagar, International Book Distri, 2003,

Mohd. Amanullah : *Veterinary Biochemistry and Biotechnology*, International Book, Delhi, 2009.

N. K. Singh and Harkirat Singh : *Diagnostic Veterinary Parasitology*, New India Publishing Agency, Delhi, 2013.

P. Kinjavdekar, H.P. Aithal and A.M. Pawde : *Anaesthesia and Analgesia for Veterinary Graduates*, Satish Serial Publishing House, Delhi, 2013.

P. Srinivasan : *Veterinary Anatomy Of the Ox*, Bio-Green Books, Delhi, 2012.

Index

A

B

C

D

E